MAYO CLINIC
Guide to
SELF-CARE

Answers for Everyday Health Problems

Philip T. Hagen, M.D.
Editor in Chief

Third Edition

Mayo Clinic
Rochester, Minnesota
Jacksonville, Florida
Scottsdale, Arizona

Published by Mayo Clinic Health Information.

Library of Congress Control Number 2001 132728

ISBN 1-893005-19-4

Printed in the United States of America

Third Edition

5 6 7 8 9 10

Preface

This book comes to you as a complimentary benefit of your membership in Thrivent Financial for Lutherans. It is one way in which we can demonstrate our concern for your overall well-being and that of your family.

We want to be a resource for you and your family in the areas of financial security, wellness and care for others.

In an ongoing effort to help you meet those needs, we solicit information on the benefits our members find most helpful. Over and over again, we hear that you are interested in anything that can help you achieve and maintain good health. In response, we are pleased to send you this edition of the *Mayo Clinic Guide to Self-Care*.

We believe that healthy people develop a collection of resources in their quest for good health. Those resources may include friends, professional people and health information materials. We hope you will use this book as one important resource in a complete approach to caring for yourself.

In compiling this book, the health professionals at Mayo Clinic chose to focus on how to prevent illness, how to detect illness before it becomes a serious, costly problem, and how to avoid unnecessary trips to the clinic or emergency room.

Also included are sections on The Healthy Consumer, You and Your Health Care Provider, Dealing with the Health Care System, Vitamin and Mineral Supplements, and a discussion of Alternative Medicine and Your Health.

If you want an easy-to-understand source for information about your health, this book is it. We are pleased to provide the *Mayo Clinic Guide to Self-Care* to help improve your health and your quality of life.

Patrick Snow, MD
Vice President and Chief Medical Director
Thrivent Financial for Lutherans

Editorial Staff

Editor in Chief
Philip Hagen, M.D.

Associate Medical Editor
Charles Kennedy, M.D.

Managing Editors
Ralph Heussner, Jr.
David Swanson

Editorial Production
LeAnn Stee

Creative Director
Daniel Brevick

Illustration
John Hagen
Christopher Srnka

Editorial Assistants
Margery Lovejoy
Roberta Schwartz
Renée Van Vleet

Design
Stewart Koski
Jeffrey Satre

Contributing Writers
Harvey Black
Katie Colón
Terry Jopke
Lynn Madsen
Lee Ann Martin
Catherine LaMarca Stroebel
Jeremiah Whitten

Editorial Research
Anthony Cook
Deirdre Herman
Michelle Hewlett
Brian Laing

Proofreading
Miranda Attlesey
Donna Hanson

Indexing
Larry Harrison

Contributing Editors and Reviewers

Julie Abbott, M.D.
Susan Ahlquist, R.N.
Steven Altchuler, M.D.
Deborah Anderson, R.N., C.N.P.
Gregory Anderson, M.D.
Linda Arneson, P.T.
Patricia Barrier, M.D.
Thomas Beniak
A. Renée Bergstrom, M.Ed.
Donna Betcher, R.N.
Allen Bishop, M.D.
Judith Blomgren, R.N.
Gerald Christenson, R.Ph.
Patricia Conrad, R.N.
Michael Covalciuc, M.D.
Edward Creagan, M.D.
Bradford Currier, M.D.
Albert Czaja, M.D.
Wyatt Decker, M.D.
David Dodick, M.D.
Lisa Drage, M.D.
Joseph Duffy, M.D.
Brooks Edwards, M.D.
Frederick Edwards, M.D.
Rokea el-Azhary, M.D.
David Fabry, Ph.D.
Richard Fairley, M.D.
Richard Finlayson, M.D.
Sherine Gabriel, M.D.
Mary Gallenberg, M.D.
Gerald Gau, M.D.
James Graham, D.P.M.

Daniel Hall-Flavin, M.D.
Paul Hardwig, M.D.
Peg Harmon, R.N.
J. Taylor Hays, M.D.
Donald Hensrud, M.D.
Ruth Hicks
Daniel Hurley, M.D.
Richard Hurt, M.D.
Douglas Husmann, M.D.
Robert Jacobson, M.D.
Patricia Jensen, R.N.
Robert Johnson, M.D.
Ruth Johnson, M.D.
Mary Jurisson, M.D.
Darlene Kelly, M.D.
Sandra Kelley, R.N.
Debra Koppa, C.P.N.P.
Lois Krahn, M.D.
Barbara Kreinbring, R.N.
Teresa Kubas, R.D.
Kristine Kuhnert, R.D.
David Larson, M.D.
Edward Laskowski, M.D.
James Li, M.D.
Mary Madden, R.N.
Deb McCauley, R.N.P.
Mary Jane McHardy, M.S.
Peggy Menzel, R.N.
Linda Miller, M.D.
Sara Miller, R.N.P.
Robin Molella, M.D.
Robert Morse, M.D.

Margaret Moutvic, M.D.
Lee Nauss, M.D.
Jennifer Nelson, R.D.
Marilynn Olney, M.D.
Eric Olson, M.D.
David Patterson, M.D.
Jerald Pietan, M.D.
Gregory Poland, M.D.
Carroll Poppen, P.A.
Russell Rein, M.H.A.
Randall Roenigk, M.D.
Jeffrey Rome, M.D.
Jane Ryan
Arnold Schroeter, M.D.
Jacalyn See, R.D.
Marilyn Smith, R.N.
Ray Squires, Ph.D.
Robert Stroebel, M.D.
Jerry Swanson, M.D.
Jill Swanson, M.D.
Sandra Taler, M.D.
Robert Trousdale, M.D.
Richard Van Dellen, M.D.
Abinash Virk, M.D.
Laurie Jo Vlasak, R.N.
Roger Warndahl, R.Ph.
Floyd Willis, M.D.
Donna Wohlhuter, R.N.
Alan Wright, M.D.
Katherine Zahasky, R.N.

Introduction

Mayo Clinic Guide to Self-Care provides reliable, practical, easy-to-understand information on more than 150 common medical conditions and issues relating to your health.

No book can replace the advice of your physician or other health care providers. Instead, our intent is to help you manage some common medical problems safely at home or at work. The information you'll find may help you avoid a trip to the clinic or emergency room. Or we'll let you know when you need to visit a medical professional.

How the Book Is Organized

Most chapters in *Mayo Clinic Guide to Self-Care* begin with a general discussion of the health topic, sometimes including signs and symptoms and a summary of the cause. Next look for self-care and prevention suggestions highlighted in blue shading. Under the heading "Medical Help," you are advised when to see a physician or other health care provider and what kind of treatment you might expect. When there is special information for children, you'll see a "Kids' Care" heading. Finally, articles with gray shading are short pieces with information on related medical topics.

Listed below are summaries of the eight sections that make up *Mayo Clinic Guide to Self-Care*.

Urgent Care

Emergencies are rare and usually require the care of a medical professional. There are some things you can do before medical help arrives, however, to stabilize the person who is in the emergency situation and prepare him or her for treatment. Areas covered include how to perform cardiopulmonary resuscitation (CPR), how to help someone who is choking or having a heart attack or a brain attack (stroke) and how to deal with a variety of common problems, such as bleeding, animal bites, frostbite, puncture wounds and toothache.

We encourage you to take a certified first-aid course to learn the lifesaving techniques you may need in the event of an emergency.

General Symptoms

General symptoms are medical conditions that tend to affect your entire body rather than a specific body part or system. General symptoms might include fatigue, fever, dizziness, pain, sleeplessness, sweating and unexpected weight changes. In this section, we explain the common causes for each of these seven general symptoms. We also provide self-care information on how to treat these symptoms and advice on when to seek medical care.

Common Problems

This section, the largest single section of the book, examines common problems in areas such as your eyes, ears, nose, skin, stomach, throat, back and limbs. You'll also find chapters on women's and men's health issues. We offer simple remedies for problems such as sore throat, common cold, stomach pain, ingrown toenail and black eye.

Specific Conditions

In this section, we offer general guidelines on the prevention and management of common conditions for which there is limited opportunity for self-care. If you have any of these conditions, see your health care provider for proper diagnosis and treatment.

Mental Health

Here we offer helpful information on how to deal with a variety of addictive behaviors. We also discuss other mental health issues, such as anxiety, domestic abuse and memory loss. We explain the difference between depression and the "blues," how to cope with the loss of a loved one and how to tell whether someone may be contemplating suicide. *(continued next page)*

Staying Healthy

This section is filled with practical information on how to establish and maintain a healthy lifestyle. You'll find tips on nutrition, weight control, exercise, stress management and prevention of injury and illness.

Your Health and the Workplace

This section focuses on ways to improve your health and well-being at your place of employment.

We begin by addressing common problems such as back pain and carpal tunnel syndrome, then we deal with issues of safety and injury prevention. Balancing work and home is a familiar challenge. We offer practical tips to save your sanity and help you cope with "morning madness." You'll find an expanded discussion of stress. We deal with burnout and coworker conflict. We address time management and hostility and gossip. You'll find healthful ways to handle a demanding workload and tips on listening more effectively.

Workplace technology is on the increase. We help you cope with some of the health challenges posed by routine use of a computer.

We end with practical discussions of pregnancy and work and retirement planning.

The Healthy Consumer

In this section, we give you tips on topics such as how to talk to your physician, what you can learn from your family's medical history, home medical testing kits and what you should include in a home first-aid kit. We also discuss the use of common medications, and we provide easy-to-understand descriptions of cold remedies and over-the-counter pain medications.

Do you travel for business or pleasure? We end with a comprehensive review of what you need to know before you pack your bags.

Children and Adolescent Health

We address the major medical conditions likely to affect your child during his or her preteen years in this book. But the book is not a comprehensive resource for every childhood illness. Many of our chapters include a section on "Kids' Care," which provides information regarding specific concerns. We summarize well-child immunizations in our Staying Healthy section and give many safety tips for children throughout the book. We also discuss how to identify and cope with alcohol and tobacco use in teenagers. If you have a question about an issue dealing with your child's health, check our index. You'll probably find an entry.

A Few Words About How We Speak

When doctors talk to their patients, doctors understand clearly the message they intend to convey. But often their patients do not. In this book, we use conversational English because it's the way people talk to each other. You won't find many, if any, technical terms.

One term you will see is "health care provider." We use this phrase because, in addition to "doctor" and "physician," the term health care provider includes medical personnel such as physician's assistants, nurse-practitioners and certified nurse-midwives.

About Mayo Clinic

Mayo Clinic evolved from the frontier practice of Dr. William Worrall Mayo, and the partnership of his two sons, William J. and Charles J. Mayo, in the early 1900s. Pressed by the demands of their busy surgical practice in Rochester, Minn., the Mayo brothers invited other physicians to join them, pioneering the private group practice of medicine. Today, with more than 2,400 physicians and scientists at its three major locations in Rochester, Minn., Jacksonville, Fla., and Scottsdale, Ariz., Mayo Clinic is dedicated to providing comprehensive diagnosis, accurate answers and effective treatments and to being a dependable source of health information for patients and the public.

With its depth of knowledge, experience and expertise, Mayo Clinic occupies an unparalleled position as a health information resource. Since 1983, Mayo Clinic has published reliable health information for millions of consumers through award-winning newsletters, books and online services. Revenue from the publishing activities supports Mayo Clinic programs, including medical education and research.

Table of Contents

Urgent Care

- CPR
- Choking
- Heart Attack
- Stroke (Brain Attack)
- Poisoning Emergencies
- Severe Bleeding
- Shock
- Allergic Reactions
- Bites
- Burns
- Cold Weather Problems
- Cuts, Scrapes and Wounds
- Eye Injuries
- Food-Borne Illness
- Heat-Related Problems
- Poisonous Plants
- Tooth Problems
- Trauma

Emergencies don't happen often, but when they do there's not much time to seek out information. To react effectively, you must know what action to take when a person appears injured, seriously ill or in distress. Your skills may never be required. However, you could someday be the link between life and death for another human being.

Take a certified first-aid training course to learn life-saving skills such as CPR, the Heimlich maneuver and dealing with a heart attack, shock and traumatic injury. Check with your local Red Cross, county emergency services, public safety office or the American Heart Association for information on first-aid courses in your community.

CPR

CPR (cardiopulmonary resuscitation) involves a combination of mouth-to-mouth rescue breathing and chest compression. CPR keeps oxygenated blood flowing to the brain and other vital organs until appropriate medical treatment can restore a normal heart rhythm.

Before starting CPR, you must assess the situation. Is the person conscious or unconscious? If the victim appears unconscious, tap or shake his or her shoulder and ask loudly, "Are you OK?" If the person does not respond, think of the ABCs (see below), and get help by calling 911. If you cannot leave the scene, have someone else call.

A: Airway. Your first action is to open the airway, which may be obstructed by the back of the tongue or the epiglottis (the flap of cartilage that covers the windpipe) (see steps 1 and 2 below).

B: Breathing. Mouth-to-mouth rescue breathing is the quickest way to get oxygen into a person's lungs (see steps 3 and 4 below).

C: Circulation. Chest compressions replace the heartbeat when it has stopped. Compressions help maintain some blood flow to the brain, lungs and heart (see step 6 on page 3). You must perform rescue breathing anytime you perform chest compressions.

The following six steps and illustrations demonstrate the CPR technique.

1. Position the victim so you can check for breathing and signs of circulation by laying the victim flat on a firm surface.

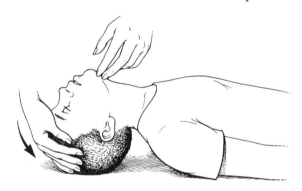

2. Open the victim's airway; tilt the head back by lifting on the chin with one hand while pushing down on the forehead with the other hand.

3. Determine whether the victim is breathing by simultaneously listening for breath sounds, feeling for air motion on your cheek and ear, and looking for chest motion.

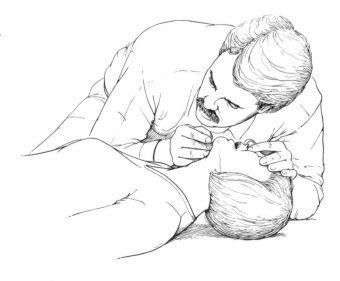

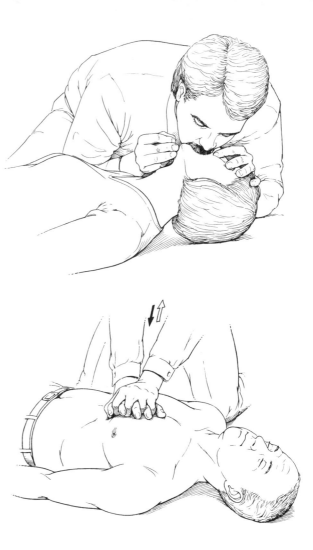

4. *If the victim is not breathing, pinch the person's nostrils closed, make a seal around the mouth and breathe into his or her mouth twice. If the victim's chest doesn't rise when you breathe into his or her mouth, the airway is probably blocked. Attempt to reopen the airway by tilting the head and lifting the chin, then breathe into the victim's mouth again.*

5. *After you deliver two rescue breaths, or if you are unable to get the chest to rise, look for signs of circulation: breathing, coughing or movement.*

6. *If there are no signs of circulation, begin chest compressions. The heel of one hand should be located in the middle of the breastbone, right between the nipples. Place the heel of your other hand on top of your first hand. To make best use of your weight, keep your elbows straight and your shoulders positioned directly above your hands. Push down 1 1/2 to 2 inches at a rate of 100 times a minute. The "pushing down" and "letting up" phase of each cycle should be equal in duration. Don't "jab" down and relax. After every four cycles of 15 compressions and two breaths, recheck for signs of circulation and breathing. Continue the rescue maneuvers as long as there is no pulse or breathing. If the victim has signs of circulation but is not breathing, continue only rescue breaths at a rate of one rescue breath every five seconds.*

CPR for Infants

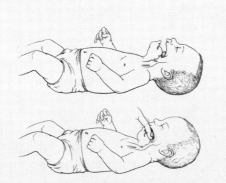

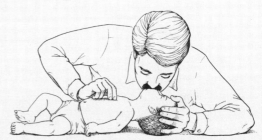

Before giving mouth-to-mouth resuscitation to an infant, tilt the child's head back to open the airway (top). Then, if visual inspection reveals a foreign object in the mouth, remove the object with a sweep of your finger (bottom). Be careful not to push the food or object deeper into the child's airway.

To perform CPR on a baby, cover the mouth and nose with your mouth. Give two rescue breaths. Check for signs of circulation in response to the two rescue breaths (breathing, coughing or movement). Give one breath for every five chest compressions. Compress the chest 1/2 to 1 inch at least 100 times a minute, using only two fingers.

Choking

Choking occurs when the respiratory passage in the throat or windpipe is blocked. This situation requires emergency treatment to prevent unconsciousness or death. Choking, heart disease or other conditions may cause the heart and breathing to stop. To save the life of the person, breathing and blood circulation must be restored immediately (see previous chapter on CPR).

Recognizing and Clearing an Obstructed Airway

Choking is often the result of inadequately chewed food becoming lodged in the throat or windpipe. Most often, solid foods such as meats are the cause.

Commonly, persons who are choking have been talking while simultaneously chewing a chunk of meat. False teeth also may set the stage for this problem by interfering with the way food feels in the mouth while it is being chewed. Food cannot be chewed as thoroughly with false teeth as with natural teeth because less chewing pressure is exerted by false teeth.

Panic is an accompanying sensation. The choking victim's face often assumes an expression of fear or terror. At first, he or she may turn purple, the eyes may bulge and he or she may wheeze or gasp.

If some food "goes down the wrong pipe," the coughing reflex often will resolve the problem. In fact, a person is not choking if he or she is able to cough freely, has normal skin color and is able to speak. If the cough is more like a gasp and the person is turning blue, the individual is probably choking.

If in doubt, ask the choking person whether he or she can talk. If the person is capable of speech, then the windpipe is not completely blocked and oxygen is reaching the lungs. A person who is choking is unable to communicate except by hand motions.

The universal sign for choking is a hand clutched to the throat, with thumb and fingers extended. A person who displays this requires emergency treatment and should never be left unattended.

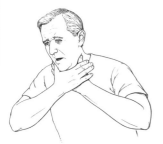

A person who is choking is unable to communicate except by hand motions. Often the hand and arm motions are uncoordinated. It is important to remember that the universal sign for choking is hands clutched to the throat, with thumbs and fingers extended.

The Heimlich Maneuver

The Heimlich maneuver is the best known method of removing an object from the airway of a person who is choking. You can use it on yourself or someone else. These are the steps:

1. Stand behind the choking person and wrap your arms around his or her waist. Bend the person slightly forward.

2. Make a fist with one hand and place it slightly above the person's navel.

3. Grasp your fist with the

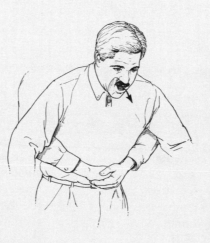

other hand and press hard into the abdomen with a quick, upward thrust. Repeat this procedure until the object is expelled from the airway.

If you must perform this maneuver on yourself, position your own fist slightly above your navel. Grasp your fist with your other hand and thrust upward into your abdomen until the object is expelled, or lean over the back of a chair to produce this effect.

Heart Attack

Half of all people who have heart attacks wait 2 hours or longer before seeking treatment. And half — 300,000 Americans each year — die before reaching the hospital.

Among those who survive to deal with recovery, most of the permanent damage to the heart occurs during the first hour. If you're having a heart attack, what you don't do could kill you.

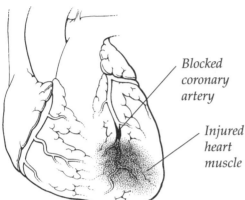

Blocked coronary artery

Injured heart muscle

A heart attack occurs when arteries supplying your heart with blood and oxygen become blocked. With each passing minute, more tissue is deprived of oxygen and deteriorates or dies. Restoring blood flow within the first hour when most damage occurs is critical to survival.

Why Is the First Hour Critical?

A heart attack is injury to heart muscle caused by a loss of blood supply. An attack occurs when arteries supplying your heart with blood and oxygen become blocked.

A blood clot that forms in an artery narrowed by buildup of cholesterol and other fatty deposits usually causes the blockage. Without oxygen, cells are destroyed, causing pain or pressure, and heart function is impaired.

A heart attack is not a static, one-time event. It's a dynamic process that typically evolves over 4 to 6 hours. With each passing minute, more tissue is deprived of oxygen and deteriorates or dies.

Minutes Matter

The main way to prevent progressive damage is to treat early with clot-dissolving medications or angioplasty. "Clot-busters," such as tissue-plasminogen activator (tPA) and streptokinase, dissolve the clot and restore blood flow. In a University of Washington study, 75 percent of people survived heart attacks with little or no heart damage when clot-dissolving therapy was started within 70 minutes of onset of symptoms.

Emergency angioplasty, a procedure available at large medical centers, also widens blocked arteries, letting blood flow more freely to your heart. As with use of clot-dissolving drugs, if angioplasty is delayed beyond 2 hours, benefits are substantially reduced.

In the initial minutes, a heart attack also can trigger ventricular fibrillation. This unstable heart rhythm produces an ineffective heartbeat, causing insufficient blood flow to vital organs. Without immediate treatment, ventricular fibrillation can lead to sudden death.

Be Alert to Symptoms

During a heart attack, many people waste precious minutes because they don't recognize symptoms or they deny them. Many people also delay calling for help because they're afraid to risk the embarrassment of a "false alarm."

A heart attack generally causes chest pain for more than 15 minutes. But a heart attack also can be "silent" and have no symptoms.

About half of heart attack victims have warning symptoms hours, days or weeks in advance. The earliest predictor of an attack may be recurrent chest pain that's triggered by exertion and relieved by rest.

The American Heart Association lists these warning signs of a heart attack. Be aware that you may not have all of them, and that symptoms may come and go.

- Uncomfortable pressure, fullness or squeezing pain in the center of your chest, lasting more than a few minutes.
- Pain spreading to your shoulders, neck or arms.
- Light-headedness, fainting, sweating, nausea or shortness of breath.
  If you have diabetes, you may have fewer or more atypical symptoms.

Emergency Treatment

In a heart attack emergency, you have to make crucial decisions under stress. Even if you ultimately make wise choices, you waste valuable minutes weighing your options. Whether you suspect a heart attack or think it's just indigestion, act immediately. Take these steps:

- **Call 911 first.** The 911 operator contacts the emergency medical services (EMS) system. In areas without 911 service, call the emergency medical response system. It's usually better to call these emergency numbers first. Calling your doctor may add unnecessary time.

  When you call, describe symptoms such as severe shortness of breath or chest pain. This ensures a priority dispatch of EMS responders trained in basic and advanced cardiac life support.

  Most EMS units carry portable defibrillators. Restoring normal heart rhythm by delivering electrical shocks to the heart is critical to early treatment and survival. Many police and fire rescue units also carry defibrillators and may respond before an ambulance.

- **Begin CPR.** If the person is unconscious, a 911 dispatcher may advise you to begin CPR (mouth-to-mouth breathing and chest compression). Even if you're not trained, a dispatcher can instruct you in CPR until help arrives. (See page 2 for more on CPR.)

- **Decide on fastest method of transport.** A dispatcher automatically notifies the closest well-equipped EMS unit. Ideally, EMS responders should reach you within 4 to 5 minutes. If you live in a rural area, however, you may get someone to the hospital faster by driving. If you think you're having a heart attack, ask someone to drive you. Never drive yourself.

- **Go to the nearest emergency cardiac care facility.** Identify, in advance, the nearest center staffed 24 hours a day with physicians trained to provide emergency cardiac care.

- **Chew aspirin.** Aspirin inhibits blood clotting, which helps maintain blood flow through a narrowed artery. When taken during a heart attack, aspirin can decrease death rates by about 25 percent. Take a regular-strength aspirin and chew it to speed absorption.

  Clot-dissolving drugs and angioplasty improve your chances of surviving a heart attack once treatment begins. But successful treatment begins early. Recognize symptoms and act quickly.

Stroke (Brain Attack)

In the United States, stroke is the third-leading cause of death and the leading cause of adult disability; only cardiovascular disease and cancer cause more annual deaths. Every year, about 700,000 Americans experience a stroke. About 160,000 of these people die. For each decade of life after 55, your risk of stroke doubles.

You can reduce your chances of having a stroke by recognizing and changing certain lifestyle habits. If you're at high risk, drugs such as aspirin and a surgical procedure called carotid endarterectomy (kuh-ROT-id end-ahr-tur-EK-tuh-me) may prevent a major stroke.

If you do have a stroke, early treatment may minimize damage to your brain and subsequent disability. Today, 70 percent of people who have a stroke remain independent; 10 percent recover completely.

A "Brain Attack"

A stroke is a "brain attack." Seek immediate medical assistance, just as you would for a heart attack. Every minute counts. The longer a stroke goes untreated, the greater the damage and potential disability. Success of treatment may depend on how soon care is given.

Your brain has 100 billion nerve cells and trillions of nerve connections. Although it's only 2 percent of your body weight, it uses approximately 25 percent of your body's oxygen and other nutrients. Because your brain can't store these nutrients as muscles can, it requires a constant flow of blood to keep working properly.

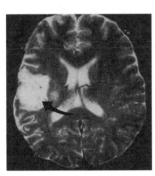

In this magnetic resonance imaging (MRI) scan, the arrow points to an area of brain tissue damaged by a stroke.

A stroke occurs when this blood supply is altered and brain tissue is starved of blood. Within 4 minutes of being deprived of essential nutrients, brain cells begin to die.

There are two main types of stroke:

- **Ischemic:** About 80 percent of strokes are caused by atherosclerosis (buildup of cholesterol-containing fatty deposits called plaque). Growth of plaque roughens the inside of your artery. The irregular surface can cause turbulent blood flow around the buildup—like a boulder in a rushing stream—and trigger development of a clot.

  Temporary and, usually, brief symptoms stemming from the disruption in blood supply describe a transient ischemic attack (TIA). During a TIA, your body may release enzymes that dissolve the clot quickly and restore blood flow.

- **Hemorrhagic:** This type of stroke occurs when a blood vessel in your brain leaks or ruptures. Blood from the hemorrhage spills into the surrounding brain tissue, causing damage. Brain cells beyond the leak or rupture are deprived of blood and also are damaged.

  One cause of a hemorrhagic stroke is an aneurysm. This "ballooning" from a weak spot in a blood vessel wall develops with advancing age. Some aneurysms also may form as a result of a genetic predisposition. The most common cause of a hemorrhagic stroke is high blood pressure (hypertension).

  Hemorrhagic strokes are less common than ischemic strokes — but more often deadly. About 40-50 percent of people who have hemorrhagic strokes die, compared with about 20 percent for ischemic strokes. Strokes that occur in young adults are typically hemorrhagic.

Can You Prevent a Stroke?

You can't change some risk factors for stroke. Other predictors of a stroke are manageable with medications and changes in lifestyle. Because some of these risk factors don't always cause symptoms, however, you may not know you have them.

Risk factors that can be controlled are described below:

- **High blood pressure:** About 40 percent of strokes may be due to high blood pressure (hypertension), defined as a systolic pressure more than 140 mm Hg and a diastolic pressure more than 90 mm Hg (see page 180).
- **Cigarette smoking:** Smokers have about a 50 percent greater chance of having a stroke than nonsmokers.
- **Cardiovascular disease**: In addition to atherosclerosis, heart conditions including congestive heart failure, a previous heart attack, acute heart-valve disease or valve replacement and atrial fibrillation (an irregular and, often, rapid heartbeat) predispose you to a stroke.
- **TIA:** A TIA may last just a few minutes and cause only slight symptoms. Yet about 15 to 20 percent of people who have a stroke have had one or more TIAs. The more frequent the TIAs, the greater the possibility of a stroke.
- **Diabetes:** Diabetes doubles your risk of stroke.
- **Undesirable blood cholesterol levels:** High blood levels of low-density lipoprotein (LDL) cholesterol increase your risk of atherosclerosis. In contrast, high levels of high-density lipoprotein (HDL) cholesterol are protective because they may prevent formation of plaque.

Know the Warning Signs

If you notice one or more of these signs, call your doctor immediately. They may be signaling a possible stroke or TIA:

- Sudden weakness or numbness in your face, arm or leg on one side of your body.
- Sudden dimness, blurring or loss of vision, particularly in one eye.
- Loss of speech, or trouble talking or understanding speech.
- Sudden, severe headache—a "bolt out of the blue"—with no apparent cause.
- Unexplained dizziness, unsteadiness or a sudden fall, especially if accompanied by any of the other symptoms.

Some Risk Factors Are Beyond Your Control

You can't change these risk factors for stroke. But knowing you're at risk can motivate you to change your lifestyle to reduce your risk.

- *Family history:* Your risk is greater if your parent, brother or sister has had a stroke or TIA. It's not clear whether the increased risk is genetic or due to family lifestyles.
- *Age:* Generally, your risk of stroke increases as you get older.
- *Sex:* If you're a man, your risk is higher than a woman's until age 55. After age 55, when estrogen levels decrease during menopause, a woman's risk equals a man's.
- *Race:* Blacks are more likely to have strokes than other minority groups or whites. The increase is partly because of their greater risk of high blood pressure and diabetes.

Poisoning Emergencies

Many conditions mimic the symptoms of poisoning, including seizures, stroke and insulin reactions. If there is no indication of poisoning, do not treat the person for poisoning, but call 800-222-1222 or emergency medical help 911.

Call the poison control center immediately, even if the person looks and feels fine. Don't wait to see if symptoms arise before calling. Many toxins have delayed life-threatening effects. Early treatment may be important.

Children under 5 are often exposed to poisons because they are curious. If infants and toddlers dwell in your home, or visit, you should:
- Keep potential poisons in cabinets located up high, or with safety locks.
- Have syrup of ipecac in your home. This is a medication used to induce vomiting. It's available at any pharmacy.
- Keep the poison information line phone number (800-222-1222) easily accessible.

Emergency Treatment

Swallowed poison
Remove anything remaining in the person's mouth. Unless the victim is unconscious, having a seizure, or cannot swallow, give about 2 ounces of water to drink. Do not induce vomiting unless directed by a poison control center or a physician.

Poison in the eye
Gently flush eye for 10 minutes using slightly warm water. Pour a stream of water from a clean glass held about 3 inches above the eye.

Poison on the skin
Remove any contaminated clothing. Rinse the skin with large amounts of water for 10 minutes.

Inhaled poison
Get to fresh air as soon as possible. Avoid breathing the fumes.

If the poisoned person is unconscious, confused, having seizures or trouble breathing, call 911 or emergency medical help, or call 800-222-1222 immediately.

If the person is going to the hospital emergency department, bring the container or any information about the poison with you.

Medications as Poisons

Lifesaving medications can be killers. Overdoses of seemingly harmless medications such as aspirin and acetaminophen take many lives each year. Numerous other over-the-counter drugs are dangerous when taken in large doses.

Severe Bleeding

To stop a serious bleeding injury, follow these steps:

1. Lay the affected person down. If possible, the person's head should be slightly lower than the trunk, or the legs should be elevated. This position reduces the chances of fainting by increasing blood flow to the brain. If possible, elevate the site of bleeding.

2. Remove any obvious debris or dirt from the wound. Do not remove any objects pierced into the victim. Do not probe the wound or attempt to clean it at this point. Your principal concern is to stop the loss of blood.

3. Apply pressure directly on the wound with a sterile bandage, clean cloth or even a piece of clothing. If nothing else is available, use your hand.

4. Maintain pressure until the bleeding stops. When it does, bind the wound dressing tightly with adhesive tape or a bandage. If none is available, use a piece of clean clothing.

5. If the bleeding continues and seeps through the gauze or other material you are holding on the wound, do not remove it. Rather, add more absorbent material on top of it.

6. If the bleeding does not stop with direct pressure, you may need to apply pressure to the major artery that delivers blood to the area of the wound. In the case of a wound on the hand or lower arm, for example, squeeze the main artery in the upper arm against the bone. Keep your fingers flat; with the other hand, continue to exert pressure on the wound itself.

7. Immobilize the injured body part once the bleeding has been stopped. Leave the bandages in place and get the injured person to the emergency room as soon as possible.

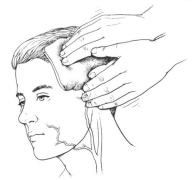

To stop bleeding, apply pressure directly to the wound using gauze or a clean cloth.

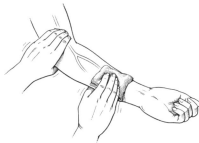

If bleeding continues despite pressure applied directly to the wound, maintain pressure and also apply pressure to the nearest major artery.

Detecting Internal Bleeding

In the event of a traumatic injury, such as an automobile crash or fall, internal bleeding may not be immediately apparent. Look for the following signs:

- Bleeding from the ears, nose, rectum or vagina, or the vomiting or coughing up of blood
- Bruising on the neck, chest or abdomen
- Wounds that have penetrated the skull, chest or abdomen
- Abdominal tenderness, perhaps accompanied by hardness or spasm of the abdominal muscles
- Fracture

Internal bleeding may produce shock. The volume of blood in the body becomes inadequate and the person may feel weak, thirsty and anxious. The skin may feel cool. Other symptoms of shock that may indicate internal bleeding include shallow and slow breathing, a rapid and weak pulse, trembling and restlessness. The person may faint and lose consciousness when standing or seated but recovers when allowed to lie down.

If you suspect internal bleeding, request emergency assistance. Treat the person for shock (see page 11). Keep the person lying quietly and comfortably. Loosen clothing but do not give the person anything to eat or drink.

Internal bleeding, especially in the abdomen, head or chest, is extremely serious and can be life-threatening. Blood loss can be considerable, even if there is no evident external bleeding.

Shock

Shock may result from trauma, heat, allergic reaction, severe infection, poisoning or other causes. Various symptoms appear in a person experiencing shock:

- The skin may appear pale or gray. It is cool and clammy.
- The pulse is weak and rapid, and breathing is slow and shallow. Blood pressure is reduced.
- The eyes lack luster and seem to stare. Sometimes the pupils are dilated.
- The person may be conscious or unconscious. If conscious, the person may feel faint or be very weak or confused. Shock sometimes causes a person to become overly excited and anxious.

Even if a person seems normal after an injury, take precautions and treat the person for shock by following these steps:

Keep the shock victim warm. Elevate legs and feet above the level of the heart to maximize flow of blood to the head.

1. Get the person to lie down on his or her back and elevate the feet higher than the person's head. Keep the person from moving unnecessarily. Observe for the signs of shock noted above.
2. Keep the person warm and comfortable. Loosen tight clothing and cover the person with a blanket. Do not give the person anything to drink.
3. If the person is vomiting or bleeding from the mouth, place the person on his or her side to prevent choking.
4. Treat any injuries (such as bleeding or broken bones) appropriately.
5. Summon emergency medical assistance immediately. Dial 911.

Anaphylaxis Can Be Life-Threatening

The most severe allergic response is called anaphylaxis. It can produce shock and be life-threatening. Although it is infrequent, each year several hundred Americans die of the reaction.

The anaphylactic response occurs rapidly. It can begin within seconds or minutes. Almost any allergen can cause the response, including insect venoms, pollens, latex, certain foods and drugs. Some people have anaphylactic reactions of unknown cause.

If you are extremely sensitive, you may notice severe hives and severe swelling of your eyes or lips or inside your throat which causes difficulty with breathing and shock. Dizziness, mental confusion, abdominal cramping, nausea or vomiting also may accompany a severe reaction.

Many people who know their specific allergies carry medication with them as an antidote to an allergic reaction. Epinephrine is the most commonly used drug. The effects of the medication are only temporary, however, and you must seek further medical attention immediately.

If you observe an allergic reaction with signs of anaphylaxis, call 911. Check to see whether the person is carrying special medication (to inhale, swallow or inject) to counter the effects of the allergic attack. CPR must be performed as a life-saving measure if there is no breathing or no pulse (see page 2).

Allergic Reactions

An allergy is a reaction to a foreign substance (called an allergen) by the body's immune system. The reaction may take many forms, including rashes, congestion, asthma and, rarely, shock or death. Common allergens include pollen (see Respiratory Allergies, page 158) and insect venom (see Bites, page 14). This chapter covers food and drug allergies.

■ Food Allergies

Food allergies may be the most misunderstood of all allergies. Two of five Americans believe they are allergic to specific foods. However, fewer than 1 percent have true food allergies.

Ninety percent of food allergies are caused by certain proteins in cow's milk, egg whites, peanuts, wheat or soybeans. Other foods that can cause problems include berries, shellfish, corn, beans and gum arabic (a thickener used in processed foods). Yellow Food Dye No. 5 may produce an allergic response. Chocolate, long thought to cause allergies (particularly among children), is actually seldom a cause of allergy.

Signs and symptoms of food allergies include the following:
- Abdominal pain, diarrhea, nausea or vomiting
- Fainting
- Hives (see page 123), swelling beneath the skin or eczema (see page 121)
- Swelling of the lips, eyes, face, tongue and throat
- Nasal congestion and asthma

Self-Care

- Avoidance is the best way to prevent an allergic reaction.
- When choosing substitute foods, be careful to select foods that provide the necessary replacement nutrients.
- If you have had a severe reaction, wear an alert bracelet or necklace (see page 13); these are available in most drugstores. Ask your doctor about carrying emergency medications.
- Learn rescue techniques, and teach them to family members and friends.

Medical Help

Food allergies can be diagnosed through a careful process that includes the following five steps:

Step 1: History of your symptoms, including when they occur, which foods cause problems, the amount of food needed to trigger symptoms and whether you have a family history of allergies.

Step 2: Food diary to track eating habits, symptoms and medication use.

Step 3: Physical examination.

Step 4: Testing: Skin prick tests using food extracts and a blood test that measures IgE (one of the body's defense proteins) can help. Neither test is 100 percent accurate. They may be more helpful in determining foods to which you are not allergic.

Step 5: Food elimination-challenge diet is the standard test because it can link symptoms to a specific food. It can't be used, however, if you have severe reactions.

For reactions to foods that are mild, your doctor may prescribe antihistamines or skin creams.

Caution	Severe reactions such as anaphylaxis (see page 11) or acute asthma are very serious because they can be life-threatening. Such reactions are rare. Most reactions are limited to rashes and hives. However, this does not mean they can be ignored. Malnutrition and conditions that suppress your immune system increase the likelihood of developing a food allergy.
Kids' Care	Children are 10 times as likely as adults to have a food allergy. As the digestive system matures, it's less apt to allow absorption of foods that trigger allergies. Children typically outgrow allergies to milk, wheat and eggs by around age 6. Severe allergies and those due to tree nuts and shellfish are more likely to be lifelong.

■ Drug Allergies

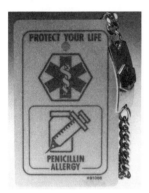

If you have a drug allergy, carry appropriate identification at all times. Drug alert necklaces and bracelets are available at drugstores.

Almost any drug can cause an adverse reaction in some people. Reactions to most drugs are not common, but they can range from merely irritating to life-threatening. Some reactions (such as rashes) are true allergic responses. Most, however, are side effects of a particular drug, typified by dry mouth or fatigue. Some are toxic effects of the drugs, such as liver damage. Still other reactions are poorly understood. Your physician will determine the nature of the reactions and what to do about them.

Penicillin and its relatives are responsible for many drug allergy reactions, ranging from mild rashes to hives to immediate anaphylaxis. Most reactions are minor rashes.

Drugs most likely to cause reactions include sulfas, barbiturates, anticonvulsants, insulin and local anesthetics. These are all common, effective, useful medications. Reactions occur in a minority of people. If you're taking one of them and not having problems, don't stop using it. In addition, contrast dyes used in some X-ray studies to help outline major organs contain iodine and may cause an allergic reaction.

Almost a million Americans, primarily adults, have reactions to a common drug, aspirin. Although not a true allergy, the response mimics one, and it can be serious.

Signs and symptoms of allergic reactions to drugs include the following:
- Wheezing and difficulty breathing
- Rash, hives, generalized itching
- Shock

Self-Care	<ul><li>Avoid drugs that cause an allergic response.</li><li>If you have a severe reaction, learn the names of related drugs.</li><li>Wear a drug-alert necklace or bracelet to indicate your allergy.</li><li>Alert physicians of your sensitivity before treatment.</li><li>Report possible reactions to your doctor. Reactions can occur days after stopping use of a drug.</li><li>Carry an antihistamine when away from home.</li></ul>
Medical Help	The most common drug reactions—rash, itching and hives—are treated with antihistamines or, occasionally, cortisone. Most drug allergies cannot be cured. The allergy to penicillin is an exception. In some cases, this sensitivity can be reduced enough so that the person can tolerate the drug. Small amounts of the drug are given in slowly increasing amounts to desensitize the immune response.

Bites: Animals, Humans, Insects and Spiders

■ Animal Bites

Domestic pets cause most animal bites. Dogs are more likely to bite than cats. However, cat bites are more likely to cause infection. The best treatment is prevention.

Self-Care

- If the bite only breaks the skin, treat it as a minor wound. Wash the wound thoroughly with soap and water. Apply an antibiotic cream to prevent infection, and cover it with a clean bandage.
- Establish whether you have had a tetanus shot within the past 5 years. If not, you should get a booster shot with any bite that breaks the skin.
- Report suspicious bites to local health authorities.
- Follow veterinary guidelines for immunization of your pets.

Medical Help

If the bite creates a deep puncture or the skin is badly torn and bleeding, apply pressure to stop the bleeding and see your doctor. If you have not had a recent tetanus shot, seek medical care. Watch for signs of infection. Swelling, redness around the wound or in a red streak extending from the site, pus draining from the wound or pain should be reported immediately to your doctor.

The Risk of Rabies

Bats, foxes, raccoons and other wild animals may carry rabies, but so can the dog, especially if it runs in the woods. Farm animals, especially cows, may carry rabies, although farm animals rarely transmit rabies to humans.

Rabies is a virus that affects the brain. Transmitted to humans by saliva from the bite of an infected animal, the rabies virus has an incubation period (the time from a bite until symptoms appear) of between 3 and 7 weeks.

Once the incubation period is over, a tingling sensation usually develops at the site of the bite. As the virus spreads, foaming at the mouth may occur because of difficulty with swallowing. Uncontrolled irritability and confusion may follow, alternating with periods of calm.

In the event of an unprovoked bite by a domestic dog, cat or farm animal, the animal should be confined and observed by a veterinarian for 7 to 10 days. Even if the bite is provoked, the animal should be confined for 10 days of observation. Contact a veterinarian if there is any sign of sickness in the animal. If a wild animal has bitten you, the animal should be killed.

■ Human Bites

There are two kinds of human bites. The first is what is usually thought of as a "true" bite—an injury that results from flesh being caught between the teeth. The second kind, called a "fight bite," occurs when a person is cut on the knuckles by an opponent's teeth. Treatment is the same in both cases. Human bites are dangerous because of the risk of infection. The human mouth is a breeding ground for bacteria.

Self-Care

- Apply pressure to stop bleeding, wash the wound thoroughly with soap and water and bandage the wound. Then visit an emergency room. Your health care provider may prescribe antibiotics to prevent infection or update your tetanus shot if you have not had one for more than 5 years.

■ Snake Bites

Triangular head
Elliptical eyes
Nostrils
Pit
Fangs

Most snakes are not poisonous. However, because a few are (including rattlesnakes, coral snakes, water moccasins and copperheads), avoid picking up or playing with any snake unless you are properly trained.

If you're bitten by a snake, it's important to determine whether the snake is poisonous. Most poisonous snakes have slit-like (elliptical) eyes. Their heads are triangular, with a depression or "pit" midway between the eyes and nostrils on both sides of the head.

Self-Care
- If the snake is not poisonous, wash the bite thoroughly, cover it with an antibiotic cream and bandage it. In general, a snake bite is more scary than dangerous.
- Check on the date of your last tetanus shot. If it has been more than 5 years and the bite broke the skin, get a tetanus booster.

Medical Help
If you suspect that the snake is poisonous, seek emergency medical assistance immediately. Apply ice to the bite if possible, but don't delay.

■ Insect Bites and Stings

Some bites or stings cause little more than an annoying itching or stinging sensation and mild swelling that disappear within a day or so. However, 15 percent of the population is sensitive to insect venom. Bees, wasps, hornets, yellow jackets and fire ants are typically the most troublesome. Mosquitoes, ticks, biting flies and some spiders also can cause problems, but these are generally milder reactions.

Symptoms of an allergic reaction usually appear within a few minutes after the sting or bite occurs. But some take hours or even days to appear. If you are mildly sensitive to the venom, hives, itchy eyes, pain and intense itching around the site of the sting or bite are common. With a delayed reaction, you may experience fever, painful joints, hives and swollen glands. You may experience both the immediate and the delayed reactions from the same bite or sting.

The most severe allergic reactions can be life-threatening. If you are extremely sensitive, you may have severe hives and severe swelling of your eyes, lips or inside your throat; the swelling of the throat can cause breathing difficulty. Dizziness, mental confusion, abdominal cramping, nausea, vomiting or fainting also may accompany a severe reaction.

Self-Care
- Remove the stinger with tweezers. Grasp it where it enters your skin, or scrape the skin with a firm edge such as a credit card. Swab the site with disinfectant.
- To reduce pain and swelling, apply ice or a cold pack.
- Apply 0.5 or 1 percent hydrocortisone cream, calamine lotion or a baking soda paste to the bite or sting several times daily until your symptoms subside.
- Take an antihistamine—diphenhydramine (Benadryl, Chlor-trimeton).

If you have experienced a severe reaction in the past:
- Always carry an allergy kit containing epinephrine.
- Obtain a medical alert bracelet.
- Train family members or friends in what to do in an emergency.

Medical Help

If your reaction to an insect bite is severe (shortness of breath, tongue swelling, hives), see your doctor or go to the emergency room immediately.

The most severe allergic reactions to bee stings can be life-threatening. If you experience any breathing problems, swelling of the lips or throat, faintness, confusion, rapid heartbeat or hives after a sting, seek emergency care. Less severe allergic reactions include nausea, intestinal cramps, diarrhea or swelling larger than 2 inches in diameter at the site. See your physician promptly if you experience any of these symptoms.

Your doctor may prescribe shots that can help desensitize your body to insect venom, and an emergency kit containing antihistamine tablets and a syringe filled with epinephrine (adrenaline). Keep the medicine fresh; regularly check the shelf-life.

■ Spider Bites

Black widow (viewed from below)

Brown recluse (viewed from above)

Only a few spiders are dangerous to humans. Two are the black widow (*Latrodectus mactans*), known for the red hourglass marking on its belly, and the brown recluse (*Loxosceles reclusa*), with its violin-shaped marking on its top.

Both prefer warm climates and dark, dry places where flies are plentiful. They often live in outdoor toilets. You may not notice if you're bitten because bites may feel like a pinprick. But within hours, swelling and breathing problems can occur. Sometimes the black widow bite causes muscle cramping, tingling or weakness.

Seek emergency care immediately. In the meantime, apply a cloth dampened with cold water or filled with ice to the bite. If the bite is on a limb, you can help slow the venom's spread by placing a snug bandage above the bite and applying ice.

■ Tick Bites

By and large, ticks are harmless, but they can be a threat to human health. Some ticks carry infections, and their bite can transmit bacteria that cause illnesses such as Lyme disease (caused by the deer tick, see below) or Rocky Mountain spotted fever. Your risk of contracting one of these diseases depends on what part of the United States you live in, how much time you spend in wooded areas and how well you protect yourself.

Self-Care

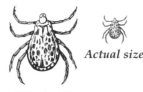

Actual size

Deer tick

Actual size

Wood tick

- When walking in wooded or grassy areas, wear shoes, long pants tucked into socks and long-sleeved shirts. Try to stick to trails, and avoid walking through low bushes and long grass.
- Tick-proof your yard by clearing brush and leaves; keep woodpiles in sunny areas.
- Check yourself and your pets often for ticks after being in wooded or grassy areas. Showering immediately after leaving these areas is a good idea, because ticks often remain on your skin for many hours before biting.
- Insect repellents often repel ticks. Use products containing DEET or permethrin. Be sure to follow label precautions.
- If you find a tick, remove it with tweezers by gently grasping it near its head or mouth. Do not squeeze or crush the tick, but pull carefully and steadily. Once you have the entire tick removed, apply antiseptic to the bite area.
- When you discard a tick, bury, burn or flush it.
- If you've developed a rash or are sick after a tick bite, bring the tick to your doctor's office.

Burns

Burns can be caused by fire, the sun, chemicals, hot liquids or objects, steam, electricity and other means. They can be minor medical problems or life-threatening emergencies.

Burn Classifications

Distinguishing a minor burn from a more serious burn involves determining the degree of damage to the tissues of the body. The following three classifications and illustrations will help determine your response.

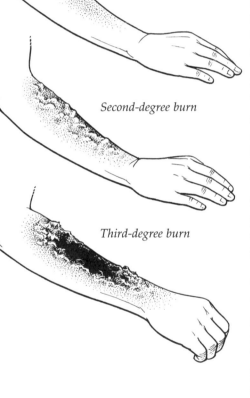

First-degree burn

Second-degree burn

Third-degree burn

First-Degree: Minor

The least serious burns are those in which only the outer layer of skin (epidermis) is burned. The skin is usually reddened, and there may be swelling and pain. However, the outer layer of skin has not been burned through. Unless such a burn involves substantial portions of the hands, feet, face, groin, buttocks or a major joint, it may be treated as a minor burn with the self-care remedies listed on page 18. Chemical burns may require additional follow-up. If the burn was caused by exposure to the sun, see Sunburn, page 19.

Second-Degree

When the first layer of skin has been burned through and the second layer of skin (dermis) also is burned, the injury is termed a second-degree burn. Blisters develop, and the skin takes on an intensely reddened appearance and becomes splotchy. Severe pain and swelling are accompanying symptoms.

If a second-degree burn is limited to an area no larger than 2 to 3 inches in diameter, follow the home remedies listed on page 18. If the burned area of the skin is larger, or if the burn is on the hands, feet, face, groin, buttocks or a major joint, seek urgent care immediately.

Third-Degree: Severe

The most serious burns involve all layers of the skin. Fat, nerves, muscles and even bones also may be affected. There are usually areas that are charred black or appear a dry white. There may be severe pain or, if nerve damage is substantial, no pain at all. You must take immediate action in all cases of third-degree burns.

Emergency Treatment: All Major Burns

Seek emergency treatment immediately for major burns. Dial 911. Until an emergency unit arrives, follow these steps:
- **Do not remove burnt clothing**, but do make sure that the victim is not still in contact with smoldering materials.
- **Make certain that the burn victim is breathing.**
- **Cover the area of the burn** with a cool, moist sterile bandage or with a clean cloth.

Self-Care: **Minor Burns Only**	For minor burns, including second-degree burns limited to an area no larger than 2 to 3 inches in diameter, take the following action: • **Cool the burn.** Hold the burned area under cold running water for 15 minutes. If this step is impractical, immerse the burn in cold water or cool it with cold compresses. Cooling the burn reduces swelling by carrying heat away from the skin. • **Consider a lotion.** Once a burn is completely cooled, a lotion, such as one that contains aloe vera, or moisturizer prevents drying and increases your comfort. For sunburn, try 1 percent hydrocortisone cream or an anesthetic cream. • **Bandage a burn.** Cover the burn with a sterile gauze bandage. (Fluffy cotton may be irritating.) Wrap it loosely to avoid putting pressure on burned skin. Bandaging keeps air off the area, reduces pain and protects blistered skin. • **Take over-the-counter pain relievers** (see page 265). • Minor burns will usually heal in about 1 to 2 weeks without further treatment, but watch for signs of infection.
Caution	**Do not use ice.** Putting ice directly on a burn can cause frostbite and further damage your skin. **Do not break blisters.** Fluid-filled blisters protect against infection. If blisters break, wash the area with mild soap and water, then apply an antibiotic ointment and a gauze bandage. Clean and change dressings daily.

■ Chemical Burns

Self-Care	• **Make sure the cause of the burn has been removed.** Flush the chemicals off the skin surface with cool running water for 20 minutes or more. (If the burning chemical is a powder-like substance such as lime, brush it off your skin before flushing.) • **Treat the person for shock (see page 11).** Symptoms include fainting, pale complexion or breathing in a notably shallow fashion. • **Remove clothing or jewelry** that has been contaminated by the chemical. • **Wrap the burned area** with a dry, sterile dressing (if possible) or a clean cloth. • **Rewash the burn** for several more minutes if the victim complains of increased burning after the initial washing. **Prevention** • When using chemicals, always wear protective eyewear and clothing. • Know about the chemicals you use. • At work, read appropriate Material Safety Data Sheets, or call your local poison control center listed in your telephone book to learn more about the substance.
Medical Help	Minor chemical burns usually heal without further treatment. However, seek emergency medical assistance (1) if the chemical burned through the first layer of skin and the resulting second-degree burn covers an area more than 2 to 3 inches in diameter or (2) if the chemical burn occurred on the hands, feet, face, groin, buttocks or a major joint. If you are unsure if a given compound is toxic, call a poison control center.
Caution	Common household cleaning products, particularly those that contain ammonia or bleach, and garden chemicals can cause serious harm to the eyes or skin. Read labels. They contain instructions for proper use and treatment recommendations.

Mayo Clinic Guide to Self-Care

■ Sunburn

Although the sun provides a welcome change from gray winter months, it can damage your skin and increase your risk of skin cancer. Symptoms of sunburn usually appear within a few hours after exposure, bringing pain, redness, swelling and occasional blistering. Because a large area is often exposed, a sunburn can cause headache, fever and fatigue.

Self-Care

- Take a cool bath or shower. Adding one-half cup of cornstarch, oatmeal or baking soda to your bath may provide some relief.
- Leave water blisters intact to speed healing and avoid infection. If they burst on their own, apply an antibacterial ointment on the open areas.
- Take over-the-counter pain relievers (see page 265).
- Avoid products containing benzocaine (an anesthetic) because they can cause allergic reactions in many people.

Prevention

- If you plan to be outside, avoid the hours of 10 a.m. to 3 p.m., when the sun's ultraviolet (UV) radiation is at its peak. Cover exposed areas, wear a broad-brimmed hat and use a sunscreen with a sun protection factor (SPF) of at least 15.
- Protect your eyes. Sunglasses that block 95 percent of UV radiation are adequate. But you may need lenses that block 99 percent if you spend long hours in the sun, have had cataract surgery or are taking a prescription medication that increases your sensitivity to UV radiation.

Medical Help

If your sunburn begins to blister or you feel ill, see your physician. Oral cortisone such as prednisone is occasionally helpful.

Caution

Sunburn may not slow you down too much, but a lifetime of overexposure to the sun's UV radiation can damage your skin and increase your risk for skin cancer. If you have severe sunburn or immediate complications (rash, itching or fever), contact your physician.

■ Electrical Burns

Any electrical burn should be examined by a physician. An electrical burn may appear minor, but the damage can extend deep to the tissues beneath the skin. A heart rhythm disturbance, cardiac arrest or other internal damage can occur if the amount of electrical current that passed through the body was large.

Sometimes the jolt associated with the electrical injury can cause a person to be thrown or to fall, and fractures or other associated injuries can result.

Cold Weather Problems

◼ Frostbite

Cover your face if you feel the effects of frostbite.

Frostbite can affect any area of your body. Your hands, feet, nose and ears are most susceptible because they are small and often exposed.

In subfreezing temperatures, the tiny blood vessels in your skin tighten, reducing the flow of blood and oxygen to the tissues. Eventually, cells are destroyed.

The first sign of frostbite may be a slightly painful, tingling sensation. This often is followed by numbness. Your skin may be deathly pale and feel hard, cold and numb.

Frostbite can damage deep layers of tissue. As deeper layers of tissue freeze, blisters often form. Blistering usually occurs over 1 to 2 days.

Persons with atherosclerosis or who are taking medication for a heart condition may be more susceptible to frostbite.

Self-Care

- Carefully and gradually rewarm frostbitten areas. If you are outside, place your hands directly on the skin of warmer areas of your body. Warm your hands by tucking them into your armpits; if your nose, ears or face is frostbitten, warm the area by covering it with your warm hands (but try to keep them protected).
- If possible, immerse your hands or feet in water that is slightly above normal body temperature (100 to 105 F) or that feels warm to someone else.
- Do not rub the affected area. Never rub snow on frostbitten skin.
- Do not smoke cigarettes. Nicotine causes your blood vessels to constrict and may limit circulation.
- If your feet are frostbitten, elevate them after rewarming.
- Don't use direct heat (such as heating pads).
- Do not rewarm an affected area if there is a chance that it will refreeze.

Follow-Up

Frostbitten areas will turn red and throb, or they will burn with pain as they thaw. Even with mild frostbite, normal sensation may not return immediately. When frostbite is severe, the area will probably remain numb until it heals completely. In extreme cases, healing can take months, and the damage to your skin can permanently change your sense of touch. In severe cases, in which infection is present after the affected area has been rewarmed, antibiotics may be necessary. Bed rest and physical therapy may be appropriate. Do not smoke cigarettes during recovery. Once you've had frostbite—no matter how mild—you're more likely to have it again.

Emergency Treatment

If numbness remains during rewarming, seek medical care immediately. A person with frostbite on the extremities also may have hypothermia (see page 21).

Kids' Care

Watch for signs of chilling or cold injury while your child is outside. Watch for wet chinstraps on caps or snowsuits because the skin under the strap can easily freeze. Teach older children the signs of cold injury and have them keep a close watch for changes in skin color on their younger friends.

Teach your child to avoid touching cold metal with bare hands and licking extremely cold metal objects.

Mayo Clinic Guide to Self-Care

How to Prevent Cold Weather Injuries

- **Stay dry.** Your body loses heat faster when your skin is dampened by rain, snow or perspiration.
- **Protect yourself from the wind.** Wind robs more heat from your body than cold air alone. Exposed skin is particularly affected by wind.
- **Wear clothing that insulates,** shields and "breathes." Layers of light, loose-fitting clothing trap air for effective insulation. As an outer layer, wear something that's water-repellent and windproof.

- **Cover your head, neck and face.** Wear two pairs of socks and boots tall enough to cover your ankles. Mittens protect your hands better than gloves.
- If a part of your body becomes so cold that it is starting to feel numb, take the time to rewarm it before continuing your activity.
- Don't touch metal with bare skin—cold metal can absorb heat quickly.
- Plan for trips and outdoor activities. Carry emergency equipment (see page 226).

■ Hypothermia

Under most conditions, your body maintains a healthy temperature. However, when exposed for prolonged periods to cold temperatures or a cool, damp environment, your body's control mechanisms may fail to keep your body temperature normal. When more heat is lost than your body can generate, hypothermia can result. Wet or damp clothing can increase your chances of hypothermia.

Falling overboard from a boat into cold water is a common cause of hypothermia. An uncovered head or inadequate clothing in winter is another frequent cause.

The key symptom of hypothermia is a body temperature that drops to less than 94 F. Signs include shivering, slurred speech, an abnormally slow rate of breathing, skin that is cold and pale, a loss of coordination and feelings of tiredness, lethargy or apathy. The onset of symptoms is usually slow; there is likely to be a gradual loss of mental acuity and physical ability. The person experiencing hypothermia, in fact, may be unaware that he or she is in a state requiring emergency medical treatment.

The elderly, the very young and very lean people are at particular risk of hypothermia. Other conditions that may predispose you to hypothermia are malnutrition, heart disease, underactive thyroid and excessive consumption of alcohol.

Emergency Treatment

- After getting the person out of the cold, change the victim into warm, dry clothing. If going indoors is not possible, the person needs to be out of the wind, have the head covered and be insulated from the cold ground.
- Seek emergency medical assistance. While waiting for help to arrive, monitor the person's breathing and pulse. If either has stopped or seems dangerously slow or shallow, initiate CPR immediately (see page 2).
- In extreme cases, once the victim has arrived at a medical center, blood rewarming, similar to the procedure in a heart bypass machine, is sometimes used to restore normal body temperature quickly.
- If emergency care is not available, warm the person with a bath at 100 to 105 F (warm to the touch but not hot). Give warm liquids.
- Companions may be able to share body heat.

Caution

Do not give the victim alcohol. Give warm nonalcoholic drinks (unless he or she is vomiting).

Cuts, Scrapes and Wounds

Everyday cuts, scrapes or wounds often don't require a trip to the emergency room. Yet proper care is essential to avoid infection or other complications. The following guidelines can help you in caring for simple wounds. Puncture wounds may require medical attention.

■ Simple Wounds

Self-Care

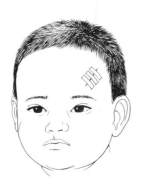

A strip or two of surgical tape (Steri-Strips) may close a minor cut, but if the mouth of the wound is not easily closed, seek a physician's care. Proper closure also will minimize scarring.

- **Stop the bleeding.** Minor cuts and scrapes usually stop bleeding on their own. If not, apply gentle pressure with a clean cloth or bandage.
- **Keep the wound clean.** Rinse with clear water. Clean the area around the wound with soap and a washcloth. Keep soap out of the wound. Soap can cause an irritation. If dirt or debris remains in the wound after washing, use clean tweezers to remove the particles. Apply alcohol to the tweezers before use. If debris remains embedded in the wound after cleaning, contact your health care provider, and don't attempt to remove it by yourself. Thorough wound cleaning also reduces the risk of contracting tetanus (see page 23).
- Hydrogen peroxide, iodine or an iodine-containing cleanser may be used in the area around the wound. However, these substances are irritating to living cells and should not be used in the wound itself.
- **Consider the source.** Puncture wounds or other deep cuts, animal bites or particularly dirty wounds put you at risk for tetanus infection (see page 23). If the wound is serious, you may require an additional tetanus booster even if you received your last one within the past 10 years. A booster is given for dirty or deep wounds if you have not had one in the previous 5 years.
- **Prevent infection.** After you clean the wound, apply a thin layer of an antibiotic cream or ointment (such as Neosporin or Polysporin) to help keep the surface moist. The products don't make the wound heal faster, but they can discourage infection and allow your body's healing factors to close the wound more efficiently. Be aware that certain ingredients in some ointments can cause a mild rash in some people. If a rash appears, stop using the ointment.
- **Cover the wound.** Exposure to air will speed healing, but bandages can help keep the wound clean and keep harmful bacteria out. Blisters that are draining are vulnerable and should be covered until a scab forms.
- To help prevent infection, **change the dressing** at least once a day or whenever it becomes wet or dirty. If you're allergic to the adhesive used in most bandages, switch to adhesive-free dressings or sterile gauze and paper tape. These supplies generally are available at pharmacies.

Medical Help

If bleeding persists—if the blood spurts or continues to flow after several minutes of pressure—emergency care is necessary.

Are stitches needed? A deep (all the way through the skin), gaping or jagged-edged wound may require stitches to hold it together for proper healing. A strip or two of surgical tape may close a minor cut, but if the mouth of the wound is not easily closed, seek medical care. Proper closure also minimizes scarring (see page 23).

Mayo Clinic Guide to Self-Care

Caution
Watch for signs of infection. Every day that a wound remains unhealed, the risk of infection increases. See your health care provider if your wound isn't healing steadily or if you notice any redness, drainage, warmth or swelling.

A Shot in the Arm: Tetanus Vaccine

A cut, laceration, bite or other wound, even if minor, can lead to a tetanus infection. The result can be lockjaw that occurs days or even weeks later. Lockjaw, or tetanus, is a stiffness of jaw muscles and other muscles. It may be followed by a range of other symptoms and could lead to convulsions, breathing problems and even death.

Tetanus bacteria usually are found in the soil but can occur virtually anywhere. If their spores enter a wound beyond the reach of oxygen, they germinate and produce a toxin that interferes with the nerves controlling your muscles.

Active immunization is vital for everyone in advance of an injury. The tetanus vaccine usually is given to children as a DTP shot. Adults generally need a tetanus booster every 10 years. If the wound is serious, your physician may recommend an additional booster even if your last one was within 10 years. A booster is given if you have a deep or dirty wound and your most recent booster was more than 5 years ago. Boosters should be given within 2 days of the injury.

■ Puncture Wounds

A puncture wound does not usually result in excessive bleeding. Often, in fact, little blood flows and the wound seems to close almost instantly. These features, however, do not mean that treatment is unnecessary.

A puncture wound—such as stepping on a nail or being stuck with a tack—can be dangerous because of the risk of infection. The object that caused the wound may carry spores of the tetanus or other bacteria, especially if the object has been exposed to soil. Follow the same self-care steps and advice on seeking medical help listed on page 22, but a deep, contaminated puncture wound may need to be cleaned by a physician.

What About Scarring?

No matter how you treat them, most deep wounds that penetrate beyond the first layer of skin form a scar when healed. Even superficial wounds can form a scar if infection or re-injury occurs. Following the guidelines on page 22 may help avoid these complications.

When a healing wound is exposed to sunlight, it can darken permanently. This darkening can be prevented by covering the area with clothing or sunblock (sunscreen protection factor more than 15) whenever you are outside during the first 6 months after the wound occurs.

A scar usually thickens about 2 months into the healing process. Within 6 months to a year, it should become thinner and be even with your skin surface.

A large, jagged scar that continues to enlarge is called a keloid, an abnormal growth of scar tissue. Surgical incisions, vaccinations, burns or even a scratch can cause keloids. The tendency to develop keloids is often inherited, and they're more common on deeply pigmented skin than on white skin.

Keloids are harmless. But if they itch or look unattractive, doctors can remove small keloids by freezing them with liquid nitrogen, then injecting with cortisone. Sometimes they stop growing, but they rarely disappear by themselves.

Ask a dermatologist or plastic surgeon to evaluate your scar and advise treatment.

Eye Injuries

Consider some common objects in your home—paper clips, pencils, tools and toys. Used without care, they pose a threat to your windows on the world—your eyes.

The topic of eye injuries offers a "bad news-good news" scenario. Eye injuries are common, and some are serious. Fortunately, you can prevent the vast majority of these injuries by taking simple steps (see page 76 for common eye problems).

■ Corneal Abrasion (Scratch)

The most common types of eye injury involve the cornea—the clear, protective "window" at the front of the eye. The cornea can be scratched or cut by contact with dust, dirt, sand, wood shavings, metal particles or even an edge of a piece of paper. Usually the scratch is superficial, and this is called a corneal abrasion. Some corneal abrasions become infected and result in a corneal ulcer, which is a serious problem.

Everyday activities can lead to corneal abrasions. Examples are playing sports, doing home repairs or being scratched by children who accidentally brush your cornea with a fingernail. Other common injuries to the cornea include "splash accidents"—contact with chemicals ranging from antifreeze to household cleaners.

Because the cornea is extremely sensitive, abrasions can be painful. If your cornea is scratched, you might feel like you have sand in your eye. Tears, blurred vision, sensitivity or redness around the eye can suggest a corneal abrasion.

Self-Care

In case of injury, seek prompt medical attention. Other immediate steps you can take are to:
- Run lukewarm tap water over the eye, or splash the eye with clean water. Many work sites have eye-rinse stations for this purpose. Rinsing the eye may wash out the offending foreign body. The technique is described on page 25.
- Blink several times. This movement may remove small particles of dust or sand.
- Pull the upper eyelid over the lower eyelid. The lashes of the lower eyelid can "brush" the foreign body from the undersurface of the upper eyelid.

Caution

- If abrasion was caused by an object in the eye, refer to page 25.
- Don't apply patches or ice packs to the eye. If you do get an object within the eye itself—typically when hammering metal on metal—do not press on the eyeball.
- Don't rub your eye after an injury. This action can worsen a corneal abrasion.

■ Chemical Splash

If a chemical splashes into your eye, flush it with water immediately. Any source of clean drinking water will do. It is more important to begin flushing than it is to find sterile water. Flushing water may dilute the chemical. Continue to flush the eye for at least 20 minutes, particularly if your eye is exposed to household cleaners that contain ammonia. After washing the eye thoroughly, close the eyelid and cover it with a loose, moist dressing. Then seek emergency medical assistance.

■ Object in the Eye

Children and adults alike occasionally get foreign objects in their eyes. You can take appropriate steps in some cases to remove the object. In other situations, you need to see a health care provider.

Clearing the Eye

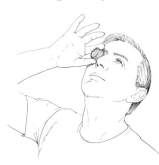

To remove a small object from your eye, flush the eye with a small amount of clean water using a small cup.

Your Own Eye

If no one is nearby to help you, try to flush the eye clear. Using an eyecup or small juice glass, wash your eye with clean water. Position the glass with its rim resting on the bone at the base of your eye socket and pour the water in, keeping the eye open. If you do not succeed in clearing the eye, seek emergency medical help.

Someone Else's Eye

- Do not rub the eye. Wash your hands before examining the eye. Seat the person in a well-lighted area.
- Locate the object in the eye visually. Examine the eye by gently pulling the lower lid downward and instructing the person to look upward. Reverse the procedure for the upper lid. Hold the upper lid and examine the eye while the person looks downward. If you find that the foreign object is embedded in the eyeball, cover the person's eye with a sterile pad or a clean cloth. Do not try to remove the object.
- If the object is large and makes closing the eye difficult, cover it with a paper cup taped to the face and forehead. Seek emergency medical assistance immediately.
- If the object is floating in the tear film or on the surface of the eye, you may be able to flush it out or remove it manually. While holding the upper or lower lid open, use a moistened cotton swab or the corner of a clean cloth to remove the object by lightly touching it. If you are unable to remove the object easily, cover both eyes with a soft cloth and seek emergency medical assistance.
- If you do succeed in removing the object, flush the eye with an eye irrigating solution or with water.
- If pain, vision problems or redness persists, seek emergency medical care.

Common Sense Can Save Your Sight

- **Wear goggles** while working with industrial chemicals, power tools and even hand tools. Some of the most serious eye injuries occur while people are using hammers. Also wear a safety helmet when appropriate.
- **Wear safety glasses** for sports such as racquetball, basketball, squash or tennis. Also wear appropriate headgear, such as batter's helmets for baseball and face masks for hockey.
- **Carefully follow the instructions for using detergents,** ammonia and cleaning fluids. When using fluids that come in spray containers, point nozzles away from your eyes at all times. Store household chemicals safely and out of children's reach.
- **Supervise children at play.** Remove toys that could lead to an eye injury. Examples are BB guns, plastic swords or spring-loaded toys that shoot darts. Don't allow children to have fireworks.
- **Don't lean over a car battery** when attaching jumper cables.
- **Pick up rocks and sticks** before mowing your lawn. While mowing, watch for trees with low-hanging branches.
- **Carefully follow your physician's instructions** for removing and applying contact lenses. Also, investigate any pain or red eye that occurs while you're wearing contact lenses.

Food-Borne Illness

Food-borne illness is a growing problem in the United States. The major reasons for this problem are an increase in restaurant dining and more centralized food processing.

All foods naturally contain small amounts of bacteria. But when food is poorly handled, improperly cooked or inadequately stored, bacteria can multiply in great enough numbers to cause illness. Parasites, viruses and chemicals also can contaminate food, but food-borne illness from these sources is less common.

If you eat contaminated food, whether you'll become ill or not depends on the organism, the amount of exposure, your age and your health. As you get older, immune cells may not respond as quickly and effectively to infectious organisms. Young children are at increased risk of illness because their immune systems haven't developed fully. Conditions such as diabetes and AIDS and cancer treatment also reduce your immune response, making you more susceptible to food-borne illness.

Food poisoning can cause various ailments. If you become ill within 1 to 6 hours after consuming contaminated food or water, you probably have a common type of food poisoning. Symptoms include nausea, vomiting, diarrhea or stomach pain.

Self-Care

- Rest and drink plenty of liquids.
- Don't use antidiarrheal medications because they may slow elimination of the bacteria and toxins from your system.
- Mild to moderate illness often resolves on its own within 12 hours.

Medical Help

If the symptoms last more than 12 hours, or if you have severe symptoms or belong to one of the high-risk groups noted above, see your physician.

Caution

Botulism is a potentially fatal food poisoning. It results from eating foods containing a toxin formed by certain spores in food. Botulism toxin is most often found in home-canned foods, especially green beans and tomatoes. Symptoms usually begin 12 to 36 hours after eating the contaminated food. Symptoms include headache, blurred or double vision, muscle weakness and eventually paralysis. Some people report nausea, vomiting, constipation, urinary retention and reduced salivation. These symptoms require immediate medical attention.

Handling Food Safely

- **Plan ahead.** Thaw meats and other frozen foods in the refrigerator, not on the countertop.
- **When shopping,** don't buy food in cans or jars with dented or bulging lids.
- **When preparing food,** wash your hands with soap and water. Rinse produce thoroughly or peel off the skin or outer leaves. Wash knives and cutting surfaces frequently, especially after handling raw meat and before preparing other foods to be eaten raw. Launder dishcloths and kitchen towels frequently.
- **When cooking,** use a meat thermometer. Cook red meat to an internal temperature of 160 F, poultry to 180 F. Cook fish until it flakes easily with a fork. Cook eggs until the yolks are firm and no longer runny.
- **When storing food,** always check expiration dates. Use or freeze fresh red meats within 3 to 5 days after purchase. Use or freeze fresh poultry, fish and ground meat within 1 to 2 days. Refrigerate or freeze leftovers within 2 hours of serving.

Troublesome Bacteria and How You Can Stop Them

Keep hot food hot. Keep cold food cold. Keep everything—especially your hands—clean. Follow these three basic rules and you're less likely to become ill from the troublesome bacteria listed here.

Bacteria	How Spread	Symptoms	To Prevent
Campylobacter jejuni	Contaminates meat and poultry during processing if feces contact meat surfaces. Other sources: unpasteurized milk, untreated water	Severe diarrhea (sometimes bloody), abdominal cramps, chills, headache. Onset within 2 to 11 days. Lasts 1 to 2 weeks	Cook meat and poultry thoroughly. Wash knives and cutting surfaces after contact with raw meat. Don't drink unpasteurized milk or untreated water
Clostridium perfringens	Meats, stews, gravies. Commonly spread when serving dishes don't keep food hot enough or food is chilled too slowly	Watery diarrhea, nausea, abdominal cramps. Fever is rare. Onset within 1 to 16 hours. Lasts 1 to 2 days	Keep foods hot. Hold cooked meats above 140 F. Reheat to at least 165 F. Chill foods quickly. Store in small containers
Escherichia coli 0157:H7	Contaminates beef during slaughter. Spread mainly by undercooked ground beef. Other sources: unpasteurized milk, unpasteurized apple cider, human stools, contaminated water	Watery diarrhea may turn bloody within 24 hours. Severe abdominal cramps, nausea, occasional vomiting. Usually no fever. Onset within 1 to 8 days. Lasts 5 to 8 days	Cook beef to internal temperature of 160 F. Don't drink unpasteurized milk or unpasteurized apple cider. Wash hands after bathroom use
Salmonella	Raw or contaminated meat, poultry, milk; contaminated egg yolks. Survives inadequate cooking. Spread by knives, cutting surfaces or an infected person who practices poor hygiene	Severe diarrhea, watery stools, nausea, vomiting, temperature 101 F or more. Onset within 6 to 72 hours. Lasts 1 to 14 days	Cook meat and poultry thoroughly. Don't drink unpasteurized milk. Don't eat raw or undercooked eggs. Keep cutting surfaces clean. Wash hands after bathroom use
Staphylococcus aureus	Spread by hand contact, coughing and sneezing. Grows on meats and prepared salads, cream sauces, cream-filled pastries	Explosive, watery diarrhea, nausea, vomiting, abdominal cramps, light-headedness. Onset within 1 to 6 hours. Lasts 1 to 2 days	Don't leave high-risk foods at room temperature for more than 2 hours. Wash hands and utensils before preparing food
Vibrio vulnificus	Raw oysters and raw or undercooked mussels, clams, whole scallops	Chills, fever, skin lesions. Onset 1 hr to 1 wk. Fatal in 50 percent of cases	Don't eat raw oysters. Make sure all shellfish is thoroughly cooked

Heat-Related Problems

Under normal conditions, your body's natural control mechanisms—skin and perspiration—adjust to the heat. However, those systems may fail when you are exposed to high temperatures for prolonged periods.

Heat Cramps

Heat cramps are painful muscle spasms. They usually occur after vigorous exercises and profuse perspiration. Your abdominal muscles and ones you use during exercise are most frequently affected.

Heat Exhaustion

Signs of heat exhaustion include an increased temperature, faintness, rapid heartbeat, low blood pressure, an ashen appearance, cold, clammy skin and nausea. Symptoms often begin suddenly, sometimes after excessive perspiration and inadequate fluid intake.

Heatstroke

Elderly and obese people are particularly at risk of heatstroke. Other risk factors include dehydration, alcohol use, heart disease, certain medications and vigorous exercise. People born with an impaired ability to sweat are particularly at risk. Signs of heatstroke include rapid heartbeat, rapid and shallow breathing, confusion and either increased or lowered blood pressure. Fainting can be the first sign in the elderly. A victim may stop sweating, but this is not a reliable sign.

Self-Care

For Heat Cramps
- Rest briefly; cool down.
- Eat salty foods.
- Drink water with a teaspoon of salt per quart.

For Heat Exhaustion
- If you suspect heat exhaustion, get the person out of the sun and into a shady spot or air-conditioned location. Then, lay the person down and elevate his or her feet slightly. Loosen or remove the clothing.
- Give cold (not ice) water to drink, or give an electrolyte-containing drink such as one of the popular sports drinks.

Medical Help

If you suspect heatstroke, get emergency help immediately, move the victim out of the sun and into a shady spot or air-conditioned space and give the victim a sponge bath.

Monitor victims of heat exhaustion carefully. Although less dangerous than heatstroke, heat exhaustion can quickly become heatstroke.

Tips to Beat the Heat

- **Stay out of the sun.** Avoid going outside during the hottest part of the day, noon to 4 p.m.
- **Limit activity.** Reserve vigorous exercise or activities for early morning or evening.
- **Dress properly.** Wear light-colored, light-weight, loose-fitting clothing that breathes.
- **Drink lots of liquids.** (Avoid alcohol and caffeine.)
- **Avoid hot and heavy meals.**

Poisonous Plants

Poison ivy

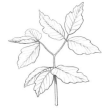

Poison oak

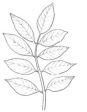

Poison sumac

When it comes to poison oak and ivy, it's wise to heed these words of advice: "Leaves of three, let them be."

With their leaves usually grouped three to a stem, poison ivy and poison oak are two of the most common causes of an allergic skin reaction called contact dermatitis.

Contact with poison ivy and poison oak usually causes red, swollen skin, blisters and severe itching. This reaction typically develops within 2 days after exposure, but it can develop as soon as a few hours. The rash usually reaches its peak after about 5 days, and it is usually gone within 1 to 2 weeks.

The rash is caused by exposure to resin, a colorless, oily substance contained in all parts of these plants. Resin transfers easily from clothing or from pet hair to your skin. Burning the plants is also hazardous because inhaling the smoke can cause internal and external reactions.

It takes only a tiny amount of resin to cause a reaction. Poison ivy and other rashes do not develop as a result of merely being near the plant, nor does the rash spread as a result of washing or scratching open rash blisters. The resin is not present in blister fluid. However, it can be spread by accidentally rubbing the resin on other areas of the skin before all the resin is washed off.

Besides poison ivy and oak, other plants also can cause the reaction. They include sumac, heliotrope (found in the deserts of the Southwest), ragweed (both the leaves and pollen), daisies, chrysanthemums, sagebrush, wormwood, celery, oranges, limes and potatoes.

Self-Care

- Washing the harmful resin off the skin with soap within 5 or 10 minutes after exposure may avert a skin reaction.
- Do not try to remove the resin by taking a bath. Bathing can spread the resin to other areas of your body.
- Wash any clothing or jewelry that may have been in contact with the plant. Note: Footwear and shoelaces also should be washed.
- Try not to scratch. Take cool showers.
- Over-the-counter preparations (calamine lotion or hydrocortisone cream) can ease itching. Or, apply a paste of baking soda or Epsom salts and water.
- Creams and lotions do not help much when the blisters open, but they can be used again when the blisters close.
- Do not apply alcohol because this tends to make the itching worse. Cover open blisters with a sterile gauze to prevent infection.
- To avoid exposure, learn to recognize poisonous plants and wear protective clothing when appropriate. Poison ivy leaves are oval or spoon-shaped. Poison oak leaves resemble oak leaves. The colors of the leaves of these plants change with the seasons, from green in the summer to orange and red in the fall.

Medical Help

If you have a severe reaction, or when your eyes, face or genital area is involved, contact your health care provider, who may prescribe cortisone or an antihistamine, either orally or topically.

Tooth Problems

■ Toothache

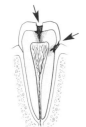

Dental cavities can lead to toothaches.

In most children and adults, tooth decay (cavities, also called caries) is the primary cause of toothaches. Tooth decay mainly is caused by bacteria and carbohydrates. Bacteria are present in a thin, almost invisible film on your teeth called plaque.

Tooth decay takes time to develop, often a year or two in permanent teeth but less in primary teeth. Acid formation occurs within the first 20 minutes after you eat.

The decay-producing acid that forms in plaque attacks the tooth's outer surface. The erosion caused by the plaque leads to the formation of tiny cavities (or openings) in the tooth surface. The first sign of decay may be a sensation of pain when you eat something sweet, very cold or very hot.

Self-Care

Until you are able to get to the dentist, try these self-care tips:
- Try flossing to remove any food particles wedged between the teeth.
- Suck on an ice cube placed in the area of irritation.
- Use an over-the-counter pain reliever.
- Over-the-counter antiseptics containing benzocaine will offer temporary relief. Oil of cloves (eugenol) can relieve pain. It is available at most pharmacies.
- Prevention is the best way to avoid tooth decay and cavities.

Caution

Swelling, pain when you bite, a foul-tasting discharge and redness indicate infection. See your dentist as soon as possible. If you have fever with the pain, seek emergency care.

■ Tooth Loss

Whenever a tooth is accidentally knocked out, appropriate emergency medical care is required immediately. Today, permanent teeth that are knocked out sometimes can be reimplanted if you act quickly. A broken tooth, however, cannot be reimplanted.

Emergency Treatment

If a permanent tooth is knocked out, save the tooth and consult your dentist immediately. If it is after office hours, call your dentist at home. If he or she is unavailable, go to the nearest emergency room.

Successful reimplantation depends on several factors: prompt insertion (within 30 minutes if possible; no longer than 2 hours after loss) and proper storage and transportation of the tooth. Keeping it moist is essential.

Self-Care

To preserve the tooth until you get to the dentist:
- Handle the tooth by the top (crown) only.
- Do not rub it or scrape it to remove dirt.
- Gently rinse the tooth in a glass of tap water, but not under the faucet.
- Try to replace the tooth in the socket and bite down gently on gauze or a moistened tea bag to help keep it in place.
- If the tooth cannot be replaced in the socket, immediately place it in milk, your own saliva or a warm, mild saltwater solution.

Trauma

Trauma is any injury sustained as a result of external force or violence. A broken bone, a severe blow to the head and a knocked-out tooth are all considered trauma.

Fractures, severe sprains, dislocations and other serious bone and joint injuries also are trauma emergencies and usually require professional medical care.

■ Dislocations

A dislocation is an injury in which the ends of bones in a joint are forced from their normal positions. In most cases, a blow, fall or other trauma causes the dislocation.

The indications of a dislocation include the following:
● An injured joint that is visibly out of position, misshapen and difficult to move
● Swelling and intense pain at a joint

The dislocation should be treated as quickly as possible, but do not try to return the joint to its proper place. Splint the affected joint in the position it is in. Treat it as you would a fracture. Seek immediate medical attention.

For more information on dislocations, see page 93.

■ Fractures

A fracture is, simply, a broken bone. It requires immediate medical attention.

If you suspect a fracture, the proper approach is to protect the affected area from further damage. Do not try to set the broken bone. Instead, immobilize the area with a splint. Also keep joints above and below the fracture immobilized.

If bleeding occurs along with the broken bone, apply pressure to stop the bleeding. If possible, elevate the site of bleeding to lessen the blood flow. Maintain pressure until the bleeding stops.

If the person is faint, pale or breathing in a notably shallow, rapid fashion, use the treatment steps for shock: lay the person down, elevate the legs and cover with a blanket or something for warmth.

Signs of a fracture are as follows:
● Swelling or bruising over a bone
● Deformity of the affected limb
● Localized pain that is intensified when the affected area is moved or pressure is put on it
● Loss of function in the area of the injury
● A broken bone that has poked through adjacent soft tissues and is sticking out of the skin

For more information on fractures, see page 89.

■ Sprains

A sprain occurs when a violent twist or stretch causes a joint to move outside its normal range. A sprain is the result of overstretched ligaments. Tearing of the ligaments may occur. The usual indications of a sprain are the following:

- Pain and tenderness in the affected area
- Rapid swelling and possible discoloration of the skin
- Impaired joint function

Most minor sprains can be treated at home. However, if a popping sound and immediate difficulty in using the joint accompany the injury, seek emergency medical care.

For more information on sprains, see page 88.

■ Head Injuries

Most head injuries are minor. The skull provides the brain with considerable protection from injury. Only 10 percent of all head injuries require hospitalization. Simple cuts and bruises can be treated with basic first aid techniques.

The serious types of head injuries that require emergency medical care are listed below. In all cases of worrisome head injury, do not move the neck because it may have been injured.

Concussion: When the head sustains a hard blow as the result of being struck or from a fall, a concussion may result. The impact creates a sudden movement of the brain within the skull. A concussion involves a loss of consciousness. Victims are often described as dazed. Loss of memory, dizziness and vomiting also may occur. Partial paralysis and shock are other possible symptoms.

Blood clot on the brain: This occurs when a blood vessel ruptures between the skull and the brain. Blood then leaks between the brain and skull and forms a blood clot (hematoma), which presses on the brain tissue. Symptoms occur from a few hours to several weeks after a blow to the head. There may be no open wound, bruise or other outward sign. Symptoms include headache, nausea, vomiting, alteration of consciousness and pupils of unequal size. There may be progressive lethargy, unconsciousness and death if the condition is not treated.

Skull fracture: This type of injury is not always apparent. Look for the following:

- Bruising or discoloring behind the ear or around the eyes
- Blood or clear, watery fluids leaking from the ears or nose
- Pupils of unequal size
- Deformity of the skull, including swelling or depressions

Emergency Treatment

Seek emergency medical care if any of the following symptoms are apparent:

- Severe head or facial bleeding
- Change in level of consciousness, even if only briefly
- Irregular or labored breathing
- Vomiting

Caution

- Until emergency help arrives, keep the person lying down and quiet in a dimmed room. Observe the person for vital signs: breathing, heartbeat and alertness. Stop any bleeding by applying firm pressure.

Mayo Clinic Guide to Self-Care

General Symptoms

- **Dizziness and Fainting**
- **Fatigue**
- **Fever**
- **Pain**
- **Sleep Disorders**
- **Sweating and Body Odor**
- **Unexpected Weight Changes**

Fatigue...fever...dizziness...pain...
sleep disorders...sweating...unex-
pected weight changes. In medicine, these conditions are called
"general symptoms" because
they tend to affect your whole
body rather than a particular
body part or system. In this
section, we explain the common
causes for each of seven general
symptoms and provide self-care
information and advice on when
to seek medical care.

Dizziness and Fainting

Dizziness has many causes. Fortunately, most dizziness is mild, brief and harmless. It can be caused by many things, including medications, infections and stress. The word "dizziness" actually describes various sensations.

Vertigo and Imbalance

Vertigo is the sensation that you or your surroundings are rotating. You may feel that the room is spinning, or you may sense the rotation within your own head or body. Vertigo usually is associated with problems in your inner ear. The inner ear has an ultrasensitive device for sensing movement. Viral illness, trauma or other disturbance can result in the device sending a false message to your brain.

Imbalance is the sensation that you must touch or hold onto something to maintain your balance. Severe imbalance may make it difficult to stand without falling.

Light-Headedness and Fainting

Light-headedness includes feelings of being woozy, floating or near fainting. Fainting is a sudden, brief loss of consciousness. It occurs when your brain doesn't receive enough blood and the oxygen it carries. Although frightening, fainting generally isn't a reason for alarm. Once you are lying flat, blood flows to your brain and you regain consciousness within about a minute. Fainting may be caused by medical disorders, including heart disease, severe coughing spells and circulatory problems. In other cases, fainting may be related to the following:

- Medications for high blood pressure and erratic heartbeats
- Excessive sweating that results in loss of sodium and dehydration
- Extreme fatigue
- Upsetting news or an unexpected or unusual stress such as the sight of blood

A rapid drop in blood pressure, called *postural hypotension*, occurs when you get up quickly from a sitting or reclining position. Everyone experiences this reaction to a mild degree. You feel light-headed or slightly faint, and it usually passes within seconds. When it leads to fainting or blackouts, it's more serious. It often occurs after a hot bath or in people taking medications to control blood pressure.

Self-Care

- If your vision darkens or you feel faint, lower your head. Lie down and elevate your legs slightly to return blood to the heart. If you can't lie down, lean forward and put your head between your knees.

Prevention

- Stand and change positions slowly—particularly when turning from side to side or when changing from lying down to standing. Before standing up in the morning, sit on the edge of the bed for a few minutes.
- Stand still for a minute or two before you start to walk.
- Pace yourself. Take breaks when you are active in heat and humidity. Dress appropriate to the conditions to avoid overheating.
- Drink enough fluids to avoid dehydration and assure good circulation.
- Avoid smoking, alcohol and illegal drugs.
- Don't drive a car or operate dangerous equipment if you feel dizzy.
- Don't climb or descend staircases.
- Check medications. You may need to ask your doctor about adjustments.

Mayo Clinic Guide to Self-Care

Medical Help

Mild symptoms that persist for weeks or months may be due to serious nervous system diseases. Because problems of dizziness and balance can have many different causes, making a diagnosis usually requires a complete medical history and several tests.

Treatments for sudden onset of vertigo include avoiding positions or movements that cause dizziness, sedatives, antinausea drugs and a positioning treatment your doctor may suggest.

Contact your health care provider if:
- The condition is severe, prolonged (more than a few days or a week) or recurrent
- You are taking drugs for high blood pressure
- You have black tarry stools, blood in your stools or other signs of blood loss
  Seek emergency medical care if:
- You faint when you turn your head or extend your neck, or if fainting is accompanied by symptoms such as pain in the chest or head, trouble with breathing, numbness or continuing weakness, irregular heartbeat, blurred vision, confusion or trouble with talking
- The symptoms listed above are present on awakening
- Someone faints without warning
- This was the person's first fainting spell and there were no obvious reasons for it
- The person was injured during the faint

Until medical help arrives, do the following: If the person is lying down, position him or her on the back. Watch the airway—people often vomit after fainting. If you believe the person is about to vomit, roll him or her onto the side. Listen for breathing sounds and check for a pulse. (If they are absent, the problem is more serious than fainting, and CPR, see page 2, must be started.) Raise the legs above the level of the head. If a person faints and remains seated, quickly lay him or her flat. Loosen tight clothing.

How Your Body Maintains Balance

Maintaining balance requires a complex networking of several different parts of your body. To maintain balance, your brain must coordinate a constant flow of information from your eyes, muscles and tendons, and inner ear. All of these parts of the body work together to help keep you upright and provide you with a sense of stability when you are moving.

Many problems with dizziness are caused by problems within your inner ear. However, problems in any part of the system that controls your balance can cause dizziness and imbalance.

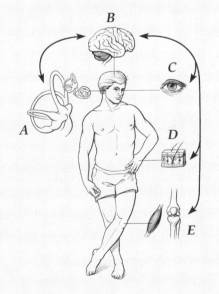

A. *The inner ear contains our primary balance structure.*

B. *The brain relays and interprets information to and from the body.*

C. *The eyes record the body's position and surroundings.*

D. *When we touch things, sensors in our skin give us information about our environment.*

E. *Muscles and joints report bodily movement to the brain.*

Fatigue

Almost everyone experiences fatigue at some time. After putting in a long weekend of yard chores or a hectic day with the children or at the office, it's natural to feel tired. This kind of physical and emotional fatigue is normal, and you can usually restore your energy with rest or exercise.

If you feel tired all the time, or if the exhaustion is overwhelming, you might start to worry that your condition is more serious than just fatigue. However, when fatigue is not accompanied by other symptoms, a specific cause often can't be determined. A common cause of chronic fatigue is lack of regular exercise (deconditioning). This problem can be remedied easily by gradually increasing your activity and beginning an exercise program.

Fatigue can be the result of physical or emotional problems. Physical fatigue is usually more pronounced later in the day, and it often resolves with a good night's sleep. Emotional fatigue often peaks first thing in the morning and gets better as the day progresses.

Common Causes

Common causes of physical fatigue include the following:
- Poor eating habits
- Lack of sleep
- Being out of shape
- Warm working or living quarters
- Carbon monoxide poisoning
- Over-the-counter medications, including pain relievers, cough and cold medicines, antihistamines and allergy remedies, sleeping pills and motion sickness pills
- Prescription drugs such as tranquilizers, muscle relaxants, sedatives, birth control pills and blood pressure medications
- Dehydration

Fatigue also can be an early symptom of these conditions:
- A low red blood cell count (anemia)
- Low thyroid activity (hypothyroidism)
- Various acute or chronic infections
- Heart disease
- Sleep disorder
- Electrolyte imbalance (when the levels of salts in your blood such as sodium, potassium and other minerals are too high or too low)
- Cancer
- Diabetes
- Alcoholism
- Rheumatoid arthritis

Most of these illnesses are accompanied by other symptoms such as muscle aches, pain, nausea, fever, weight loss, cold sensitivity or shortness of breath.

Common causes of emotional fatigue include:
- Overextending yourself, especially if you can't say "no"
- Boredom or lack of stimulation from family, friends or coworkers
- A major crisis (losing a spouse or a job), a move or a family difficulty
- Depression
- Loneliness
- Unresolved past emotional issues
- Repressing anger instead of expressing it

Mayo Clinic Guide to Self-Care

Self-Care

Before you talk to a health care provider, consider the possibility that your fatigue is related to an explainable cause that can be remedied with some of the following lifestyle changes:

- Get an adequate night's sleep—6 to 8 hours of uninterrupted sleep.
- Give yourself a break. Ask others to pitch in.
- Organize your schedule, and prioritize activities.
- Rest and relax—unwind. Do something fun.
- Exercise more, starting gradually. Walk instead of watching television. If you are older than 40, consult your doctor before beginning a vigorous exercise program.
- Increase your exposure to fresh air at home and at work.
- Eat a balanced diet. Steer clear of high-fat foods.
- Lose weight if you are overweight.
- Drink plenty of water (2 or more quarts per day to avoid dehydration).
- Review your medications (over-the-counter and prescription) to determine if fatigue is a side effect.
- Quit smoking.
- Reduce or eliminate your use of alcohol.
- If you have problems at your job, find ways to resolve them. (See Keeping Stress Under Control, page 224, and Stress Relievers, page 239.)

Medical Help

If fatigue persists even when you rest enough, and it lasts for 2 weeks or longer, you may have a problem that requires medical care. See your health care provider.

Kids' Care

Children and young adults rarely complain of fatigue. If they do, it's usually a sign that they have an acute infection, or that one is developing. Consult your physician.

What Is Chronic Fatigue Syndrome?

Chronic fatigue syndrome is a poorly understood, flu-like condition that can completely drain your energy and may last for years. People who were previously healthy and full of energy experience intense fatigue, pain in joints and muscles, painful lymph glands and headaches.

Experts haven't yet determined the causes of chronic fatigue syndrome, although there are likely to be many. Theories include infections, hormonal imbalances and psychological, immunologic or neurologic abnormalities. In one study, researchers found that some people with the syndrome had a low blood pressure disorder triggering the fainting reflex.

Treatment for chronic fatigue syndrome is aimed at relieving your symptoms. Anti-inflammatory pain relievers, such as ibuprofen, often are prescribed, but they rarely help. Low doses of certain antidepressants may help relieve pain and the depression that often is present with a chronic illness. Because people with chronic fatigue syndrome may become deconditioned, perpetuating the fatigue, physical therapy is crucial. It can help prevent or decrease the muscle weakness that is caused by prolonged inactivity. You may benefit from counseling to help you deal with the illness and the limitations it creates.

Fever

Even when you're well, your temperature varies, and that variation is normal. We consider 98.6 F (37 C) a healthy body temperature. But, your "normal" temperature may differ by a degree or more.

In the morning your temperature is generally lower, and in the afternoon it's somewhat higher. Check your family members' temperatures when they're healthy. Discover their "normal" range.

What Is the Cause?

Fever itself is not an illness, but it is often a sign of one. A fever tells you that something is happening inside your body.

Most likely, your body is fighting an infection caused by either bacteria or a virus. The fever may even be helpful in fighting the infection. Rarely, it's a sign of a reaction to a medicine, an inflammatory condition or too much heat. Sometimes you don't know why you have a fever. But don't automatically try to lower your temperature. Decreasing it may mask symptoms, prolong an illness and delay identifying the cause.

You usually will know what caused a fever in a day or two. If you think it's something other than a viral illness, consult your health care professional. Other common causes of fever include the following:

- An infection, such as urinary tract infection (frequent or painful urination), strep throat or tonsillitis (often with a sore throat), sinus infection (pain above or beneath the eyes) or bronchitis (cough and chest congestion) dental abscess (tender area in the mouth)
- Infectious mononucleosis, accompanied by fatigue
- An illness you picked up in a foreign country
- Heat exhaustion or severe sunburn

Caution

Never give a child or young adult aspirin for a fever unless directed by your doctor. Rarely, aspirin causes a serious or even fatal disease called Reye's syndrome if given during a viral infection.

Self-Care

Drink plenty of water to avoid dehydration (because the body loses more water with a fever) and get enough rest.

- **For children and adults with temperatures less than 102 F (38.9 C):**
  - Normally, avoid using medicine for a new fever in this range.
  - Wear comfortable, light clothing and cover yourself with only a sheet or light blanket
- **For children and adults with temperatures between 102 F (38.9 C) and 104 F (40 C):**
  - Give adults or children acetaminophen (Tylenol or generic brand) or ibuprofen (Advil, Motrin or generic), according to the label instructions. Adults may use aspirin instead. Do not give children aspirin.
- **For children and adults with temperatures more than 104 F (40 C):**
  - Give adults or children acetaminophen (Tylenol or generic) or ibuprofen (Advil, Motrin or generic), following the manufacturer's instructions. Adults may use aspirin instead.
  - A sponge bath of lukewarm water may bring the temperature down.
  - Recheck the temperature every half hour.

Fahrenheit		Centigrade
105	Seek medical help	40.6
104		40
103	Caution	39.4
102		38.9
101	Self-care	38.3
100		37.8
99	Normal	37.2
98	range	36.7
97		36.1
96		35.6

Mayo Clinic Guide to Self-Care

Medical Help

Call your health care provider about a fever in any of the following situations:
- Your temperature is more than 104 F (40 C)
- A baby younger than 3 months whose temperature is 100.5 F (38 C) or higher
- Your temperature has been more than 101 F (38.3 C) for more than 3 days

A fever is only one sign of the illness. Tell the physician what contagious diseases people around you have, including flu, colds, measles or mumps.

Call your health care provider **immediately** if any of these symptoms accompany a fever:
- A severe headache
- Severe swelling of the throat
- Unusual eye sensitivity to bright light
- Significant stiff neck and pain when you bend your head forward
- Mental confusion
- Persistent vomiting
- Difficulty breathing
- Extreme listlessness or irritability
- A bulging soft spot on a baby's head

Kids' Care

An unexplained fever is a greater cause for concern in children than in adults. A rapid rise or fall in temperature causes a seizure in about 1 in 20 children younger than 4. It generally lasts less than 10 minutes. It usually causes no permanent damage. If a seizure occurs, lay your child on his or her side and hold the child to prevent trauma. Don't place anything in the mouth or try to stop the seizure. Promptly seek medical attention to determine the cause of the seizure and any necessary treatment.

Sometimes a fever accompanies teething. Fever with ear pulling often indicates a middle ear infection. Ask your doctor about fevers associated with shots.

It's usually easier to give medications in liquid form. For a small child, use a syringe with measurements on the side and a bulb on the tip. Gently squirt the medicine in the back corners of the child's mouth.

Encourage children to drink ample water, juice and sugared pop or to eat frozen ice pops.

Taking Temperatures

Several types of thermometers are available: glass thermometers, electronic thermometers and tympanic (ear) thermometers. Disposable temperature strips are often inaccurate.

Learn to read your thermometer, following these steps:
- Clean it with soapy, cool water or alcohol.
- To prepare a glass thermometer for use, hold it firmly between two fingers. Flick your wrist to shake the indicator to less than 98.6 F (37 C), ideally down to 92 F.
- **Oral thermometer:** Place the bulb under your tongue. Close your mouth for 3 minutes.

Remove the thermometer and rotate it slowly until you can read the temperature.
- You also can use an oral thermometer for an armpit reading (hold the arms across the chest). Wait 5 minutes. Add 1° to the temperature to convert to an approximate oral temperature.
- **Rectal thermometer** (for infants): Place a dab of petroleum jelly on the bulb. Lay your child on his or her stomach. Carefully insert the bulb 1/2 to 1 inch into the rectum. Hold the bulb and child still for 3 minutes. Subtract 1° from the temperature to convert to an approximate oral temperature.

Pain

Physical pain is a part of life. Perhaps you've slammed your finger in a door, burnt your hand touching the hot handle of a pan on the stove or twisted your ankle while playing your favorite sport. The result is a sensation of pain.

A great deal of the pain you experience in life may be intense, but it is usually short-lived. It may last only moments or might continue for days or weeks, depending on the severity of the injury and how long it takes to heal. Most of the time, however, the pain eventually does go away. This type of temporary pain is known as **acute pain**.

When pain lasts long after the normal healing process, or when there does not seem to be any past injury or bodily damage causing ongoing pain, it is known as **chronic pain.** Generally, chronic pain is considered to be pain that lasts more than 3 months. A 1996 survey of employees in the United States indicated that more than two-thirds of workers have chronic or repeated episodes of pain—more than 80 million people. This type of pain resulted in employees taking nearly 50 million sick days during 1995.

Chronic pain can be overwhelming. But you can learn ways to manage your pain so that your life can be more fulfilling and enjoyable, and you can still carry out your daily activities. Your attitude about your pain, along with medications and therapies, can help you to control it. An important part of managing your pain is understanding it.

Why Doesn't the Pain Stop?

When your body is injured or infected, special nerve endings in your skin, joints, muscles or internal organs send messages to your brain telling it that there has been damage or unpleasant stimulus to your body. Certain nerve fibers instantaneously tell your brain where the pain is, how badly it hurts and how it feels (such as, it is sharp, burning or throbbing). Your brain then "reads" these pain signals and sends back a message to stop you from doing whatever is causing the pain. If you are touching something hot, for example, your brain will send a message to your muscles to contract so that you will pull back your hand.

Your brain also sends a message to your nerve cells to stop sending pain signals once the cause of the pain goes away (for example, when your injury starts to heal). But sometimes this mechanism fails, like a gate that is blocked open. For some reason, your nervous system continues to fire pain signals to your brain for months or even years after the injury heals, or even when there has been no bodily damage. The result is chronic pain.

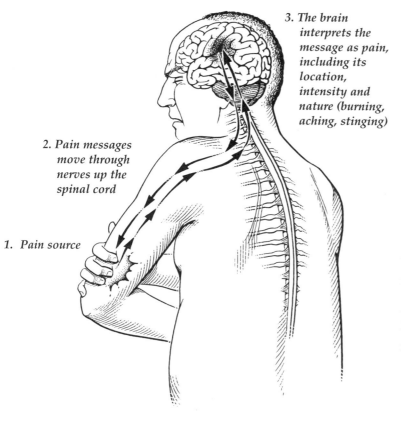

3. The brain interprets the message as pain, including its location, intensity and nature (burning, aching, stinging)

2. Pain messages move through nerves up the spinal cord

1. Pain source

The Role of Emotions in Pain

There is no exact definition for pain. Everybody perceives it differently. Pain is not only a physical experience but also an emotional one. Part of how you interpret and react to your pain is the result of your personal experience and upbringing.

If you learned to ignore or work through pain, for example, it may have less of an effect on you than if you grew up in a family where people talked a lot about the pain they were in and how much they were suffering.

When you experience pain for a long time, it can also increase your level of frustration and irritability and can lead to feelings of depression. You might also fall into a "sick role." This feeling of being a victim of your pain might bring you more attention and relieve you of some responsibilities, but eventually it also can cause you to become more inactive and isolated and even increase your perception of pain. This pain behavior can become a habit. Stress and unhappiness also tend to amplify pain and lessen your tolerance to pain. Finding positive ways to cope with your pain can have physical and emotional benefits.

■ Common Forms of Chronic Pain

Chronic pain is often debilitating, but still treatable. Many techniques exist. The key to pain control is a careful review of causes and a coordinated approach to management. Early and effective treatment of acute pain, such as after an operation or after a bout of shingles, often can prevent chronic pain. But, if you have chronic pain, there's still hope. Some of the common forms of chronic pain are listed below.

Low back: More people have low back pain than any other form of chronic pain. It is caused most frequently by muscular stress or wear due to overuse, injury or poor body mechanics. (See Back and Neck, page 50.)

Cancer: Most of the pain you experience with cancer results from the pressure of a growing tumor or the spreading of tumor cells into bones, tissues or other organs. As a result, the pain can increase as the illness progresses. Although they often relieve pain, radiation treatment or chemotherapy also can generate pain. In addition, pain can become worse if you are anxious or depressed. (See Cancer, page 168.)

Headache: The most common type of head pain is the so-called tension headache. However, doctors are not certain this is caused by actual muscle tension. The start or worsening of tension headaches is not always related to stressful events. The throbbing pain of migraine headaches may be related to changes in the blood vessels in your head. Genetics, medications, alcohol, certain foods, exertion and anxiety or depression may provoke this kind of headache. (See Headache, page 82.)

Arthritis: Arthritis is the general name for affliction of the joints. Osteoarthritis usually affects cartilage in joints of the knees, hands, hips and spine. Rheumatoid arthritis involves inflammation of tissue around and in the joints and typically affects the hands and feet. (See Arthritis, page 161.)

Rheumatism: Although the term is no longer used, rheumatism, when confined to the joints, is classified as arthritis.

Neuropathic: This pain is caused by damage to your nervous system, often after a stroke or long-term diabetes. It can be one of the most difficult types of pain to treat. Some people experience severe, stabbing pain in the cheek, lips, gums or chin on one side of the face. Another form of pain related to nerve damage follows an attack of shingles, which usually affects older adults. It causes burning, searing pain.

Stimulating Your Natural Pain Killers

Studies show that aerobic exercise can stimulate the release of endorphins, your body's own natural pain killers. Endorphins are morphine-like pain relievers that send "stop pain" messages to your nerve cells. Duration of exercise seems to be more important than intensity. Doing low-intensity aerobic exercises for 30 to 45 minutes at a time 5 or 6 days a week may produce an effect. Be sure to build up slowly. Even 3 or 4 days of exercise a week may have some effect.

If you begin an exercise program more vigorous than walking, you should have a medical evaluation if:

- You are older than 40
- You have been sedentary
- You have risk factors for coronary artery disease (see page 176)
- You have chronic health problems

Self-Care

Once serious diseases have been excluded or treated, ask your doctor about the following options:

- **Stay active.** Focus on the things you can do. Try new hobbies and activities. Exercise daily. An activity that initially causes some pain doesn't necessarily cause further damage or worsen chronic pain. If you have arthritis, exercise can improve the range of motion in your joints. Exercises for your back and abdominal muscles may help relieve or even prevent back pain. Begin slowly. Work up to 20 to 30 minutes three or four times a week.
- **Focus on others.** When you pay more attention to the needs of others, you focus less on your own difficulties. Get involved in community, church or other volunteer activities.
- **Accept your pain.** Don't deny or exaggerate how you feel, but be clear and honest with others about your current capabilities. Be practical about what you can accomplish, and let people know when you are overcommitted.
- **Stay healthy**. Eat and sleep on a regular schedule.
- **Relax.** Muscle tension increases your awareness of pain. Traditional techniques such as massage or enjoying a whirlpool bath can promote muscle relaxation and general comfort. Learn relaxation skills, such as controlled-breathing exercises and visualization. (See Keeping Stress Under Control, page 224.)
- **Keep a pain diary.** A pain diary can be helpful when you are communicating with your doctor about pain.
  - Write a detailed description of your pain while you are having it.
  - Describe the location, intensity and frequency of your pain and what makes your pain better or worse.
  - Use words such as stinging, penetrating, dull, throbbing, achy, nagging or gnawing to describe the quality of your pain.
  - Note what days or time of day the pain is better or worse.

Medical Help

You should see a physician again if pain does not lessen in 4 to 6 weeks, if the pain changes in character or if you have new symptoms.

Mayo Clinic Guide to Self-Care

Using Pain-Relieving Medications Safely

Some over-the-counter medications can be effective for relieving chronic pain. Drugs such as aspirin, ibuprofen and acetaminophen can provide pain relief by stopping the production of certain hormones in your nervous system which carry pain signals to your brain.

Follow these recommendations for using pain medications safely at home:

- Read the label and follow all instructions, cautions and warnings. Never use more than the maximal recommended dose.
- Unless a doctor recommends it, adults should not use pain medication for more than 10 days in a row. The limit for children and teenagers is 5 days.
- Don't take aspirin during the last 3 months of pregnancy unless your doctor recommends it. Aspirin can cause bleeding in both the mother and the child. Children should not take aspirin unless directed to do so by a physician.
- If you are allergic to aspirin, check with your doctor or pharmacist about which pain relievers you can use safely.
- For more on pain medications, see page 264.

■ Chronic Pain Programs

When standard treatments for chronic pain have failed, you may benefit from a pain clinic or pain management center. Before entering a program, you should undergo a thorough physical examination to exclude an unrecognized problem (such as diabetes or cancer) that may be responsible for your pain. Chronic pain programs may use one or a combination of the following treatment approaches:

Comprehensive: Physical and occupational therapy, behavior modification, group interaction, educational experiences, biofeedback and counseling are the mainstays of this type of program. This treatment approach emphasizes the elimination of medications and the initiation of physical activity to gain independence from chronic pain.

Symptom-oriented: This approach focuses on a single form of pain, such as headaches or backache. Clinics that use this approach typically offer an array of treatments that address a specific type of pain.

Treatment-oriented: This type of program emphasizes specific forms of therapy, such as neurosurgery or nerve blocks, which may be appropriate courses of treatment for several types of pain.

Chronic pain programs may offer both inpatient and outpatient services. They usually have a multidisciplinary approach, which means many specialists are involved with the patient's care. When inquiring about a program, ask about its success rate, insurance coverage and follow-up services.

FOR MORE INFORMATION
- American Pain Society, 4700 W. Lake Avenue, Glenview, IL 60025-1485; (847) 375-4715, toll free (877) 734-8758, or E-mail info@ampainsoc.org.
- American Chronic Pain Association, P.O. Box 850, Rocklin, CA 95677; (916) 632-0922, fax (916) 632-3208, or E-mail ACPA@pacbell.net; Internet address: http//www.theacpa.org.

Sleep Disorders

■ Insomnia

The most common of 60 or more sleep disorders is insomnia. Insomnia includes difficulty going to sleep, staying asleep or going back to sleep when you awaken early. It may be temporary or chronic. Insomnia is a symptom, not a disease.

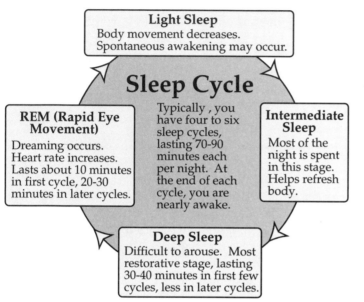

Sleep Cycle

Light Sleep
Body movement decreases. Spontaneous awakening may occur.

REM (Rapid Eye Movement)
Dreaming occurs. Heart rate increases. Lasts about 10 minutes in first cycle, 20-30 minutes in later cycles.

Typically , you have four to six sleep cycles, lasting 70-90 minutes each per night. At the end of each cycle, you are nearly awake.

Intermediate Sleep
Most of the night is spent in this stage. Helps refresh body.

Deep Sleep
Difficult to arouse. Most restorative stage, lasting 30-40 minutes in first few cycles, less in later cycles.

Common causes include the following:
- Stress related to work, school, health or family concerns
- Depression
- Use of stimulants (caffeine or nicotine), herbal supplements and over-the-counter and prescription medications
- Alcohol
- Change in environment or work schedule
- Long-term use of sleep medications
- Chronic medical problems, including fibromyalgia or complex diseases of the nerves and muscles
- Behavioral insomnia, which may occur when you worry excessively about not being able to sleep well and try too hard to fall asleep. Most people with this condition sleep better when they're away from their usual sleep environment.

Self-Care

- Establish and follow a ritual for going to bed.
- Avoid afternoon or evening naps.
- Avoid strenuous exercise right before bedtime. However, moderate exercise 4 to 6 hours before bedtime is helpful.
- Set aside a "worry time" during the day.
- Don't take work materials to bed.
- Take a warm bath 1 to 2 hours before bedtime.
- Drink a glass of milk, warm or cold. A light snack is fine, but don't eat a large snack or meal or consume alcohol close to bedtime.
- Keep your sleeping environment dark, quiet and comfortably cool. If necessary, use eye covers.
- Try relaxation exercises (see page 225).
- Lower or eliminate use of stimulants. Avoid beverages and medications with caffeine.
- Do not smoke before bedtime.
- If you still can't sleep, get up. Stay up until you feel tired, and then return to bed. But, as a result, do not shift your rising time.
- Keep a sleep diary. If, after a week or two, you still can't sleep, see your physician. Tests may uncover the cause of your insomnia.

Kids' Care

Bedwetting (enuresis) is the most common reason children ages 3 to 15 wake up at night. Contact the National Enuresis Society (1-800-NES-8080) for helpful suggestions.

Nightmares may be a response to stress or trauma that occurs during waking hours. Calmly reassure your child after an incident.

Night terrors generally occur between ages 3 and 5, and they tend to run in families. Sleepers may awaken screaming, with no recollection of a dream. Emotional tension increases night terrors.

Sleepwalking may include opening doors, going to the bathroom, dressing or undressing. This runs in families and is most common in children ages 6 to 12.

Should You Nap, or Not?

The urge for a mid-day snooze is built into your body's biologic clock. This typically occurs between 1 p.m. and 4 p.m., as indicated by a slight dip in your body temperature.

Napping is not a substitute for a full night's sleep. Don't nap if sleeping at night is a problem. If you find a nap refreshes you and doesn't interfere with nighttime sleep, try these ideas:

- **Keep it short.** A half-hour nap is ideal. Naps longer than an hour or two are more likely to interfere with your nighttime sleep.
- **Take a mid-afternoon nap.** Naps at this time produce a physically invigorating slumber.
- **If you can't nap, just rest.** Lie down and keep your mind on something else.

Other Sleep Disorders

Recurrent episodes of breathing stoppage during sleep (sleep apnea): People with this problem snore and stop breathing for short periods, from which they emerge with a jerk or gasp. Sleep apnea may occur when an upper airway is blocked by relaxation of tissues of the soft palate or by enlarged adenoids or nasal polyps. If you have these symptoms, see your doctor. It may help to lose weight, sleep on your stomach or side, avoid consuming alcohol before bedtime and use nasal decongestants, but only under the guidance of a physician.

Grinding or clenching your teeth during sleep (bruxism) may be associated with stress. Your dentist can check whether your bite needs adjustment and provide you with a plastic guard to prevent further damage. Attempt to deal with the source of your tension. Learn relaxation skills (see page 225).

Excessive sleepiness may be controlled by getting plenty of sleep at night, taking a daytime nap and eating light or vegetarian meals, especially before important activities. Use caffeinated drinks (coffee, tea and colas) to keep you awake. If you still need help, your physician may prescribe a stimulant after appropriate testing.

Restless legs is the irresistible urge to move your legs and can occur shortly after you go to bed or throughout the night, interfering with your ability to get to sleep or stay asleep. Stress often makes the condition worse. Get up and walk around. Try muscle relaxation techniques and a warm bath before bedtime. If your condition is severe, see your physician.

FOR MORE INFORMATION

- National Sleep Foundation, 1522 K Street NW, Suite 500, Washington, DC 20005; (202) 347-3471.

General Symptoms

Sweating and Body Odor

Sweating is the body's normal response to the buildup of body heat. Sweating varies widely from person to person. Many women perspire more heavily during menopause. Drinking hot beverages, or those containing alcohol or caffeine, can cause temporary increases in sweating.

For most of us, sweating is only a minor nuisance. But for some people, sweaty armpits, feet and hands are a major dilemma. Sweat is basically odorless, but it may take on an unpleasant or offensive odor when bacteria multiply and break down the body's secretions into odor-causing by-products. Sweating and odor may be influenced by mood, activity, hormones and some foods, such as caffeine.

A "cold sweat" is usually the body's response to a serious illness, anxiety or severe pain. A cold sweat should receive immediate medical attention if there are signs of light-headedness or chest and stomach pains.

Self-Care

- **Wear clothing made of natural materials,** especially cotton, next to the skin.
- **Bathe daily.** Antibacterial soaps may help, but they can be irritating.
- **Try over-the-counter products,** such as antiperspirant sprays and lotions, that contain aluminum chlorhydrate or buffered aluminum sulfate.
- **For sweaty feet,** choose shoes made of natural materials that breathe, such as leather. Wear the right socks. Cotton and wool socks can help keep your feet dry because they absorb moisture. Socks made of acrylic, a synthetic material, keep moisture away from your feet. Change your socks or hosiery once or twice a day, drying your feet thoroughly each time. Dry your feet thoroughly after a bath. Microorganisms thrive in the damp spaces between your toes. Use over-the-counter foot powders to help absorb sweat. Air out your feet. Go without shoes when it's sensible. But when you can't, slip out of them from time to time. Women should try pantyhose with cotton soles.
- **For sweaty armpits,** use antiperspirants. If irritation remains a problem, a 0.5 percent hydrocortisone cream (available without prescription) can help.
- **Apply antiperspirants nightly** at bedtime to sweaty palms or soles of feet. Try perfume-free antiperspirants.
- **Try iontophoresis.** This procedure, in which a low current of electricity is delivered to the affected body part with a battery-powered device, may help. However, it may be no more effective than a topical antiperspirant.
- **Eliminate caffeine and other stimulants** from your diet, as well as foods with strong odors such as garlic and onions.

Medical Help

Your doctor may recommend a prescription antiperspirant. For a few people, surgery may help. The operation removes the troublesome sweat glands. However, this is appropriate for only a few people who have persistent soreness and irritation caused by antiperspirants or excessive sweating.

Consult your doctor if there's an increase in sweating or nighttime sweating without an obvious cause. Infections, thyroid gland dysfunction and certain forms of cancer may produce unusual sweating patterns.

Excessive sweating associated with shortness of breath requires immediate action. This could be a sign of a heart attack.

Occasionally, a change in odor signals a disease. A fruity smell may be a sign of diabetes, or an ammonia-like smell could be a sign of liver disease.

Mayo Clinic Guide to Self-Care

Unexpected Weight Changes

In most cases, the reasons for change in weight are obvious. Changes in diet or activity are the usual explanations. However, physical illness also can affect your weight. An unexpected weight change of 5 to 10 percent of your body weight (7 1/2 to 15 pounds for a 150-pound person, or 3.4 to 6.8 kilograms for a 68-kilogram person) in 6 or fewer months is significant. If you lose or gain weight and can't point to a reason, or if you are losing or gaining weight very rapidly, talk to your health care provider.

■ Weight Gain

Are you overweight? Refer to the discussion of normal weight and body mass indicator on page 206.

Weight gain is the most common scenario in adulthood. It's usually a gradual creep—a few pounds a year. Careful diet and regular exercise can stop this trend. If you've experienced a rapid gain, consider these possible causes:

1. Diet changes—increased intake of alcohol or soda, a new favorite high-fat food such as ice cream, sweet rolls or fried foods, increased snacking, a switch to fast foods or prepared foods.
2. Decrease in activity—an injury restricting movement, a switch from an active to a sedentary job or a change in a routine such as using stairs or walking to work.
3. New medication—some medicines may contribute to weight gain. Some antidepressants and some hormones, including estrogen, progesterone and cortisone, may produce weight gain.
4. Changes in mood—excessive anxiety, stress or depression can affect activity and food intake. (See Depression and the "Blues," page 198.)
5. Fluid retention—medical conditions such as heart or kidney failure or thyroid conditions cause fluid buildup. Have you noted puffiness of the tissues—tight rings or shoes, progressive swelling of the ankles as the day progresses, unusual shortness of breath or new, frequent trips to the bathroom at night?

Self-Care

If item 1 or 2 listed above applies to you, change your diet and increase your activity. (See Weight: What's Healthy for You?, page 205.) Wait 4 to 6 weeks to see if the changes work. If they don't affect your weight, or if item 3, 4 or 5 applies to you, then see your doctor.

■ Weight Loss

Unexplained weight loss of 5 to 10 percent of your body weight over 6 or fewer months is usually cause for concern, but occasionally it's not. Consider the following causes:

1. Change in diet—skipping meals, eating on the run, a significant reduction in fat intake, a change in meal preparation methods, a change in routines around meal-time, eating alone.
2. Change in activity—job change, from sedentary to active, new exercise program, busy or hectic schedule, seasonal variation.
3. New medication—some antidepressants, stimulants—prescription or over-the-counter (caffeine, herbals).

General Symptoms

4. Mood changes—anxiety, stress and depression also can cause weight loss (see page 198).
5. Other conditions—dental problems; uncontrolled diabetes with thirst or increased urination; hyperthyroidism (overactive thyroid gland); digestive disorders such as malabsorption or ulcer with abdominal pain; inflammatory bowel diseases, such as Crohn's or colitis, causing diarrhea and bloody stools; infections such as HIV, AIDS or tuberculosis; cancer of many types.

Self-Care

If item 1 or 2 listed above applies to you, but none of the other items seem to fit, modify your diet. Eat three balanced meals. For snacks, or when you can't eat a good meal, try a nutritional supplement drink. Instant breakfasts are simple, fairly balanced and less expensive than prepared supplements. If you haven't reversed the weight loss trend in 2 weeks, or if item 3, 4 or 5 seems to fit, see your doctor without delay.

Kids' Care

Weight loss or failure to grow in children may be caused by a digestive problem that prevents important nutrients from being digested or absorbed. Loss of these nutrients can lead to bony changes and other problems. Your child also may have an eating disorder. If your child has unexplained weight loss, consult your child's health care provider.

Eating Disorders: Anorexia Nervosa and Bulimia Nervosa

Anorexia nervosa is an eating disorder that can lead to drastic weight loss as a result of self-imposed semistarvation. A person with bulimia nervosa is often at normal weight but uses binge-eating and purging as a means of weight control. Both disorders are most common in adolescent girls and young women, but they also can occur in males and older individuals.

The number of people affected by anorexia and bulimia has increased as society has placed more emphasis on being thin and attractive. Decreasing this emphasis and not placing unrealistic expectations on adolescents may be steps in curbing this trend. If you suspect an eating disorder in yourself or others, contact your health care provider.

Anorexia Nervosa

Symptoms and signs:

- Misperception of body image—you see yourself as being fatter than you are
- Unrealistic fear of becoming fat
- Excessive dieting and exercise
- Significant weight loss or failure to gain weight during a period of growth
- Refusal to maintain a normal body weight
- Absence of menstrual periods
- Preoccupation with food, calories and food preparation

The cause of anorexia nervosa is unclear, but biologic and psychological factors may be involved. Total recovery is possible if the disorder is diagnosed early. Left untreated, anorexia can lead to death. Treatment involves psychotherapy, diet counseling and family counseling in most cases. Hospitalization may be needed in severe cases.

Bulimia Nervosa

Symptoms and signs:

- Recurrent episodes of binge eating
- Self-induced vomiting or laxative abuse
- Weight usually within fairly normal range
- Fear of becoming fat

Bulimia involves eating large amounts of food and then purging by vomiting or abusing laxatives. It is also a form of semistarvation. Purging depletes water and potassium from the body and can lead to death. People with bulimia often become depressed because they realize that their eating is abnormal. Treatment usually includes behavior modification, psychotherapy and, in some cases, antidepressant medication. Hospitalization may be needed if the disorder is out of control and there are physical complications.

Mayo Clinic Guide to Self-Care

Common Problems

- Back and Neck
- Digestive System
- Ears and Hearing
- Eyes and Vision
- Headache
- Limbs, Muscles, Bones and Joints
- Lungs, Chest and Breathing
- Nose and Sinuses
- Skin, Hair and Nails
- Throat and Mouth
- Men's Health
- Women's Health

Most pains and ailments are not serious. Often, simple remedies in combination with time can help resolve the problem and save you a trip to the doctor. Of course, if the problem persists or if simple remedies don't help, you need to seek medical care.

This section is organized by body system. Each chapter includes several illnesses or symptoms with appropriate self-care advice and directives on when to see your doctor. Sidebar articles (with light gray shading in the background) address related topics or offer insight into medical issues. We pay special attention to children's health where appropriate throughout the section.

Back and Neck

Almost everyone has a back problem at some time. Back pain sends many people to health care providers each year. Fortunately, you can do things to prevent back problems. And you can do them most effectively if you know a little bit about your back.

Your back supports your body. It holds and protects your spinal cord and nerves that send signals back and forth from your brain to the rest of your body. And it serves as a place of attachment for muscles and ligaments of the back.

A Bit of Anatomy

Your spine, or so-called backbone, is not one bone, but many. If you look at a healthy spine from the side, it curves inward at your neck and lower back and outward at your upper back and pelvis.

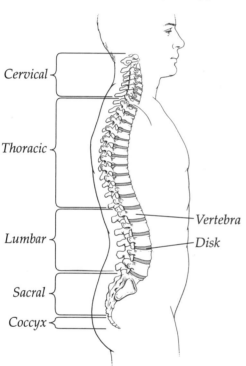

Cervical

Thoracic

Lumbar

Sacral

Coccyx

Vertebra

Disk

Vertebrae: The backbone, or vertebral column, is composed of bones called vertebrae, which are held together by tough, fibrous bands called ligaments. The normal adult vertebral column consists of 7 cervical (neck) vertebrae, 12 thoracic (middle back) vertebrae, and 5 large lumbar (lower back) vertebrae. The lumbar vertebrae are the largest because they bear most of the body weight. The sacrum, made from five vertebrae that are fused together, is below the lumbar vertebrae. The last three vertebrae, also fused together, are called the coccyx or tailbone.

Spinal cord: The spinal cord, part of the central nervous system, extends from the base of the skull to the lower back. Two nerves (called spinal nerves) are sent out at each vertebral level. In the upper lumbar part of the back where the spinal cord ends, a group of nerves (called the cauda equina) continue down the spinal canal. The spinal nerves exit from openings (foramina) on either side of the vertebrae, one leading to the right side of the body and the other to the left. In all, there are 31 pairs of these spinal nerves in the back and neck.

Disks: Between the vertebrae, and close to the point of exit of each pair of spinal nerves, are intervertebral discs. These disks serve as cushions or "shock absorbers" between the vertebrae, preventing the hard and bony vertebrae from hitting one another when we walk, run or jump. A disk is made up of a ring of tough, fibrous tissue that has a jelly-like substance in the center. Damaged outer disk rings may result in a protruded, herniated or ruptured disk (see page 53). This produces pressure on nerves or surrounding tissues, causing pain. (A disk does not actually "slip" because it is firmly attached between the vertebrae.)

Muscles: Muscles are like elastic bands up and down your back which support your spine. They contract or relax to help you stand, twist, bend or stretch. Tendons connect muscles to bones. The muscles of your abdomen and trunk support, protect and move your spine.

With age your spine may become stiff and lose its flexibility. Disks become worn, and the spaces between your vertebrae narrow. These changes are part of the aging process, but they are not necessarily painful. Vertebrae sometimes develop jutting bone spurs, which also may or may not produce pain. As the cartilage that cushions joints wears out, bones rub together and you experience the pain of arthritis. But often it's hard to pinpoint the cause of back pain because of the back's complexity.

■ Common Back Problems

Your lower back carries most of your weight. It's the site of most back pain for people between the ages of 20 and 50. But strains and sprains can injure any part of your neck or back. The most common sources of back pain are one or more strained (overstretched) muscles or sprained (overstretched) ligaments. The cause may be:

- Improper lifting (see Lifting Properly, page 54)
- A sudden, strenuous physical effort; an accident, sports injury or fall
- Lack of muscle tone
- Excess weight, especially around your middle
- Your sleeping position, especially if you sleep on your stomach
- A pillow that forces your neck into an awkward angle
- Sitting in one position a long time; poor sitting and standing postures
- Holding the telephone with your shoulder
- Carrying a heavy briefcase, purse or shoulder bag or backpack
- Sitting with a thick wallet in your back pocket
- Holding a forward-bending position for a long time
- Daily stress and tension
- Normal or excessive weight gain during pregnancy

Your lower back, a pivot point for turning at your waist, is vulnerable to muscle strains.

"No Pain, No Gain" —Not True!

You may become sore immediately after you've injured a muscle, or it may take several hours before it feels sore. An injured muscle may uncontrollably tighten or "knot up" (a muscle spasm). Your body is telling you to slow down and prevent further injury. A severe muscle spasm may last 48 to 72 hours, followed by days or weeks of less severe pain. Strenuous use of an injured muscle during the next 3 to 6 weeks may bring back the pain. However, most back pain is gone in 6 weeks.

As you age, muscle tone tends to decrease, and your back is more prone to aches or injury. Maintaining your flexibility and strength and keeping your abdominal muscles strong are your best bets to avoid back problems. Spending 10 to 15 minutes a day doing gentle stretching and strengthening exercises can help.

Self-Care

Healing will occur most quickly if you can continue your usual activities in a gentle manner while avoiding what may have caused the pain in the first place. Avoid long periods of bed rest, which can worsen your pain and make you weaker.

With proper care of a strain or sprain, you should notice steady improvement within the first 2 weeks. Most back pain is much better in 6 weeks. Sprained ligaments or severe muscle strains may take up to 12 weeks to heal. Once you have back pain, you're more prone to experience repeated painful episodes.

Follow these home care steps:
- Use cold packs initially to relieve pain. Wrap an ice pack or a bag of frozen vegetables in a piece of cloth. Hold it on the sore area for 15 minutes four times a day. To avoid frostbite, never place ice directly on your skin.
- You may be most comfortable lying with your back on the floor, hips and knees bent and legs elevated. Get plenty of rest, but avoid prolonged bed rest—more than a day or two may slow recovery. Moderate movement keeps your muscles strong and flexible. Avoid the activity that caused the sprain or strain. Avoid heavy lifting, pushing or pulling, repetitive bending and twisting.

Common Problems

Self-Care

- After 48 hours, you may use heat to relax sore or knotted muscles. Use a warm bath, warm packs, a heating pad or a heat lamp. Be careful not to burn your skin with extreme heat. But if you find that cold provides more relief than heat, you can continue using cold, or try a combination of the two methods.
- Gradually begin gentle stretching exercises. Avoid jerking, bouncing or any movements that increase pain or require straining.
- Use over-the-counter pain medications (see page 265).
- Massage may be helpful, especially for muscle spasms, but avoid placing any pressure directly on your spine.
- If you must stand or sit much of the day, you may consider using a support brace or corset. Worn properly, they may relieve your pain and provide warmth, comfort and support. However, relying on this type of support for a long time, rather than using your muscles, may actually weaken your muscles.

Medical Help

If your back or neck pain hasn't improved noticeably after 72 hours of self-care, contact your health care provider.

Seek medical care *immediately* if your pain:
- Is severe or tearing in quality.
- Results from a fall or blow to your back. Do not try to move someone who has severe neck pain or can't move his or her legs after an accident. Moving the person can cause further injury.
- Produces weakness or numbness in one or both legs.
- Is new and is accompanied by an unexplained fever.
- Results from an injury that causes pain from your neck to shoot down your arms and legs.
- You also need to seek medical care *immediately* if you have one of the following conditions: poorly controlled blood pressure, cancer, an abdominal aortic aneurysm or a sudden loss of bowel or bladder control.

The nerves to most of your body travel through your back. Sometimes, back or neck pain may be caused by a problem somewhere else in your body. Your physician may do testing to determine the cause of your pain.

Kids' Care

Low back pain is unusual in children before their teen years. Common causes for back pain are sports injuries or falls. Be sure that your children's athletic programs:
- Use the proper protective equipment
- Have competent coaches
- Use sufficient warmup and conditioning activities

If your injured child has not been unconscious, can move freely and has no numbness or weakness, use the self-care tips listed on page 51. Be careful to avoid excessive heat or cold. Check proper children's doses for over-the-counter medicines. Do not give children aspirin.

If the pain is unrelated to an injury or other known cause, your health care provider may want to check for an infection (especially if your child has a fever) or for factors in your child's development which may cause the pain. Girls often experience lower back pain with their menstrual period.

Warning signs of serious back problems in children younger than 11 include constant pain that lasts for several weeks or occurs spontaneously at night; pain that interferes with school, play or sports; and pain that occurs with stiffness and fever.

Less Common Back Problems

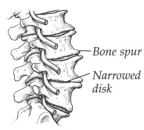

Osteoarthritis

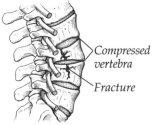

Osteoporosis

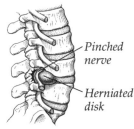

Herniated disk

Back and neck problems often don't result from a single incident. They may be the product of a lifetime of stress and strain for your back and neck. If you have chronic back pain, your health care provider may look for the following conditions:

Osteoarthritis affects nearly everyone older than 60. An imbalance of enzymes may promote deterioration of cartilage, the protective tissue that covers the surface of vertebral joints. Disks between vertebrae become worn and the spaces between the bones narrow. Bony outgrowths called spurs also develop. Gradually, your spine stiffens and loses flexibility.

Osteoporosis is the weakening of your bone structure as the amount of calcium in your bones decreases. Weakened vertebrae become compressed and fracture easily. Modern drugs and hormone replacement therapy may slow or halt this process, once considered inevitable for women older than 50.

Herniated or so-called slipped disk occurs when normal wear and tear or exceptional strain causes a disk to rupture. Bulging of disks is common and often painless. It becomes painful when excessive bulging or fragments of the disk herniate or break off and place pressure on nearby nerves. This condition may lead to leg pain (sciatica, named for the sciatic nerve that extends down the back of each leg from your buttock to your heel). Symptoms from herniated disks may resolve over weeks.

Fibromyalgia is a chronic syndrome that produces achy pain, tenderness and stiffness in the muscles and joints where tendons attach to your bones. Pain is usually worse after inactivity and improves with movement.

Some back and neck problems are complex. Rarely is surgery the answer. Surgery is usually reserved for times when a nerve is pinched severely and threatens to cause permanent weakness or is affecting bowel or bladder control. Back pain without nerve injury is rarely a reason for surgery.

Back Injuries in the Workplace

You can avoid many back problems by following these guidelines (see Exercises for Office Workers, page 232, and Coping With Technology, page 243, for other ideas):
- Change positions often.
- Avoid high heels. If you stand for long periods, rest one foot on a small box or stool from time to time.
- Use adjustable equipment. Find comfortable (rather than extreme) positions.
- Don't bend continuously over your work. Hold reading materials at eye level.
- Avoid excessive repetition. Take frequent, short breaks to stretch or relax— even 30 seconds every 10 to 15 minutes helps.
- Avoid unnecessary bending, twisting and reaching.
- Stand to answer your phone. If you are on the phone a lot, get a headset.
- Adjust your chair so your feet are flat on the floor. Change leg positions often.
- Use a chair that supports your lower back's curve or place a rolled towel or pillow behind your lower back. The seat of your chair should not press on the back of your thighs or knees.
- Lift objects properly (see page 54).
- Carry objects close to the body at about waist level.

◼ Preventing Common Backaches and Neck Pains

Regular exercise is your most powerful weapon against back and neck problems. Proper exercise can help you:

- Maintain or increase flexibility of muscles, tendons and ligaments
- Strengthen the muscles that support your back
- Increase muscle strength in your arms, legs and lower body to reduce the risk of falls and other injuries and allow optimal posture for lifting and carrying
- Improve your posture
- Increase bone density
- Shed excess pounds that stress your back

If you're over 40 or have an illness or injury, check with your health care professional before you begin an exercise program. If you're out of condition, start slowly and increase gradually. Exercises that are good for your back include the following:

- Abdominal and leg strengthening exercises.
- Nonjarring exercise on a stationary bike, treadmill or cross-country skiing machine. Bicycling is good, but be sure your bike seat and handlebars are properly adjusted to keep you in a comfortable position.
- If you have back problems or are out of shape, avoid activities that involve quick stops and starts and a lot of twisting. High-impact activities on hard surfaces— like jogging, tennis, racquetball or basketball—may add wear and tear to your back. Avoid contact sports.

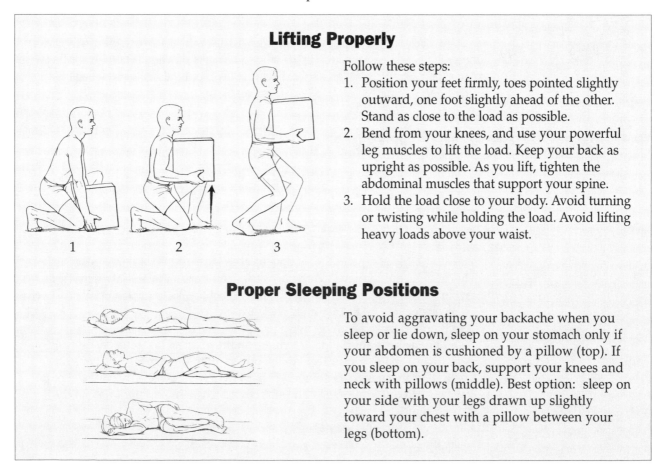

Lifting Properly

Follow these steps:
1. Position your feet firmly, toes pointed slightly outward, one foot slightly ahead of the other. Stand as close to the load as possible.
2. Bend from your knees, and use your powerful leg muscles to lift the load. Keep your back as upright as possible. As you lift, tighten the abdominal muscles that support your spine.
3. Hold the load close to your body. Avoid turning or twisting while holding the load. Avoid lifting heavy loads above your waist.

Proper Sleeping Positions

To avoid aggravating your backache when you sleep or lie down, sleep on your stomach only if your abdomen is cushioned by a pillow (top). If you sleep on your back, support your knees and neck with pillows (middle). Best option: sleep on your side with your legs drawn up slightly toward your chest with a pillow between your legs (bottom).

■ Your Daily Back Routine

Here are basic exercises to stretch and strengthen your back and supporting muscles. Try to work 15 minutes of exercise into your daily routine. (If you've hurt your back before, or if you have other health problems such as osteoporosis, get medical advice before exercising.)

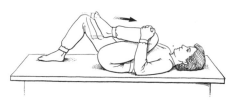

Knee to shoulder stretch: *Lie on your back on a firm surface with your knees bent and feet flat. Pull your left knee toward your chest with both hands. Hold for 15 to 30 seconds. Return to starting position. Repeat with opposite leg. Repeat with each leg three or four times.*

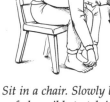

Chair stretch: *Sit in a chair. Slowly bend forward toward the floor until you feel a mild stretch in your back. Hold for 15 to 30 seconds. Repeat three or four times.*

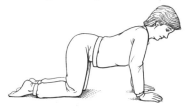

"Cat" stretch: *Step 1. Get down on your hands and knees. Slowly let your back and abdomen sag toward the floor.*

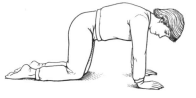

"Cat" stretch: *Step 2. Slowly arch your back away from the floor. Repeat several times.*

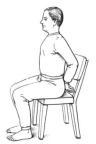

Shoulder blade squeeze: *Sit upright in a chair. Keep your chin tucked in and your shoulders down. Pull your shoulder blades together and straighten your upper back. Hold a few seconds. Return to starting position. Repeat several times.*

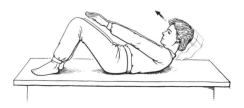

Half sit-up: *Lie on your back on a firm surface with your knees bent and feet flat. With your arms outstretched, reach toward your knees with your hands until your shoulder blades no longer touch the ground. Do not grasp your knees. Hold for a few seconds and slowly return to the starting position. Repeat several times.*

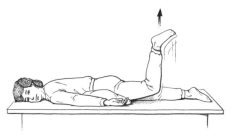

Leg lifts: *Step 1. Lie face down on a firm surface with a large pillow under your hips and lower abdomen. Keeping your knee bent, raise your leg slightly off the surface and hold for about 5 seconds. Repeat several times.*

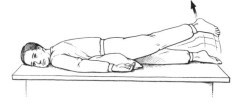

Leg lifts: *Step 2. With your leg straight, repeat the exercise. Raise one leg slightly off the surface and hold for about 5 seconds. Repeat several times.*

Common Problems

Digestive System

Your digestive tract is an extremely complex system. Problems can occur anywhere along this tract, upsetting its delicate balance. Because of the complexity of this system, you should not attempt to diagnose new problems, such as unexplained pain or bleeding, on your own.

Digestion begins when you chew your food. The food is broken into smaller pieces by your teeth and, at the same time, is mixed with saliva secreted by your salivary glands. Your saliva contains an enzyme that begins to change starches (carbohydrates) into sugars.

Food is propelled down your esophagus to the stomach and then on through the intestines by muscular contractions. This process, called digestion, is aided by digestive juices (acid, bile and enzymes) from the stomach, pancreas and gallbladder. They break down food and allow the nutrients to be absorbed. Undigestible food and bacteria are eliminated as feces from the rectum.

Gastrointestinal tract

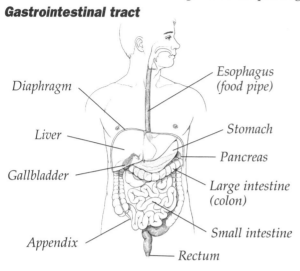

Diaphragm

Liver

Gallbladder

Appendix

Esophagus
(food pipe)

Stomach

Pancreas

Large intestine
(colon)

Small intestine

Rectum

◼ Abdominal Pain

Pain in your abdomen can occur anywhere along your digestive tract, from your mouth or throat to your pelvis and rectum. In some cases, pain can signal a mild problem such as overeating. In others, it can be an early warning sign of a more serious disorder that may require medical treatment.

Fortunately, many forms of discomfort respond well to a combination of self-care and supervised medical treatment. See the following pages if your pain accompanies any of these conditions: constipation, page 58; diarrhea, page 59; excessive gas, page 60; gastritis, page 61; or hemorrhoids, page 62.

Caution

Although most abdominal pains are not serious, you should not attempt to diagnose the source of new or unexplained pain. Seek medical attention if you experience any of the following: intense pain lasting longer than a minute or pain that seems to be worsening; pain accompanied by shortness of breath or dizziness; pain accompanied by a temperature of 101 F or more.

What Is Appendicitis?

Your appendix is a worm-shaped structure that projects out from the large intestine. This tiny structure can become inflamed, swollen and filled with pus. This condition is called appendicitis.

Appendicitis typically causes acute pain that starts around your navel and settles in the lower right side of your abdomen. These symptoms generally progress over 12 to 24 hours. You also may experience a loss of appetite, nausea, vomiting and the urge to have a bowel movement or pass gas.

Although appendicitis can affect people of all ages, it usually occurs between the ages of 10 and 30.

An infected appendix may burst and cause a serious infection. Seek immediate medical attention if you suspect you have appendicitis.

Mayo Clinic Guide to Self-Care

Colic

Generations of families have dealt with colic. This frustrating and largely unexplainable condition affects babies who otherwise seem healthy. Colic usually peaks at 6 weeks of age and disappears in the baby's third or fourth month.

Colic is a difficult experience for everyone. One doctor describes colic as "when the baby's crying—and so is Mom."

Although the term "colic" is used widely for any fussy baby, true colic is determined by the following:

- **Predictable crying episodes:** A colicky baby cries at about the same time each day, usually in the evening. Colic episodes may last minutes or 2 or more hours.
- **Activity:** Many colicky babies pull their legs to their chests or thrash around during crying episodes as if they are in pain.
- **Intense or inconsolable crying:** Colicky babies cry more than usual and are extremely difficult—if not impossible—to comfort.

Doctors call colic a "diagnosis of exclusion," which means other possible problems are ruled out before determining the baby has colic. The parent of a colicky infant, therefore, can be assured that the crying is probably not a sign of a serious medical problem.

Studies of colic have focused on several possible causes: allergies, an immature digestive system, gas, hormones, mother's anxieties and handling. Still, it is unclear why some babies have colic and others don't.

Self-Care

If your health care provider determines that your baby has colic, these measures may help you and your child find some relief:

- Lay your baby tummy-down on your knees or arms and sway your baby gently and slowly.
- Rock, cuddle or walk your baby. Avoid fast, jiggling movements.
- Play a steady, uninterrupted "white noise" near your baby. Motors with soft noise, such as a clothes dryer, may work.
- Put your baby in an infant swing.
- Give your baby a warm bath or lay him or her tummy-down on a warm water bottle.
- Try singing or humming while walking with or rocking the baby. A soothing song can have a quieting effect on both parent and baby.
- Take your baby for a car ride.
- Leave your baby with someone else for 10 minutes and walk alone.

Medical Help

At this time, there are no medications to relieve colic safely and effectively. In general, consult with your health care provider before giving your baby any medication.

If you are worried that your baby is sick or if you or others caring for the baby are becoming frustrated or angry because of the crying, call your doctor or bring the baby to the office or emergency department.

Common Problems

■ Constipation

This common problem is often misunderstood and improperly treated. Technically speaking, constipation is the passage of hard stools fewer than three times a week. You also may experience a bloated sensation and occasional crampy discomfort. The normal frequency for bowel movements varies widely—from three bowel movements a day to three a week.

Constipation is a symptom, not a disease. Like a fever, this problem can occur when one of many factors slows the passage of food through your large bowel. These factors include inadequate fluid intake, poor diet, irregular bowel habits, age, lack of activity, pregnancy and illness. Various medications also can cause constipation.

Although constipation may be extremely bothersome, the condition itself usually is not serious. If it persists, however, constipation can lead to complications such as hemorrhoids and cracks or tears in the anus called fissures.

Self-Care

To lessen your chances of constipation:
- Try to eat on a regular schedule, and eat plenty of high-fiber foods, including fresh fruits, vegetables and whole-grain cereals and breads.
- Drink 8 to 10 glasses of water or other liquids daily.
- Increase your physical activity.
- Don't ignore the urge to have a bowel movement.
- Try fiber supplements such as Metamucil, Konsyl, Fiberall or Citrucel.
- Do not rely on laxatives (see below).

Medical Help

Contact your doctor if your constipation is severe or if it lasts longer than 3 weeks. In rare cases, constipation also may signal more serious medical conditions such as cancer, hormonal disturbances, heart disease or kidney failure.

Kids' Care

Constipation is not usually a problem among infants, especially if they are breast-feeding. A healthy breast-fed infant may have as few as one bowel movement a week.

Young children sometimes experience constipation because they neglect to take time to use the bathroom. Toddlers also may become constipated during toilet training because of a fear or unwillingness to use the toilet. However, as few as one bowel movement a week may be normal for your child.

If constipation is a problem, have your child drink plenty of fluids to soften stools. Warm baths also may help relax your child and encourage bowel movements.

Avoid use of laxatives in children unless advised by your doctor.

Excessive Use of Laxatives Can Be Harmful

Habitual or excessive use of laxatives can actually be harmful and make your constipation worse. Overusing these medications can:
- Cause your body to flush out necessary vitamins and other nutrients before they are absorbed. This process disrupts your body's normal balance of salts and nutrients.
- Interfere with other medications you are taking.
- Induce lazy bowel syndrome, a condition in which your bowels fail to function properly because they have begun to rely on the laxative to stimulate elimination. As a result, when you stop using laxatives, your constipation may worsen.

Diarrhea

This unpleasant disorder affects adults an average of four times a year. Symptoms include loose, watery stools, often accompanied by abdominal cramps.

There are many causes, most of which are not serious. The most common is a viral infection of your digestive tract. Bacteria and parasites also can cause diarrhea. These organisms cause your bowel to lose excess water and salts as diarrhea.

Nausea and vomiting may precede diarrhea that is caused by an infection. In addition, you also may notice cramping, abdominal pain and other flu-like symptoms, such as low-grade fever, achy or cramping muscles and headache. Bacterial or parasitic infestations sometimes cause bloody stools or a high fever.

Infection-induced diarrhea can be extremely contagious. You can catch a viral infection by direct contact with an infected person. Food and water contaminated with bacteria or parasites also spread diarrheal infections.

Diarrhea can be a side effect of many medications, particularly antibiotics. In addition, the artificial sweeteners sorbitol and mannitol found in chewing gum and other sugar-free products can cause diarrhea. About 40 to 50 percent of healthy people may have difficulty digesting these sweeteners. Chronic or recurrent diarrhea may signal a more serious underlying medical problem such as chronic infection or inflammatory bowel disease.

Self-Care

Although uncomfortable, diarrhea caused by infections typically clears on its own without antibiotics. Over-the-counter medications such as Imodium, Pepto-Bismol and Kaopectate may slow diarrhea, but they won't speed your recovery. Take these measures to prevent dehydration and reduce symptoms while you recover:

- Drink at least 8 to 16 glasses (2 to 4 quarts) of clear liquids, including water, clear sodas, broths and weak tea.
- Add semisolid and low-fiber foods gradually as your bowel movements return to normal. Try soda crackers, toast, eggs, rice or chicken.
- Avoid dairy products, fatty foods or highly seasoned foods for a few days.
- Avoid caffeine and nicotine.

Medical Help

Contact your health care provider if diarrhea persists beyond 1 week or if you become dehydrated (excessive thirst, dry mouth, little or no urination, severe weakness, dizziness or light-headedness). You also should seek medical attention if you have severe abdominal or rectal pain, bloody stools, a temperature of more than 101 F or signs of dehydration despite drinking fluids.

Your physician may prescribe antibiotics to shorten the duration of diarrhea caused by some bacteria and parasites. However, not all diarrhea caused by bacteria requires treatment with antibiotics, and antibiotics don't help viral diarrhea, which is the most common kind of infectious diarrhea.

Kids' Care

Diarrhea can cause infants to become dehydrated. Contact your health care provider if diarrhea persists for more than 12 hours or if your baby:

- Hasn't had a wet diaper in 8 hours
- Has a temperature of more than 102 F
- Has bloody stools
- Has a dry mouth or cries without tears
- Is unusually sleepy or drowsy or unresponsive

Common Problems

■ Excessive Gas and Gas Pains

Belching

Belching and burping are normal ways to get rid of the air you swallow every time you eat or drink. Belching removes gas from your stomach by forcing it into your esophagus and then out your mouth. Swallowing too much air can cause bloating or frequent belching. If you belch repeatedly when not eating, you may be swallowing air as a nervous habit.

Passing Gas

Most intestinal gas (flatus) is produced in the colon. Usually the gas is expelled during a bowel movement. All people pass gas (called flatulence), but some people produce an excessive amount of gas that bothers them throughout the day. Intestinal gas is composed primarily of five substances: oxygen, nitrogen, hydrogen, carbon dioxide and methane. The foul odor usually is the result of small traces of other gases such as hydrogen sulfide and ammonia and other substances. Swallowed air makes up a small fraction of intestinal gas. Carbonated drinks may release carbon dioxide in the stomach and may be a source of gas.

Gas Pains

Sharp, jabbing or crampy pains in your abdomen may be caused by the buildup of gas. They are often intense, but brief (less than 1 minute). They often occur in the right lower and left upper abdomen and change locations quickly. You may notice a "knotted" feeling in your abdomen. Passing gas sometimes relieves these pains.

Any of the sources of intestinal gas or diarrhea can lead to gas pains. Gas pains can occur when your intestines have difficulty breaking down certain foods or when you have a gastrointestinal infection or diarrhea.

Self-Care

To reduce belching and bloating, try the following tips:
- Eat slowly and avoid gulping. Eat fewer rich, fatty foods.
- Avoid chewing gum or sucking on hard candy.
- Limit sipping through straws or drinking from narrow-mouthed bottles.
- Cut down on carbonated drinks and beer.
- Don't smoke cigarettes, pipes or cigars.
- Try to control stress, which may aggravate the nervous habit of swallowing air.
- Don't force yourself to belch.
- Avoid lying down immediately after you eat.

To reduce flatulence, try the following tips:
- Identify the foods that affect you the most. Try eliminating one of these foods for a few weeks to see if your flatulence subsides: beans, peas, lentils, cabbage, radishes, onions, brussels sprouts, sauerkraut, apricots, bananas, prunes and prune juice, raisins, whole-wheat bread, bran cereals or muffins, pretzels, wheat germ, milk, cream, ice cream and ice milk.
- Temporarily cut back on high-fiber foods. Add them back gradually over weeks.
- Reduce dairy products. Try Lactaid or Dairy Ease for lactose intolerance.
- Try adding Beano to high-fiber foods to reduce the amount of gas they make.
- Occasional use of over-the-counter anti-gas products containing simethicone (Mylanta, Riopan Plus, Mylicon) can help. Activated charcoal pills may help.

Mayo Clinic Guide to Self-Care

Gallstones

About 1 in 10 Americans has or will have gallstones. Most gallstones produce no symptoms. Stones that block the ducts linking your gallbladder with your liver and small intestine can be extremely painful and potentially dangerous.

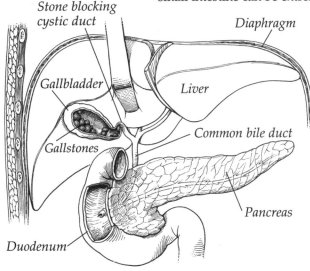

Stone blocking cystic duct

Diaphragm

Gallbladder

Liver

Common bile duct

Gallstones

Pancreas

Duodenum

Gallstones may form in your gallbladder. If a stone obstructs your cystic duct, you may experience a gallbladder attack.

Your gallbladder stores bile, a digestive fluid produced in the liver. The bile passes through ducts from the gallbladder into the small intestine and helps digest fats. A healthy gallbladder has balanced amounts of bile acids and cholesterol. When the concentration of cholesterol becomes too high, gallstones may form. They can be as small as a grain of sand or as large as a golf ball.

Gallstones can cause intense and sudden pain that may last for hours. The pain usually begins shortly after eating. It begins in your upper right abdomen and may shift to your back or right shoulder blade. Fever and nausea also may accompany the pain. After your pain subsides, you may notice a mild aching sensation or soreness in your upper right abdomen. If a gallstone blocks your bile duct, your skin and the whites of your eyes may turn yellow (jaundice). You also may develop a fever or pass pale, clay-colored stools.

The elderly and women tend to be at higher risk, especially women who are pregnant or taking estrogen or birth control pills. Your risk may also be higher if:

- You are overweight or have recently lost weight
- You have a family history of this problem or a disorder of the small intestine

Self-Care	Avoid rich, fatty foods and eat smaller meals to reduce episodes of gallbladder pain.
Medical Help	Contact your health care provider if you have recurrent or intense pain. Seek prompt medical attention if you develop yellowing skin or a fever during an attack.

Gastritis (Burning or Sour Stomach)

Gastritis is inflammation of your stomach lining. Upper abdominal discomfort, nausea and vomiting are the more common symptoms. Gastritis may cause bleeding that appears in vomit or turns your stools black. Most often, gastritis is mild and poses no danger. Gastritis may occur when acid damages your stomach lining. Excessive smoking, alcohol and medications such as aspirin also can cause gastritis.

Self-Care	• Avoid smoking, alcohol and foods and drinks that irritate your stomach. • Try taking over-the-counter antacids or medicines such as Pepcid, Tagamet and Zantac. (**Caution:** Excessive use of antacids containing magnesium can cause diarrhea. Calcium- or aluminum-based antacids can lead to constipation.) • Use pain relievers that contain acetaminophen (see page 265). Avoid aspirin, ibuprofen, ketoprofen and naproxen sodium. They can cause or worsen gastritis.
Medical Help	If your discomfort lasts longer than 1 week, contact your health care provider.

■ Hemorrhoids and Rectal Bleeding

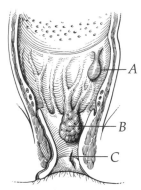

Cross-section view of anus and rectum shows the location of three common causes of rectal bleeding: (A) polyp, (B) hemorrhoids and (C) anal fissure.

More than 75 percent of Americans have problems with hemorrhoids at some time in their lives. Itching, burning and pain around the anus may signal their presence. You also may notice small amounts of bright red blood on your toilet tissue or in the toilet bowl.

Hemorrhoids occur when veins in your rectum become enlarged. They usually form over time as you strain to pass hard stools. Hemorrhoids may develop inside the anal canal or protrude outside the anal opening. Lifting heavy objects, obesity, pregnancy, childbirth, stress and diarrhea also can increase the pressure on these veins and lead to hemorrhoids. This condition seems to run in families.

In addition to hemorrhoids, bleeding from the rectum can occur for other reasons, some of which can be serious. Passing hard, dry stools may scrape the anal lining. An infection of the lining of the rectum or tiny cracks or tears in the lining of your anus called anal fissures also can cause rectal bleeding. With these types of problems, you may notice small drops of bright red blood on your stool, on your toilet tissue or in the toilet bowl.

Black, tarry stools, maroon stools or bright red blood in your stools also may signal more extensive bleeding elsewhere in your digestive tract. Small sacs that protrude from your large intestines (called diverticula), ulcers, small growths called polyps, cancer and some chronic bowel disorders can all cause bleeding.

Self-Care

Although uncomfortable, hemorrhoids are not a serious medical condition. Most hemorrhoids respond well to the following self-care measures:
- Drink at least 8 to 10 glasses of water each day and eat plenty of high-fiber foods such as wheat bran cereal, whole wheat bread, fresh fruit and vegetables.
- Bathe or shower daily to cleanse the skin around your anus gently with warm water. Soap is not necessary and may aggravate the problem.
- Stay active. Exercise. If at work or home you must sit or stand for long periods, take quick walks or breaks from work.
- Try not to strain during bowel movements or sit on the toilet too long.
- Take warm baths.
- Apply ice packs.
- For flares of pain or irritation, apply over-the-counter creams, ointments or pads containing witch hazel or a topical numbing agent. Keep in mind that these products can only help relieve mild itching and irritation.
- Try fiber supplements (Metamucil, Citrucel) to keep stools soft and regular.

Medical Help

Hemorrhoids become most painful when a clot forms in the enlarged vein. If your hemorrhoids are extremely painful, your health care provider may prescribe a cream or suppository containing hydrocortisone to reduce inflammation. Some troublesome internal hemorrhoids may require operation or other procedures to shrink or eliminate them.

Diagnosing the cause of rectal bleeding can be difficult. You should see your health care provider for evaluation. Seek immediate emergency care if you notice large amounts of rectal bleeding, light-headedness, weakness or rapid heart rate (more than 100 beats per minute).

Mayo Clinic Guide to Self-Care

■ Hernias

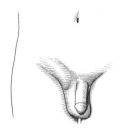

An inguinal hernia can cause a bulge at the junction of your thigh and groin. Bulges can be round or oval.

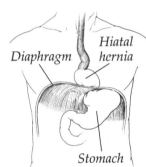

Diaphragm *Hiatal hernia* *Stomach*

In hiatal hernia, a portion of the stomach protrudes through the diaphragm into the chest cavity.

A hernia occurs when one body part protrudes through a gap into another body area. Some hernias cause no pain or visible symptoms.

Types of Hernias

Inguinal hernia is the medical name for a hernia in the groin area. It's far more frequent in men than women and accounts for 80 percent of all hernias in men. It occurs along the inguinal canal—an opening in abdominal muscles. In men, the canal is the spermatic cord's passageway between the abdominal cavity and the scrotum. In women, it's the passageway for a ligament that helps hold the uterus in place. With an inguinal hernia, you may be able to see and feel the bulge created by the protruding tissue or intestine. It's often located at the junction of your thigh and groin. Sometimes in men the protruding intestine enters the scrotum. This can be painful and cause the scrotum to swell. The first sign of an inguinal hernia may be a bulge or lump in your groin. You may notice discomfort while bending over, coughing or lifting and a "heavy" or "dragging" sensation.

A *strangulated hernia* occurs when the tissue bulging through the abdominal wall becomes pinched and the blood supply is cut off. The affected tissue dies and then swells, causing extreme pain and a potentially life-threatening situation. Seek immediate medical attention if you think you have a strangulated hernia.

A *hiatal hernia* occurs at the spot called the *hiatus,* which is an opening in your diaphragm through which your esophagus (food pipe) passes into your stomach. If this opening is too large, your stomach may protrude (herniate) through it into your chest, creating a hiatal hernia. Symptoms include heartburn, belching, chest pain and regurgitation. Hiatal hernias are common, occurring in about 25 percent of all people older than 50 years. Most hiatal hernias are minor and show no symptoms. A hiatal hernia is not painful in and of itself, but the condition allows food and acid to back up into your esophagus, causing heartburn, indigestion and chest pain in some people. Obesity aggravates these symptoms.

Self-Care	**For Inguinal Hernia** You can neither prevent nor cure a hernia through self-care. Once you've had the lump evaluated and know it's a hernia and your hernia does not cause you discomfort, you need not take any special precautions. Wearing a corset or truss may give slight relief but will not reduce a hernia or fix it. **For Hiatal Hernia** ● Lose weight if you are overweight. ● Follow self-care precautions for heartburn on page 64.
Medical Help	If your hernia is painful or bothersome, contact your health care provider to discuss whether an operation is necessary.
Caution	If you cannot reduce the hernia by lying down and pushing on the lump, the blood supply to this segment of bowel may be cut off. Symptoms of this complication include nausea, vomiting and severe pain. Left untreated, intestinal blockage or, in rare cases, a life-threatening infection may result. If you have any of these symptoms, contact your health care provider.

Common Problems

Indigestion and Heartburn

Indigestion is a nonspecific term used to describe discomfort in your abdomen which often occurs after eating. Indigestion is not a disease. It is a collection of symptoms, including discomfort or burning in your upper abdomen, nausea and a bloated or full feeling that belching may relieve.

The cause of indigestion is sometimes difficult to pinpoint. In some people, eating certain foods or drinking alcohol may trigger it.

A common form of indigestion is heartburn. Each day, as many as 10 percent of adults experience the burning sensation commonly called heartburn. Technically called gastroesophageal reflux, heartburn occurs when stomach acids back up into your esophagus (food pipe). A sour taste and the sensation of food coming back into your mouth may accompany the burning sensation behind your breastbone.

Why do these acids back up? Normally, a circular band of muscle at the bottom of your esophagus, called a sphincter, closes off the stomach but allows food to enter your stomach when you swallow. If the sphincter relaxes abnormally or becomes weakened, stomach acid can wash back up (reflux) into your esophagus and cause irritation.

Various factors can cause reflux. Being overweight puts too much pressure on your abdomen. Some medications, foods and beverages can relax the esophageal sphincter muscle or irritate the esophagus. Overeating or lying down after a meal also can encourage reflux.

Self-Care

Changing what and how you eat is the first step to prevent heartburn.
- Manage your weight. Slim down if you are overweight.
- Eat small, frequent meals.
- Avoid foods and drinks that relax the esophageal sphincter or irritate the esophagus (such as fatty foods, alcohol, caffeinated or carbonated beverages, decaffeinated coffee, peppermint, spearmint, garlic, onion, cinnamon, chocolate, citrus fruits and juices and tomato products).
- Stop eating 2 to 3 hours before you lie down or go to bed.
- Elevate the head of your bed.
- Quit smoking; eliminate nicotine use.
- Do not wear tight clothing and tight belts.
- Avoid excessive stooping or bending or heavy exertion for 1 hour after eating.
- Over-the-counter antacids can relieve mild heartburn by neutralizing stomach acids temporarily. However, prolonged or excessive use of antacids containing magnesium can cause diarrhea. Calcium- or aluminum-based products can lead to constipation.

Another type of medication such as Pepcid, Tagamet and Zantac may relieve or prevent heartburn symptoms by reducing the production of stomach acid. These medicines are available in over-the-counter and prescription strengths.

Medical Help

Most problems with indigestion and heartburn are occasional and mild. But if you have severe or daily discomfort, don't ignore your symptoms. Left untreated, chronic heartburn can cause scarring in the lower esophagus. This can make swallowing difficult. In rare cases, severe heartburn can lead to a condition called Barrett's esophagus, which may increase your risk for cancer.

Heartburn and indigestion symptoms may signal the presence of a more serious underlying disease. Contact your health care provider if your symptoms are persistent or severe, or if you have difficulty swallowing.

■ Irritable Bowel Syndrome

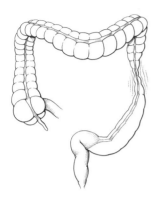

A spasm in the bowel wall may cause abdominal pain and other unpleasant symptoms commonly associated with IBS.

Irritable bowel syndrome (IBS), sometimes known as "spastic bowel" or "spastic colon," is a common medical problem that is not completely understood. IBS is annoying, painful and sometimes embarrassing, but it is not life-threatening. Some physicians rank the disorder with the common cold as the major cause of time lost from work.

Adolescents, young children and women experience this problem more than men. About one in five adult Americans has symptoms of IBS, but less than half of these people seek help.

Although experts cannot pinpoint its exact cause, IBS may be related to abnormal muscle spasms in your stomach or intestines. Stress and depression are often blamed as causes of IBS. But these emotions only aggravate the condition.

Symptoms may include abdominal pain, diarrhea, constipation, bloating, indigestion and gas. Although a bowel movement temporarily relieves the pain, you may feel as if you can't empty your bowels completely. Your stools can be ribbonlike and laced with mucus, or they can be hard, dry pellets. Often, diarrhea alternates with constipation.

Self-Care

Although no single treatment can eliminate IBS, simple diet and lifestyle measures can relieve your symptoms:

- Pay attention to what you eat. Avoid or eat smaller portions of foods that consistently aggravate your symptoms. Common irritants include tobacco, alcohol, caffeinated foods, beverages and medications, decaffeinated coffee, spicy foods, concentrated fruit juices, raw fruits and vegetables, fatty foods and sugar-free sweeteners such as sorbitol or mannitol.
- Eat high-fiber foods such as fresh fruits, vegetables and whole-grain foods. Add fiber gradually to minimize problems with gas and bloating.
- Drink plenty of fluids—at least 8 to 10 glasses a day.
- Try using fiber supplements containing psyllium, such as Metamucil or Konsyl, to help relieve your constipation and diarrhea.
- Reduce your stress through regular exercise, sports or hobbies that help you relax.
- Try over-the-counter medications such as Imodium or Kaopectate to relieve diarrhea.

Medical Help

If self-care doesn't help, your health care provider may recommend prescription medications designed to relieve muscle spasms. If depression plays a role in your symptoms, treating this problem may be helpful.

Because the symptoms of IBS mimic those of more serious medical disorders such as cancer, gallbladder disease and ulcers, you should contact your health care provider for evaluation if simple self-care measures don't help within a couple of weeks.

Common Problems

Nausea and Vomiting

Nausea and vomiting are common and uncomfortable symptoms of a wide variety of disorders, most of which are not serious.

Feeling queasy and throwing up usually signals a viral infection called gastroenteritis. Diarrhea, abdominal cramps, bloating and fever also may accompany this condition. Other causes include food poisoning, pregnancy, some medications and gastritis (see page 61).

Self-Care

If gastroenteritis is the culprit, nausea and vomiting may last from a few hours to 2 or 3 days. It is also common to have diarrhea and mild abdominal cramping. To keep yourself comfortable and prevent dehydration while you recover, try the following:
- Stop eating and drinking for a few hours until your stomach has settled.
- Try ice chips or small sips of weak tea, clear soda (Seven-Up or Sprite) and broths or noncaffeinated clear sports drinks to prevent dehydration. Consume 2 to 4 quarts (8 to 16 glasses) of liquid for no longer than 24 hours, taking frequent, small sips.
- Add semisolid and low-fiber foods gradually and stop eating if the vomiting returns. Try soda crackers, gelatin, toast, eggs, rice or chicken.
- Avoid dairy products, caffeine, alcohol, nicotine or fatty or highly seasoned foods for a few days.

Medical Help

Vomiting can lead to complications such as dehydration (if the condition is persistent), aspiration (food in the windpipe) or, in rare instances, a blood vessel in the food pipe may tear and cause bleeding. Infants, the elderly and people with suppressed immune systems are particularly vulnerable to complications. Contact your health care provider if you are unable to drink anything for 24 hours, if vomiting persists beyond 2 or 3 days, if you become dehydrated or if you vomit blood. Signs of dehydration include excessive thirst, dry mouth, little or no urination, severe weakness, dizziness or light-headedness. Vomiting also can be a warning of more serious underlying problems such as gallbladder disease, ulcers or bowel obstruction.

Kids' Care

Spitting up is an everyday occurrence for babies and usually causes no discomfort. Vomiting, however, is more forceful and disturbing to your baby and can lead to dehydration and weight loss.

To prevent dehydration, let the baby's stomach rest for 30 to 60 minutes and then offer small amounts of liquid. If you are breast-feeding, let your baby nurse smaller amounts more frequently. Offer bottle-fed babies a small amount of formula or an oral electrolyte solution such as Pedialyte or Infalyte.

If the vomiting does not recur, continue to offer small sips of liquid or the breast every 15 to 30 minutes. Contact your health care provider if vomiting persists for more than 12 hours or if your child:
- Hasn't had a wet diaper in 8 hours
- Has diarrhea or bloody stools
- Has a dry mouth or cries without tears
- Is unusually sleepy or drowsy or unresponsive

A few newborn babies have a disorder called pyloric stenosis, which can cause repeated and forceful vomiting. This condition usually appears after the third week of life. It requires medical care.

■ Ulcers

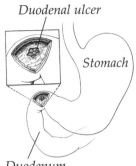

Duodenal ulcer

Stomach

Duodenum

The most common form of ulcer occurs in the duodenum and is called a duodenal ulcer.

Ulcers are sores in the inner lining of your esophagus or stomach or the uppermost section of your small intestine called the duodenum.

The cause of ulcers is not fully known. Recent research suggests that bacteria called *Helicobacter pylori (H. pylori)* play an important role, especially for duodenal ulcers. Stomach ulcers can be caused by excessive use of aspirin or aspirin-like medications. Contrary to popular belief, there is no clear evidence that emotional stress causes ulcers.

Ulcers can cause considerable distress. Symptoms may include a burning feeling beneath your breastbone in your upper abdomen, gnawing "hunger pangs" or "boring" pain and nausea. At times, ulcers also can cause belching or bloating. These symptoms typically occur when your stomach is empty. Although eating may relieve the symptoms, they often resume 1 to 2 hours later.

In severe cases, ulcers may bleed and cause you to vomit blood or pass black, tarry stools. In rare cases, an ulcer may perforate the wall of your stomach or duodenum, causing severe abdominal pain.

Self-Care

Diet, lifestyle and medication choices may help prevent or control ulcers.
- If you're using pain relievers, use acetaminophen. Aspirin, ibuprofen, ketoprofen and naproxen sodium can cause ulcer.
- Avoid alcohol and caffeinated foods, beverages and medications.
- Stop smoking.
- Eat small meals and avoid letting your stomach remain empty for long periods.
- Avoid spicy or fatty foods if they seem to make your symptoms worse.
- Take nonprescription antacids to neutralize stomach acids or medicines such as Pepcid, Tagamet or Zantac to stop the production of stomach acid.

Medical Help

Some ulcers disappear with self-care or with over-the-counter medication. If your symptoms do not improve after 1 week or if you have troublesome, recurrent ulcers, see your health care provider for further evaluation and treatment.

The diagnosis requires visualizing the ulcer with an X-ray or scope, although your doctor may treat you on the basis of your symptoms alone.

Bleeding ulcers can cause serious blood loss. Seek help immediately if you vomit blood, pass black, tarry stools or if you have severe pain.

New Treatment for Peptic Ulcers

A two-drug combination is the latest step toward simplifying the treatment of what was once a very misunderstood disease. The Food and Drug Administration allows medications such as Prilosec, Prevacid, Aciphex or Protonix, which suppress stomach acid production, in combination with an antibiotic called Biaxin for the treatment of peptic ulcers. The two drugs are used together for 14 days, followed by 14 days of treatment with the acid-suppressant alone. This treatment approach is the latest refinement in an effort to cure a common illness that was once thought to be incurable.

FOR MORE INFORMATION
- National Digestive Diseases Information Clearinghouse, 2 Information Way, Bethesda, MD 20892; (301) 654-3810.

Mayo Clinic Guide to Self-Care

Common Problems

Ears and Hearing

There's more to the ear than meets the eye. The part of your ear that's visible—your outer ear—is connected inside your head to your middle ear and inner ear, which work together to allow you to hear and help you maintain balance.

How the Ear Works

Your ear is a finely tuned organ that's specially designed to send sound impulses to your brain. When sound waves travel through the ear canal, your eardrum and the three small bones to which it is attached vibrate. This vibration moves through the middle ear to your inner ear, triggering nerve impulses to your brain, where you perceive them as sound.

Air reaches your middle ear through the eustachian tube. The middle ear must maintain the same pressure as the air outside your ear to allow your eardrum and ear bones to vibrate freely and conduct sound waves. If the middle ear has fluid in it, the eardrum and the bones can't move well. This is why an ear infection can cause temporary hearing problems.

Some common causes of ear pain and ear problems are described in this chapter.

Eardrum

Inner ear

Middle ear

Eustachian tube

Outer ear

■ Airplane Ear

The medical name for this condition is "barotrauma." Simply stated, it means an injury caused by changes in pressure. It often occurs if you fly or scuba dive with a congested nose, allergy, cold or throat infection. You may have pain in one ear, a slight hearing loss or a stuffy feeling in your ears. It is caused by your eardrum bulging outward or retracting inward as a result of a change in air pressure. Having a cold or ear infection is not necessarily a reason to change or delay a flight, however.

Self-Care	• Try taking a decongestant an hour before takeoff and an hour before landing. This may prevent blockage of your eustachian tube. • During flight, suck candy or chew gum to encourage swallowing, which helps open your eustachian tube. • If your ears plug as the plane descends, inhale and then gently exhale while holding your nostrils closed and keeping your mouth closed. If you can swallow at the same time, it is more helpful. • Remember, it is better to prevent this type of pain by following the listed suggestions rather than beginning treatment once the pain has occurred.
Medical Help	If your symptoms do not disappear within a few hours, see your physician.
Kids' Care	For babies and young children, make sure they are drinking fluids (swallowing) during ascent and descent. Give the child a bottle or pacifier to encourage swallowing. Give acetaminophen 30 minutes before takeoff to help control discomfort that may occur. Decongestants in young children are not generally recommended.

Foreign Objects in the Ear

Objects stuck in your ear can cause pain and hearing loss. Usually you know if something is stuck in your ear, but small children may not be aware of it.

Self-Care

If an object becomes lodged in the ear, follow these steps:

- Do not attempt to remove the foreign object by probing with a cotton swab, matchstick or any other tool. To do so is to risk pushing the object farther into the ear and damaging the fragile structures of the middle ear.
- If the object is clearly visible, is pliable and can be grasped easily with tweezers, gently remove it.
- Try using the pull of gravity: tilt the head to the affected side. Do not strike the victim's head, but shake it gently in the direction of the ground to try to dislodge the object.
- If the foreign object is an insect, tilt the person's head so that the ear with the offending insect is upward. Try to float the insect out by pouring mineral oil, olive oil or baby oil into the ear. It should be warm but not hot. As you pour the oil, you can ease the entry of the oil by straightening the ear canal. Pull the ear lobe gently backward and upward. The insect should suffocate and may float out in the oil bath.
- Do not use oil to remove any object other than an insect. Do not use this method if there is any suspicion of a perforation in the eardrum (pain, bleeding or discharge from the ear).

Medical Help

If these methods fail or the person continues to experience pain in the ear, reduced hearing or a sensation of something lodged in the ear, seek medical assistance.

Ruptured Eardrum

Eardrum

Rupture

An eardrum may rupture after an infection or from trauma. Signs of a ruptured, or perforated, eardrum are earache, partial hearing loss and slight bleeding or discharge from your ear. With an infection, the pain often resolves once the drum ruptures, releasing infected fluid or pus. Usually, the rupture heals by itself without complications and with little or no permanent hearing loss. Large ruptures may cause recurring infections. If you suspect that you have ruptured an eardrum, see your physician as soon as possible. Meanwhile, try the self-care tips listed here.

Self-Care

- Relieve pain with aspirin or another pain medication that is safe for you.
- Place a warm (not hot) heating pad over your ear.
- Do not flush your ear.

Medical Help

Your physician may prescribe an antibiotic to make sure that no infection develops in your middle ear. Sometimes a plastic or paper patch is placed over your eardrum to seal the opening while it heals. Your eardrum will often heal within 2 months. If it has not healed in that time, you may require a minor surgical procedure to repair the tear.

Common Problems

■ Ear Infections

To many parents of young children, coping with ear infections is almost as routine as changing wet diapers. Seven of 10 children will have at least one middle ear infection (otitis media) by age 3. One-third of these youngsters will have repeated bouts of ear infections.

A 1996 Mayo Clinic study pointed out that ear infections are increasing. According to the report, the number of office visits for ear infections in American children younger than age 2 tripled between 1975 and 1990. For children ages 2 to 5, the rate doubled.

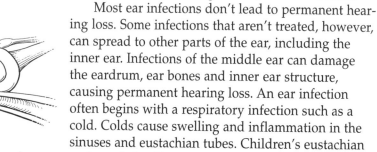

Fluid-filled middle ear creates environment for growth of bacteria.

Most ear infections don't lead to permanent hearing loss. Some infections that aren't treated, however, can spread to other parts of the ear, including the inner ear. Infections of the middle ear can damage the eardrum, ear bones and inner ear structure, causing permanent hearing loss. An ear infection often begins with a respiratory infection such as a cold. Colds cause swelling and inflammation in the sinuses and eustachian tubes. Children's eustachian tubes are shorter and narrower than adults. This size makes it more likely that inflammation will block the tube completely, trapping fluid in the middle ear. This trapped fluid causes discomfort and creates an ideal environment for bacteria to grow. The result is a middle ear infection.

Self-Care

- Consider an over-the-counter pain reliever such as ibuprofen or acetaminophen. (If your child is younger than 2, consult your health care provider.)
- Eardrops with a local anesthetic may help reduce pain. They won't prevent or stop an infection. They should **not** be used if there is drainage from the ear.
- To administer eardrops, warm the bottle slightly in water and place the child on a flat surface (not in your arms or on your lap), ear up, to insert the eardrops; then insert a small cotton wick to retain the eardrops.
- Place a warm (not hot), moist cloth or heating pad (on lowest setting) over the ear.

Medical Help

Contact your doctor if pain lasts more than a day or is associated with fever. Ear infections usually are treated with antibiotics. Even if your child feels better after a few days, continue giving the medicine for the full length of time recommended (usually 10 days).

The Pros and Cons of Ear Tubes

Recurrent ear infections are sometimes treated by surgically inserting a small plastic tube through your eardrum, which allows pus to drain out of your middle ear.

For the Procedure
- It usually results in fewer infections.
- Hearing is restored.
- The operation allows ventilation of the middle ear, which decreases the risk of permanent

changes in the lining of the middle ear—changes that might occur with prolonged infection.

Against the Procedure
- It requires brief general anesthesia.
- You must avoid getting water in your ear while the tube is in place.
- In rare cases, severe scarring or a permanent hole in the eardrum may result.

Mayo Clinic Guide to Self-Care

Common Questions About Ear Infections in Kids

What are the risk factors for infections?
Although all children are susceptible to ear infections, those at higher risk are children who:

- Are male
- Have siblings with a history of recurrent ear infection
- Have their first ear infection before they are 4 months old
- Are in group child care
- Are exposed to tobacco smoke
- Are of Native American, Alaskan or Canadian Eskimo descent
- Have frequent upper respiratory tract infections
- Were bottle-fed instead of breast-fed

What are the symptoms?
In addition to an earache or a feeling of pressure and blockage in the ear, some children may experience temporary hearing loss. Be aware of other signs of an ear infection such as irritability, a sudden loss of appetite, the development of a fever a few days after onset of a cold, nausea, vomiting or a preference for sleeping in an upright position. Your child also may have discharge in the ear or may tug at the ear.

Does your child need an antibiotic?
Because most ear infections clear on their own, your health care provider may first recommend a "wait-and-see" approach, especially if your child has few symptoms. In other cases, your doctor may opt to prescribe an antibiotic to treat the infection. Within 2 to 3 days of beginning the medication, symptoms usually improve.

Be sure to follow instructions carefully for giving the antibiotic. Continue to give the medication to your child for the entire recommended time. If you stop giving your child the antibiotic when symptoms improve, you may allow stronger remaining bacteria to multiply and cause another infection. Surviving bacteria may carry genes that make them drug-resistant.

If symptoms don't go away or if your child is younger than 15 months, schedule a follow-up visit as recommended by your health care provider. If your child is older and symptoms have resolved,

a recheck may not be necessary, especially if infections have not been recurrent.

What can you do?
Although an ear infection is not an emergency, the first 24 hours are often when your child's pain and irritability are the worst. Follow the self-care tips on page 70. To make your child more comfortable, don't underestimate the benefits of extra cuddling.

What about recurrent infections?
Time and the use of antibiotics usually resolve ear infections. But sometimes ear infections can become a chronic problem. If so, ask your health care provider about preventive antibiotic therapy. Persistent fluid buildup may cause temporary or even permanent hearing loss. This can lead to delayed speech development.

Can you prevent infections?
Preventing ear infections is difficult, but consider these approaches to help reduce your child's risk:

- Breast-feed rather than bottle-feed your baby for as long as possible.
- When bottle-feeding, hold your baby in an upright position.
- Avoid exposing your child to tobacco smoke.

Do children outgrow ear infections?
As your child matures, the eustachian tubes become wider and more angled, providing a better means of draining secretions and fluid out of the ear. Although ear infections still may occur, they probably won't develop as often as during the first few years of life.

What are medical researchers working on to help treat ear infections?
In addition to antibiotics, some approaches under investigation include the use of cortisone-like medication, such as prednisone, that would reduce inflammation (more research is needed to determine when this treatment is most effective); a "one-shot" approach using an injection of a particular antibiotic when oral drug therapy is impractical; and vaccines against the influenza virus.

■ Ringing in Your Ear

A ringing or buzzing in your ear when no other sounds are present can have many causes, including ear wax, a foreign object, infection or exposure to loud noise. It also can be caused by high doses of aspirin or large amounts of caffeine. This condition, called tinnitus, uncommonly is a symptom of more serious ear disorders, particularly if it is accompanied by other symptoms such as hearing loss or dizziness.

Self-Care

- If aspirin was recommended to you in high doses (more than 12 per day), ask your doctor about alternatives. If you are taking aspirin on your own, try lower doses or another over-the-counter pain medication.
- Avoid nicotine, caffeine and alcohol, which may aggravate the condition.
- Try to determine a cause, such as exposure to loud noise, and avoid or block it if possible.
- Wear earplugs or some other form of hearing protection if you have excess noise exposure, such as when you are working with yard equipment (leaf blowers or lawn mowers).
- Some people benefit by covering up the ringing sound with another, more acceptable sound (such as music or listening to a radio as you fall asleep).
- Other people may benefit by wearing a "masker," a device that fits in your ear and produces "white" noise.

Medical Help

If tinnitus worsens, persists or is accompanied by hearing loss or dizziness, consider evaluation by your health care provider. He or she may choose to pursue further evaluation. Although most causes of tinnitus are benign, it can be a difficult and frustrating condition to treat.

■ Swimmer's Ear

This is an infection of your outer ear canal. In addition to pain or itching, you may see a clear drainage or yellow-green pus and experience temporary hearing loss. Swimmer's ear is the result of having persistent moisture in the ear or, sometimes, from swimming in polluted water. Other similar inflammations or infections may occur from scraping your ear canal when you clean your ear or from hair sprays or hair dyes. Some people are prone to bacterial or fungal infections.

Self-Care

If the aching is mild and there is no drainage from the ear, do the following:
- Place a warm (not hot) heating pad over your ear.
- Take aspirin or another pain medication (be sure to follow the label instructions).
- To prevent swimmer's ear, try to keep ear canals dry, avoid substances that might irritate your ear and don't clean inside the ear canal unless you are instructed to do so by your health care provider.

Medical Help

Seek medical care if you have severe pain or swelling of the ear, a fever, drainage from the ear or an underlying disease. Your doctor may clean your ear canal with a suction device or a cotton-tipped probe. Your doctor also may prescribe eardrops or medications to control infection and reduce pain. Keep your ear dry while it is healing.

Wax Blockage

Ear wax is part of the body's normal defenses. It traps dust and foreign objects, protects the ear canal and inhibits growth of bacteria. At times, you may produce too much ear wax, blocking your ear canal, giving you an earache or causing a rattling in your ears. You also may notice a gradual hearing loss as the wax accumulates.

Self-Care

- Soften ear wax by applying a few drops of baby oil, mineral oil or glycerin with an eyedropper twice a day for several days.
- When the wax is softened, fill a bowl with water heated to body temperature (if it is colder or hotter, it may make you feel dizzy during the procedure).
- With your head upright, grasp the top of your ear and pull upward. With your other hand, squirt the water gently into your ear canal with a 3-ounce rubber bulb syringe. Then, turn your head and drain the water into the bowl or sink.
- You may need to repeat this several times before the extra wax falls out.
- Dry your outer ear with a towel or a handheld hair dryer.
- Ear wax removers sold in stores are also effective.
- Other home wax removal methods may also be effective if wax buildup is a recurrent problem. But ask your doctor about these self-care remedies. For example, 5 to 10 drops of Colace, an over-the-counter medication (used for constipation in infants), can be very helpful but needs flushing (leave drops in for 30 minutes). Another "flusher" is a Water-Pik. A few drops of diluted vinegar (half-strength) after flushing returns the ear canal to an acid state, which suppresses bacteria growth after ears are wet. A commercial alcohol-boric acid preparation is available for the same purpose.

Caution

Your ear canal and eardrum are very delicate and can be damaged easily. Do not poke them with objects such as cotton swabs, paper clips or bobby pins.

Flushing wax out of the ears should be avoided if there has been a prior eardrum perforation or prior ear surgery, unless your doctor approves. If infection is a concern, don't flush your ears.

Medical Help

Even if the tips given above are followed, many people have difficulty washing wax out of their ears. It may be best to have this done by your health care provider. Excessive wax can be removed in a procedure similar to the one described above. A special instrument is used to either scoop the wax out of the ear or suction it out. If this is a recurring problem, your doctor may recommend using a wax-removal medication every 4 to 8 weeks.

Common Problems

■ Noise-Related Hearing Loss

Sound is measured in decibels. An average conversation is about 60 decibels. A loud conversation in a crowded building is about 70 decibels. Your ears can be damaged by prolonged exposure to noise at 90 decibels or louder.

Self-Care

If you are exposed to loud power tools or engines, loud music, firearms or other equipment that produces loud noises, you should take the following precautions:

- Wear protective earplugs or earmuffs. Use commercially made protection devices that meet federal standards (cotton balls will not work, and they could get stuck in your ears). These bring most loud sounds down to acceptable levels. You can obtain custom-molded earplugs made of plastic or rubber to effectively protect against excessive noise.
- Have your hearing tested. Early detection of hearing loss can prevent future, irreversible damage.
- Use ear protection off the job. Protect your ears from any loud recreational activities, such as loud music or concerts, trapshooting or driving snowmobiles.
- Beware of recreational risks. Sensorineural hearing loss related to recreation is becoming more common. Activities with the greatest risk are trapshooting, driving snowmobiles and some other recreational vehicles and, particularly, listening to extremely loud music. If your son or daughter listens to loud music on a headset, use this simple test to determine whether the sound is too loud: if you can identify the music being played while your child is wearing the headset, it is too loud. Tell your child to save his or her ears for a lifetime of music enjoyment.

Maximal Job Noise Exposure Allowed by Law

Duration, Hours Daily	Sound Level, Decibels
8	90
6	92
4	95
3	97
2	100
1 1/2	102
1	105
30 minutes	110
15 minutes	115

Sound Levels of Common Noises

Decibels	Noise
	Safe range
20	Watch ticking; leaves rustling
40	Quiet street noise
60	Normal conversation; bird song
80	Heavy traffic
	Risk range
85-90	Motorcycle; snowmobile
80-100	Rock concert
	Injury range
120	Jackhammer 3 feet away
130	Jet engine 100 feet away
140	Shotgun blast

Age-Related Hearing Loss

A decrease in hearing is common with age. This condition is called presbycusis. If you or a family member suspects you have more serious hearing loss, see a physician. You may be referred to a doctor who is an ear specialist or to an audiologist (a person trained in hearing evaluation). Hearing loss can sometimes be restored with medical treatment or surgery, especially if the problem is in the outer ear or middle ear. If the problem is in the inner ear, however, it is usually not treatable. A hearing aid can improve your hearing. The advice given below may help you select a hearing aid.

Before You Buy a Hearing Aid, Here's Sound Advice

Of the 25 million Americans who have some degree of hearing loss, about 5.8 million use hearing aids. The average cost of a hearing aid is $1,000. But if it helps you hear better and improves your quality of life, it's worth the money. Yet the Food and Drug Administration (FDA) reports that too often people aren't fully satisfied with their hearing aids. Consumer complaints range from improper fit to poor repair service to lack of hearing improvement.

Here are some tips for selecting a hearing aid:
- **Have a medical and hearing examination.** Before you buy a hearing aid, be examined by a physician, preferably an ear, nose and throat doctor (otolaryngologist). An FDA regulation says it's best to have this examination within 6 months before you buy a hearing aid. An examination can determine whether a medical condition will prevent you from using a hearing aid.
- **Buy from a reputable dispenser.** If you don't get a hearing test (audiogram) from a medical facility, a dispenser will give you one. This person then takes an impression of your ear, chooses the most appropriate aid and adjusts the device to fit well. These are complex tasks, and skills of dispensers vary. Also, contact the Better Business Bureau about a dispenser's complaint record. Be cautious of "free" consultations and dispensers who sell only one brand of hearing aid.
- **Be alert to misleading claims.** For years, a few manufacturers and distributors claimed their hearing aids allowed you to hear speech and eliminate background noise. But this technology doesn't exist. Some newer hearing aids subdue loud sounds and so make wearing a hearing aid in noisy places more comfortable. But no hearing aid can filter out the voice you want to hear from other voices in a crowded room.
- **Ask about a trial period.** Have the dispenser put in writing the cost of a trial and whether this amount is credited toward the final cost of the hearing aid.
- **Obtain a second hearing test.** To determine if a hearing aid really helps you hear better, have another hearing test while wearing the aid.
- **Understand the warranty.** A warranty should extend for 1 to 2 years and cover both parts and labor.

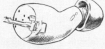

Disposable hearing aid

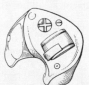

Canal aid

Low-profile aid

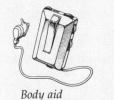

All-in-the-ear aid

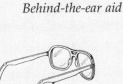

Behind-the-ear aid

Body aid

Eyeglasses aid

Eyes and Vision

Because your eyes are crucial in so many activities, eye problems usually demand attention. Luckily, many eye problems are more bothersome than serious.

Almost everyone has vision changes with age. Age also increases your risk of developing more serious eye problems. Some eye problems can't be prevented, but medications or surgery can slow or stop progression. This section covers the more common eye problems and discusses some of the issues related to declining vision.

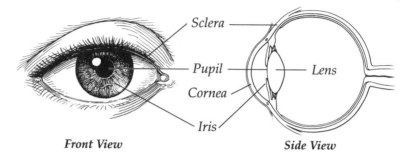

Front View   Side View

Black Eye

The so-called black eye is caused by bleeding beneath the skin around the eyes. Sometimes a black eye indicates a more extensive injury, even a skull fracture, particularly if the area around both eyes is bruised or there has been head trauma. Although most injuries are not serious, bleeding within the eye, called a "hyphema," is serious and can reduce vision and damage the cornea. In some cases, glaucoma (see page 80) also can result.

Self-Care

- Using gentle pressure, apply ice or a cold pack to the area around the eye for 10 to 15 minutes. Take care not to press on the eye itself. Apply cold as soon as possible after the injury to reduce swelling.
- Be sure there is no blood in the white and colored parts of the eye.

Medical Help

Seek medical care immediately if you experience vision problems (double vision, blurring), severe pain or bleeding in the eye or from the nose.

Taking Care of Your Eyes

- Have your vision checked regularly.
- Control chronic health conditions such as diabetes and high blood pressure.
- Recognize symptoms. Sudden loss of vision in one eye, sudden hazy or blurred vision, flashes of light or black spots or halos or rainbows around lights may signal a serious medical problem such as acute glaucoma or a stroke.

- Protect your eyes against sun damage. Buy sunglasses with UV blocking lenses.
- Eat foods containing vitamin A and beta carotene, such as carrots, yams and cantaloupe.
- Optimize your vision with the right glasses.
- Use good lighting.
- If your vision is impaired, use low-vision aids (such as magnifiers and large-type books).

Dry Eyes

Dry eyes feel hot, irritated and gritty when you blink. They may become slightly red. Tear production decreases as you age. Dry eyes usually affect both eyes, especially in women after menopause. Some medicines (such as sleeping medications, antihistamines and some drugs for high blood pressure) can cause or worsen dry eyes. Some rare medical conditions may be associated with dry eyes.

Self-Care

- Use a preservative-free artificial tear preparation such as Cellufresh.
- Because some over-the-counter eyedrops can cause drying, use them for no more than 3 to 5 days.
- Don't direct hair dryers (or other sources of air such as car heaters or fans) toward your eyes.
- Wear glasses on windy days and goggles when swimming.
- Keep your home humidity between 40 and 55 percent.
- Seek medical care if the condition persists despite the self-care efforts.

Excessive Watering

Your eyes may actually water in response to dryness and irritation. Watery eyes also commonly occur with infections such as so-called pinkeye (see page 78). They can result from an allergic reaction to preservatives in eyedrops or contact lens solutions. Watery eyes also can result from a blockage in the ducts that drain tears to the inside of your nose. Overflowing tears can cause even more eye irritation and tearing.

Self-Care

- Apply a warm compress over closed eyelids two to four times a day for 10 minutes.
- Don't rub your eyes.
- Replace mascara every 6 months. Mascara can become contaminated with skin bacteria transferred by the applicator.
- If you wear contact lenses, follow directions for wearing, cleaning and disinfecting them.

Floaters (Specks in the Eye)

The jellylike substance behind your lens (vitreous) is supported and distributed evenly within your eyeball by a fibrous framework. As you age, the fibers thicken and gather in bundles, creating the appearance of specks, hairs, or strings that move in and out of your vision. Floaters that appear gradually and become less noticeable over time are usually harmless and require no treatment. However, floaters that appear suddenly may indicate a more serious eye disorder such as hemorrhage or retinal detachment. The retina is the light-sensitive layer of tissue at the back of the eye which transmits visual images to the brain.

Medical Help

If you see a cloud of spots or a spider web, especially accompanied by flashes of light, see your eye doctor (ophthalmologist). These symptoms can indicate a retinal tear or retinal detachment, which requires prompt surgery to prevent vision loss.

Common Problems

■ Pinkeye or Red Eye

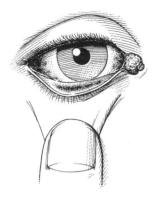

One or both eyes are red and itchy. There may be blurred vision and sensitivity to light. You may have a gritty feeling in the eye or a discharge in the eye which forms a crust during the night.

All of these are signs of a bacterial or viral infection commonly known as pinkeye. The medical term is "conjunctivitis." It is an inflammation of the membrane called the conjunctiva, which lines the eyelids and part of the eyeball.

The inflammation makes pinkeye an irritating condition, but it is usually harmless to sight. However, because it can be highly contagious, it must be diagnosed and treated early. Occasionally, pinkeye can cause eye complications.

Both viral and bacterial conjunctivitis are common among children and also affect adults. They are very contagious. Viral conjunctivitis usually produces a watery discharge, whereas bacterial conjunctivitis often produces a good deal of thick, yellow-green matter.

Allergic conjunctivitis affects both eyes and is a response to an allergen (such as pollen) rather than an infection. In addition to intense itching, tearing and inflammation of the eye, you also may experience some degree of itching, sneezing and watery discharge from the nose.

Self-Care

- Apply a warm compress to the affected eye or eyes. Soak a clean, lint-free cloth in warm water, squeeze it dry and apply it over your gently closed eyelids.
- Allergic conjunctivitis is often effectively soothed with cool compresses.

Prevention

Because pinkeye spreads easily and quickly, good hygiene is the most useful method for control. Once the infection has been diagnosed in you or a family member, the following steps may be useful to contain it:
- Keep hands away from your eyes.
- Wash hands frequently.
- Change towel and washcloth daily; don't share them.
- Wear clothes only once before washing.
- Change pillowcase each night.
- Discard eye cosmetics, particularly mascara, after a few months.
- Don't use other people's eye cosmetics, handkerchiefs or other personal items.

Medical Help

If you have any of the symptoms of pinkeye, see your physician. Your physician may culture the eye secretions to determine which form of infection you have. The physician may prescribe antibiotic eyedrops or ointments if the infection is bacterial. Viral conjunctivitis disappears on its own. If your doctor determines that you have allergic conjunctivitis, he or she may recommend medications to treat the allergy or your eye symptoms.

Kids' Care

Because the condition is contagious, keep your child away from other children. Many schools will send children with pinkeye home.

◼ Sensitivity to Glare

Glare may result when light is scattered within the eyeball. Glare may be especially bothersome in low light when your pupils are dilated (enlarged) because light is allowed into your eyes at a wider angle. Sensitivity to glare may mean a developing cataract (see page 80). To evaluate your symptoms, your health care provider may measure your vision under low, medium and high levels of glare.

Self-Care

- Reduce daytime glare by wearing polarized sunglasses with wide frames that follow your brow and opaque side shields.
- Have accurate correction for your distance vision to help minimize glare.

◼ Other Eye Problems

Drooping Eyelid

Your upper eyelid may droop if the muscles responsible for raising your eyelid weaken. Normal aging, trauma or disorders of the nerves and muscles can lead to drooping eyelid. If your eyelid interferes with vision, your ophthalmologist may recommend surgery to strengthen supporting muscles. **Caution:** A drooping eyelid that develops suddenly needs immediate evaluation and treatment. It may be associated with stroke or other acute problems of your nervous system.

Inflamed (Granulated) Eyelid

A chronic inflammation along the edges of your eyelids is called blepharitis. It may accompany dry eyes. Some people produce excess oil in glands near their eyelashes. Oil encourages growth of bacteria and causes your skin to be irritated, itchy and red. Tiny scales form along the edges of your eyelids, further irritating your skin. **Self-Care:** Apply a warm compress over your gently closed eyelids two to four times a day for 10 minutes. Immediately afterward, wash away the scales with warm water or diluted baby shampoo. If the condition is caused by an infection, your health care provider may prescribe a medicated ointment or an oral antibiotic.

Twitching Eyelid

Your eyelid takes on a life of its own—twitching at random, driving you crazy. The involuntary quivering of the eyelid muscle usually lasts less than a minute. The cause is unknown, but some people report that the painless twitching is brought on by nervous tension and fatigue. Rarely, it can be a symptom of muscle or nerve disease. Twitching eyelid is usually harmless and needs no treatment. **Self-Care:** Gentle massaging over the eyelid may help relieve the twitching.

Sty

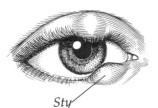

Sty

A sty is a red, painful lump on the edge of your eyelid. It is usually caused by bacterial infection in an eyelash follicle. Sties usually fill with pus and then burst in about a week. For persistent infections, your health care provider might prescribe an antibiotic cream. **Self-Care:** Apply a clean, warm compress four times a day for 10 minutes to relieve the pain and help the sty come to a point sooner. Let the sty burst on its own, then rinse your eye thoroughly.

Common Problems

■ Common Eye Diseases

Cataract

A cataract is a clouding of the normally clear lens of your eye. Lens clouding impairs vision. Some degree of cataract formation is normal as you grow older, but some exposures or conditions can accelerate the process. Long-term exposure to ultraviolet light (UV), diabetes, a previous eye injury, exposure to X-rays and prolonged use of corticosteroid drugs increase your risk. Smoking may increase your risk for cataracts, and aspirin may decrease the risk. If cataracts interfere with your daily activities, your lens can be surgically replaced. **Self-Care:** Reduce glare. Prevent or slow cataracts by wearing UV-blocking sunglasses when outside in bright sun. Ensure adequate lighting.

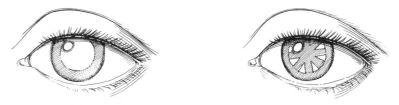

There are several forms of cataracts. Left: A nuclear cataract. Right: A wheel-spoke pattern cataract.

Glaucoma

Glaucoma involves damage to the eye (optic) nerve caused by increased pressure within the eyeball. Pressure increases when tiny pores that normally allow fluid to drain from inside your eye become blocked. Damage to the optic nerve causes your side vision to diminish slowly. Untreated, glaucoma can lead to blindness. **Caution:** Because the early symptoms can be subtle, it's important to have regular eye examinations. If diagnosed and treated early, chronic glaucoma usually can be controlled with eyedrops, oral medications or surgery. If you have symptoms such as a severe headache or pain in your eye or brow, nausea, blurred vision or rainbows around lights at night, seek immediate evaluation. Treatment may require emergency laser surgery.

Macular Degeneration

Macular degeneration blurs central vision and reduces your ability to see fine detail. It doesn't affect side vision and usually doesn't lead to total blindness. The condition occurs when tissue in the center of the retina (called the macula) deteriorates. The vision impairment is irreversible. However, when the condition is diagnosed early, laser treatment may help reduce or slow the loss of vision.

Transportation Advice for the Vision-Impaired

- Avoid stressful driving conditions—at night, in heavy traffic, in bad weather or on a freeway.
- Use public transportation or ask family members to help with night driving.
- Contact your local area agency on aging for a list of vans and shuttles, volunteer driver networks or ride-shares.
- Optimize the vision you have with the right glasses; keep an extra pair in the car.

Problems Related to Glasses, Contact Lenses

Many people begin to notice a change in their vision around age 40. Close-up objects that were once easy to see become blurred. The print in newspapers and books begins to seem smaller, and you instinctively hold reading material farther away from your eyes. The condition is presbyopia. It refers to the difficulty with near vision that develops as the lenses in your eyes become thicker and more rigid. Another symptom is eyestrain, which may include a feeling of tired eyes and a headache.

If you are already farsighted, you may notice the changes somewhat earlier and will need to have stronger corrective lenses. Even if you are nearsighted, you will experience the effects of presbyopia, and you may find yourself taking off your glasses to read small print. You may find that your eyes seem increasingly tired after reading.

Before trying over-the-counter reading glasses, first see an eye specialist to rule out other problems.

Medical Help

If you experience frequent headaches, see your ophthalmologist or optometrist, who will test your eyes and prescribe appropriate lenses, if needed.

Respond to warnings such as blurring of vision, yellowing of colors, increased sensitivity to light or loss of side vision, which could indicate cataracts or glaucoma.

Contact Lenses Versus Glasses

Contacts or glasses—which is better? Contact lenses are improving, but they are not for everyone. Certain diseases of the eye (dry eyes, previous corneal ulcers or corneas that have a loss of sensation) make wearing contact lenses inadvisable. Insertion, removal and care of contacts may be impractical for persons with arthritis of the hands, tremor from Parkinson's disease and physical disabilities from other disorders. However, contacts are preferable to glasses in some cases. For example, contact lenses offer markedly improved vision to people who are born with a malformation of the cornea. Contact lenses also offer advantages over glasses if you did not receive an artificial lens at the time of cataract removal.

Self-Care for Contact Lens Wearers
- Keep your contacts clean.
- Wash your hands before handling contacts.
- Use only commercial contact lens wetting and cleaning solutions.
- Have a pair of glasses as backup in case a problem requires you to stop wearing your contacts for a while.

Extended-Wear and Disposable Soft Contact Lenses
If you use extended-wear contact lenses, remove and sterilize them most nights. If you wear disposable lenses, do not wear them beyond the time recommended by your eye specialist. Wearing contact lenses too long without removing them may deprive your corneas of oxygen. Lack of oxygen can cause blurred vision, pain, tearing, redness and sensitivity to light. Remove your lenses at once if any of these symptoms occur. Have regular eye examinations to avoid problems that may result from extended contact wear.

FOR MORE INFORMATION
- The National Eye Institute, 2020 Vision Place, Bethesda, MD 20892-3655; (301) 496-5248; Internet address: http://www.nei.nih.gov.
- The Lighthouse Inc., 111 E. 59th St., New York, NY 10022; (800) 829-0500; Internet address: http://www.lighthouse.org.
- The local chapter of your State Society for the Blind and Visually Impaired.

Common Problems

Headache

Headaches are the most common reported medical complaint. They may point to a serious medical problem. But that situation is rare.

About 95 percent of all headaches have no underlying disease. These so-called primary headaches differ greatly. Researchers are learning more about what happens physically during a headache.

Types of Headaches

We divide primary headaches into three categories, although you may have a combination.

Tension
- Affect men and women equally
- Gradually produce a dull pain, knot or pressure in your neck, forehead or scalp

Migraine
- Pain may be severe and disabling
- Affect three times as many women as men
- May begin in your teens, rarely after 40
- May be preceded by a visual change, tingling on one side of your face or body or a specific food craving
- Often associated with nausea and sensitivity to light

Cluster
- Produce steady, boring pain in and around one eye, occurring in episodes that often begin at the same time of day or night
- Cause watering and redness of an eye and nasal stuffiness on the same side of the face
- May occur like clockwork and be linked to light or seasonal changes
- Frequently affect men, especially heavy smokers and drinkers
- May be misdiagnosed as a sinus infection or dental problem
- Usually last about 60 minutes

New Headache Theory

Research is focusing on various centers in the brain that may be involved in generating a headache. Activity in these centers causes blood vessels inside the skull to dilate and possibly become inflamed. This causes painful impulses to travel along the trigeminal nerve into the brain. The result: Headache.

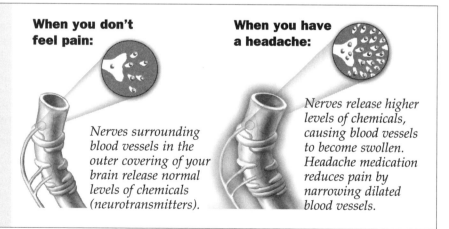

When you don't feel pain:

Nerves surrounding blood vessels in the outer covering of your brain release normal levels of chemicals (neurotransmitters).

When you have a headache:

Nerves release higher levels of chemicals, causing blood vessels to become swollen. Headache medication reduces pain by narrowing dilated blood vessels.

Self-Care	**For Occasional Tension-Type Headaches**

Self-Care

For Occasional Tension-Type Headaches

First, try massage, hot or cold packs, a warm shower, rest or relaxation techniques. If these measures don't work, try a low dose of aspirin (adults only), acetaminophen or ibuprofen. Moderate exercise may help.

For Recurrent Headaches

- Keep a headache diary. Include these factors:
  - *Severity.* Is it disabling pain, or merely annoying?
  - *Frequency and duration.* When does the headache start? Does it begin gradually or strike rapidly? Does it occur at a certain time of day? In monthly or seasonal cycles? How long does it last? What makes it stop?
  - *Related symptoms.* Can you tell it's coming? Are you nauseated or dizzy? Do you see sparkling colors or blank spots? Do you have specific hungers beforehand?
  - *Location.* Is the pain usually on one side of your head? In your neck muscles? Around one eye?
  - *Family history.* Do other family members have similar headaches?
  - *Triggers.* Can you link your headache to any particular food, activity, weather, time frame or environmental factors? (See Avoiding Headache Triggers, page 84.)
- Avoid triggers, as possible. To do so may require lifestyle changes.
- Get adequate sleep and exercise.

Special Migraine Self-Care

Begin treatment when you feel a migraine coming. This approach is your best chance to stop it early. Use acetaminophen, ibuprofen or aspirin (adults only) at the recommended dosage for pain relief. Some people can abort an attack by going to sleep in a darkened room or consuming caffeine (coffee or cola).

Medical Help

If self-care doesn't help after 1 or 2 days, see your health care provider. He or she will try to determine the type and cause of your headache, will try to exclude other possible sources of pain and may do tests. Your physician may prescribe one of many pain medications. Different medications are used for different types of headaches.

For severe migraines, your physician may prescribe a medication that mimics serotonin, a nerve chemical in your body. For frequent migraine attacks, your physician may prescribe a preventive medication to use on a daily basis.

Caution

Don't ignore unexplained headaches. Get medical attention right away if your headache:

- Strikes suddenly and severely
- Accompanies a fever, stiff neck, rash, mental confusion, seizures, double vision, weakness, numbness or speaking difficulties
- Follows a recent sore throat or respiratory infection
- Worsens after a head injury, fall or bump
- Is a new pain, and you're over 40

Common Problems

Avoiding Headache Triggers

Does a particular food, drink or activity trigger your headaches? Some people can eliminate headaches by avoiding triggers. Triggers vary among individuals. Here are some common ones:

- Alcohol, red wine
- Smoking
- Stress or fatigue
- Eye strain
- Physical or sexual activity
- Poor posture
- Changing sleeping patterns or mealtimes

- Certain foods, such as:
  - fermented, pickled or marinated food
  - bananas
  - caffeine
  - aged cheeses
  - chocolate
  - citrus fruits
  - food additives (sodium nitrite in hot dogs, sausages or lunch meat, or monosodium glutamate in processed or Chinese foods) and seasonings
  - nuts or peanut butter

  - pizza
  - raisins
  - sourdough bread
- Weather, altitude or time zone changes
- Hormonal changes during your menstrual cycle or menopause, oral contraceptive use or hormone replacement therapy
- Strong or flickering lights
- Odors, including perfumes, flowers or natural gas
- Polluted air or stuffy rooms
- Excessive noise

Kids' Care

Recurrent headaches are common during late childhood and adolescence. They rarely represent a serious problem.

Headache is associated with many viral illnesses. However, if your child frequently complains of headache, even during times when he is otherwise well, consult your physician.

Migraine headaches may occur in children and may be suspected if there is a family history of migraine. In children, this type of headache often is accompanied by vomiting, light sensitivity and sleep. Recovery follows within a few hours.

A headache may indicate stress with school, friends or family. It may be a reaction to a medication, particularly a decongestant.

If you think it's a tension-type headache, try the nonmedicating tips listed on page 83. If it occurs frequently, help your child keep a headache diary. Use acetaminophen or ibuprofen sparingly and briefly to avoid missing serious problems that the pain reliever may be masking.

If your child's headache persists, comes suddenly without explanation or gets steadily worse, call your health care provider. Also call about headaches that follow recent ear infections, toothaches, strep throat or other infections.

Be sure to tell your physician if there is any family history of migraines. That information could help lead to a diagnosis.

The Link Between Caffeine and Headaches

That morning caffeine headache can be very real, especially if you consume 4 or more cups of caffeinated drinks during the day. It may be a withdrawal headache after a night without caffeine.

But, for some headaches, caffeine may be a cure. Some kinds of headaches cause blood vessels to widen. Caffeine temporarily causes them to narrow.

So, for adults, if aspirin or acetaminophen doesn't help, use a medicine that includes caffeine. But don't overdo. Too much caffeine can cause jitteriness, rapid heart rate, sweating and, yes, withdrawal headaches.

Limbs, Muscles, Bones and Joints

Your body is amazingly intricate. You don't think about your body much when it's working fine. Somehow, everything holds together and you move about easily. But you usually do notice when there's a problem.

This chapter focuses on problems related to your limbs. Some conditions are common to many areas of your body, such as strains, sprains, broken bones, bursitis, tendinitis, fibromyalgia and gout. We address these conditions on pages 87 through 92. The remainder of the chapter provides additional information about problems related to specific limbs: shoulder; elbow; wrist, hand and fingers; hip; leg; knee; and ankle and foot. But first, here is some general information on anatomy.

Anatomy

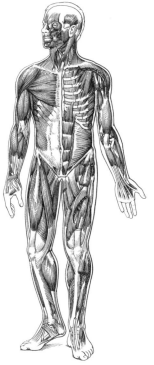

Many of your skeletal muscles are paired, enabling your body to move. Tendons connect these muscles to your bones.

Muscles and Tendons

Many of your 650 muscles help you move. Each skeletal muscle is attached to bones by bands called tendons. Pairs of muscles work together to move your bones. One muscle relaxes as its partner contracts.

If you are active, your muscles enable you to run, walk, swim, jump, climb stairs, bike, dance or mow the lawn. However, your muscles let you know when you've overdone it. They become sore and stiff.

Common causes of muscle injuries include accidents; strains; sudden, off-balance movements; overuse; and inflammation.

You can avoid many muscle and tendon aches by:
- Exercising regularly and moderately. Build up your activity gradually. You're not ready to run a marathon if you're not regularly running more than a few miles.
- Stretching your muscles gently before and after you exercise. For some people it's also helpful to use heat and massage to loosen their muscles before activity.
- Drinking plenty of water. Drinking 6 to 8 glasses of water a day maintains good hydration. But you'll need more than that when you're active, especially in the heat of summer.
- Conditioning your muscles gradually. Increase activity a little at a time.
- Strengthening your muscles with resistance exercise.
- Supporting previously injured areas with elastic tape or a brace.
- Avoiding stressing your muscles when you are tired.

Bones—Rigid, But Alive

You can't see it, but the 206 bones in your body change constantly. Proteins form the framework. Minerals, especially calcium and phosphate, fill in to give the bones strength. Because of this need for minerals, it's a good idea to consume mineral-rich milk and leafy green vegetables.

Common bone conditions include the following:
- Breaks, resulting from stress on a bone greater than it can withstand
- Bruising, usually from trauma
- Weakening through loss of minerals (osteoporosis)

A child's bones are more pliable than an adult's. When under strain or pressure, they are less likely to break. As you mature, your bones become more rigid.

Growing Pains Are Real

So-called growing pains can be very real during growth spurts. They usually occur in children's legs, often at night. They last a few hours and then go away. Growing pains usually don't hamper normal light activity.

If your child has growing pains:
- Use a warm heating pad for relief.
- Use recommended child's doses of acetaminophen or ibuprofen for pain. Don't give aspirin to children unless advised by your doctor to do so.
- Seek medical care if the area becomes swollen, hot and tender, or if your child develops a limp or unexplained fever.

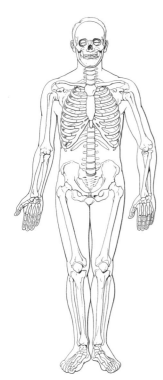

Your bones are living tissue and are always changing. They provide support for your body and function as your body's depository for important minerals.

Joints—Mechanical Masterpieces

Your bones come together at your joints. The end of each bone is covered by a layer of cartilage that glides smoothly and acts as a shock absorber. Tough bands of tissue (ligaments) hold your joints together.

Your body has several types of joints. This chapter discusses the following types:
- Hinge joints—in the ends of your fingers or your knees, for example. They allow one kind of back-and-forth movement.
- Ball and socket joints—in your shoulder or hip, for example. They allow a wide range of movement.

Causes of joint pain covered in this chapter include:
- Traumatic injuries or dislocation (when a joint is pushed out of place)
- Bursitis
- Fibromyalgia
- Gout
- Sprains

If your child has specific joint pain, you should be concerned. Call your health care provider if your child has joint pain along with:
- A fever and rash
- Swelling, stiffness, abdominal pain or unexplained weight loss
- Enlarged and tender lymph glands in the neck
- Limping or impaired normal activity

Nerves—Lines of Communication

Most of this chapter focuses on bones, muscles and joints. However, all of your limbs are wired with nerves that carry messages to and from your brain. They sense pain and also help you locate its source. They direct your movement. They let you know when your muscles are tired or injured. They may keep a muscle from working properly.

Nerves help coordinate your movement. When your body is working properly, they are in constant contact with your brain. They also help you avoid many injuries.

It's easier for you or your health care provider to identify and treat pain if you can tell how it happened. Did it follow:
- An accident
- Prolonged overuse or repetitive motions
- Inflammation
- An illness or condition elsewhere in your body

Mayo Clinic Guide to Self-Care

■ Muscle Strains: When You've Overdone It

A muscle becomes strained or "pulled"—or may even tear—when it stretches unusually far or abruptly. This type of injury often occurs when muscles suddenly and powerfully contract. A slip on the ice or lifting in an awkward position may cause a muscle strain.

Muscle strains vary in severity:
- **Mild:** causes pain and stiffness when you move and lasts a few days.
- **Moderate:** causes small muscle tears and more extensive pain, swelling and bruising. The pain may last 1 to 3 weeks.
- **Severe:** muscle becomes torn apart or ruptured. You may have significant internal bleeding, swelling and bruising around the muscle. Your muscle may not function at all. Seek medical attention immediately.

Self-Care

- Follow the instructions for P.R.I.C.E. (see below). The earlier the treatment, the speedier and more complete your recovery.
- For extensive swelling, use cold packs several times each day throughout your recovery.
- Do not apply heat when the area is still swollen.
- Avoid the activity that caused the strain while the muscle heals.
- Use over-the-counter pain medications as needed (see page 265). Avoid using aspirin in the first few hours after the strain because aspirin may make bleeding more extensive. Don't give aspirin to children.

Medical Help

Seek medical help immediately if the area quickly becomes swollen and is intensely painful. Call your health care provider if the pain, swelling and stiffness don't improve much in 2 to 3 days or if you suspect a ruptured muscle or broken bone.

P.R.I.C.E.: Your Best Tool for Muscle or Joint Injury

We refer to this information frequently throughout this section.
- **P: Protect** the area from further injury. Use an elastic wrap, a sling, splint, cane, crutches or an air cast.
- **R: Rest** to promote tissue healing. Avoid activities that cause pain, swelling or discomfort.
- **I: Ice** the area immediately, even if you're seeking medical help. Use an ice pack or slush bath for about 15 minutes each time you apply the ice. Repeat every 2 to 3 hours while you're awake for the first 48 to 72 hours. Cold reduces pain, swelling and inflammation in injured muscles, joints and connecting tissues. It also may slow bleeding if a tear has occurred.

- **C: Compress** the area with an elastic bandage until the swelling stops. Don't wrap it tightly or you may hinder circulation. Begin wrapping at the end farthest from your heart. Loosen the wrap if the pain increases, the area becomes numb or swelling is occurring below the wrapped area.
- **E: Elevate** the area above your heart, especially at night. Gravity helps reduce swelling by draining excess fluid.
- After 48 hours, if the swelling is gone, you may apply warmth or gentle heat. Heat can improve the blood flow and speed healing.
- Apply cold to sore areas after a workout, even if you are not injured, to prevent inflammation and swelling.

Common Problems

■ Sprains: Damage to Your Ligaments

Strictly speaking, a sprain occurs when you overextend or tear a ligament. Ligaments are the tough, elastic-like bands that attach to your bones and hold your joints in place.

Sometimes we use the term "sprain" any time your joint moves outside its normal range of movement. Sprains frequently are caused by twisting. They occur most often in your ankles, knees or the arches of your feet. Sprains cause rapid swelling. Generally, the greater the pain, the more severe the injury. Sprains vary in severity:

- **Mild:** your ligament stretches excessively or tears slightly. The area is somewhat painful, especially with movement. It's tender. There is not a lot of swelling. You can put weight on the joint.
- **Moderate:** the fibers in your ligament tear, but they don't rupture completely. The joint is tender, painful and difficult to move. The area is swollen and discolored from bleeding in the area.
- **Severe:** one or more ligaments tear completely. The area is painful. You can't move your joint normally or put weight on it. It becomes very swollen and discolored. The injury may be difficult to distinguish from a fracture or dislocation, which requires medical care. You may need a cast to hold the joint motionless, or an operation, if torn ligaments cause joint instability.

Self-Care

- Follow the instructions for P.R.I.C.E. (see page 87).
- Use over-the-counter pain medications (see page 265).
- Gradually test and use the joint after 2 days. Mild to moderate sprains usually improve significantly in a week, although full healing may take 6 weeks.
- Avoid activities that stress your joint. Repeated minor sprains will weaken it.

Medical Help

Seek medical care immediately if:

- You hear a popping sound when your joint is injured and you can't use it. On the way to your health care provider, apply cold.
- You have a fever and the area is red and hot. You may have an infection.
- You have a severe sprain, as described above. Inadequate or delayed treatment may cause long-term joint instability or chronic pain.

See your doctor if you are unable to bear weight on the joint after 2 to 3 days of self-care or if you don't experience much improvement in a week.

Preventing Sports Injuries

- Select your sport carefully. Don't jog if you have chronic back pain or sore knees.
- Warm up. Loosen, stretch and gradually increase your activity over 5 to 10 minutes. If you are prone to muscle pain, apply heat before you exercise.
- After exercising, cool down with muscle stretches.
- Begin a new sport gradually. Increase your level of exertion over several weeks.
- Use pain relievers with caution. It's easier to overexert and damage tissue without realizing it.
- Stop participating immediately if you think you may be injured, you become disoriented or dizzy or you lose consciousness, even briefly.
- Return gradually to full activity or switch sports until injuries heal.

Broken Bones (Fractures)

If you suspect a bone is broken, get medical care. A broken bone may or may not poke through your skin. Open fractures break through the skin. Simple fractures do not. Simple fractures are classified according to the way the bone breaks. Several varieties of simple fractures are included in the illustrations below.

| Open (Compound) | Simple | Greenstick | Transverse | Oblique | Comminuted |

Emergency Treatment

After injury or trauma, seek medical care immediately if:
- The person is unconscious or can't be moved. Call 911.
- The person is not breathing or doesn't have a pulse. Begin CPR (see page 2).
- There is heavy bleeding.
- Even gentle pressure or movement produces pain.
- The limb or joint appears deformed or the bone has pierced the skin.
- The part farthest from the heart is numb or bluish at the tip.

Self-Care

Take these precautions immediately, and seek medical care:
- Protect the area from further damage.
- If there is bleeding, try to stop it. Press directly on the wound with a sterile bandage, clean cloth or piece of clothing. If nothing else is available, use your hand. Keep pressing until the bleeding stops.
- Use a splint or sling to hold the area still. You can make a splint from wood, plastic or rolled newspaper. Place it on both sides of the bone, extending beyond the ends of the bone. Hold it firmly in place with gauze, cloth strips, tape or string, but not tight enough to stop the blood flow.
- Do not try to set the bone yourself.
- If ice is available, wrap the ice in cloth and apply it to the splinted limb.
- Try to elevate the injured area above the heart to reduce bleeding and swelling.
- If the person becomes faint or is breathing in short breaths, he or she may be in shock. Lay the person down with his or her head slightly lower than the rest of the body.

Kids' Care

The bones in your child's arms and legs have growth plates near the ends that allow bones to lengthen. If growth plates become damaged, the bone may not grow properly. Check out any possible fractures with your doctor.

■ Bursitis

Bursae

You have more than 150 bursae in your body. These tiny, fluid-filled sacs lubricate and cushion pressure points for your bones, tendons and muscles near your joints. They help you move without pain. When they become inflamed, movement or pressure is painful. This condition is called bursitis. Bursitis is commonly caused by overuse, trauma, repeated bumping or prolonged pressure such as kneeling for an extended period. It may even result from an infection, arthritis or gout. Most often, bursitis affects the shoulder, elbow or hip joint. But you also can have bursitis at your knee, heel and even in the base of your big toe.

Self-Care

- Use over-the-counter pain medications (see page 265).
- Keep pressure off the joint. Use an elastic bandage, sling or soft foam pad to protect it until the swelling goes down.
- Simple cases of bursitis usually disappear within 2 weeks. Ease the area back into activity slowly.

Prevention

- Strengthen your muscles to help protect the joint. Don't start exercising a joint that has bursitis until the pain and inflammation are gone.
- Take frequent breaks from repetitive tasks. Alternate the repetitive task with rest or other activities, even briefly.
- Cushion the joint before applying pressure (such as with kneeling or elbow pads).

Medical Help

Seek medical care if the area becomes red and hot or doesn't improve, or if you also have a fever or rash.

■ Tendinitis

Tendinitis produces pain and tenderness near a joint. You can usually associate it with a specific movement (grasping, for example). It usually means you have an inflammation or a small tear of the tendon. Tendinitis is usually the result of overuse or a minor injury. It's most common around the shoulders, elbows and knees.

Pain may cause you to limit movement. Rest is important, but so is maintaining a full range of movement. If you don't treat tendinitis carefully, tendons and ligaments around your joint may gradually stiffen over several weeks. Movement may become limited and difficult.

Self-Care

- Follow the instructions for P.R.I.C.E. (see page 87).
- Gently move the joint through its full range four times a day. Otherwise rest it. A sling or elastic bandage may help.
- Use an anti-inflammatory medication (see page 265).
- If soreness doesn't greatly improve in 2 weeks, see your health care provider.

Prevention

- Use warm-up and cool-down exercises and strengthening exercises.
- Apply heat to the area before you exercise, and apply cold afterward.
- Exercise on alternate days when starting an exercise program.

Mayo Clinic Guide to Self-Care

Medical Help	Seek medical help immediately if you have a fever and the area is inflamed.

Sometimes doctors inject a drug into tissue around a tendon to relieve tendinitis. Cortisone injections reduce inflammation and can give rapid relief of pain. These injections must be used with care, however, because repeated injections may weaken the tendon or cause undesirable side effects.

■ Fibromyalgia

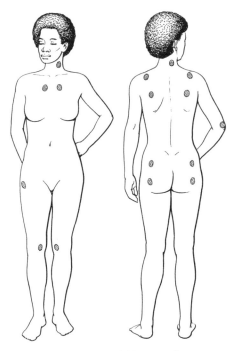

Common locations of fibromyalgia.

Persistent pain and stiffness in your muscles may have many causes. In recent years, health care providers have increasingly diagnosed a condition called fibromyalgia.

Common symptoms that lead to the diagnosis include general aches and pain and stiffness in joints and muscles. The type of pain can vary. It often affects areas where tendons attach muscles to bones. Symptoms frequently include the following:

- Widespread aching, lasting more than 3 months
- Fatigue and non-restful, non-restorative sleep
- Morning stiffness
- Tender points on the body, usually at sites of muscle attachment (see illustration)
- Associated problems such as headaches (see page 82), irritable bowel syndrome (see page 65) and pelvic pain

Fibromyalgia is a "diagnosis of exclusion." Currently, there are no laboratory tests that can be used to help make the diagnosis. Your doctor will make the diagnosis after considering other causes for your symptoms.

Emotional tension or stress may increase your likelihood of having fibromyalgia. It is more frequent in women than in men. This difference may be partially due to the fact that men may be more reluctant to see a doctor about their symptoms.

Self-Care	

- Pace yourself. Reduce your stress and avoid long hours of repetitive activity. Develop a routine that alternates work with rest.
- Develop a regular, low-impact exercise program such as walking, biking, swimming and plenty of stretching exercises. Improve your posture by strengthening supportive muscles, especially abdominal muscles (see page 55).
- Improve your sleep naturally with daily physical activity. To avoid undesirable side effects, use sleep medications sparingly, if at all.
- If necessary, use over-the-counter pain medications occasionally (see page 265).

Prevention
The best thing you can do to avoid or minimize fibromyalgia is to keep yourself in good physical condition, reduce stress and get adequate sleep.

- Try not to quit your job. Fibromyalgia seems to worsen in people who go on disability and eliminate activity entirely.
- Learn relaxation techniques. Try massage and warm baths.
- Find a support group that emphasizes maintaining health.
- Ask your family and friends for support.

Common Problems

■ Gout

Gout produces a sudden pain in a single joint, usually at the base of your big toe, although it may affect joints in your feet, ankles, knees, hands and wrists as well. The joint becomes swollen and red. Gout occurs most often in men older than 40. A fourth of persons with gout have a family history of the condition. Gout occurs when crystals of uric acid collect at a joint. Your risk of having gout increases if you are obese or have high blood pressure. Blood pressure medications that reduce your body's water content may provoke gout. Self-care measures include maintaining a reasonable weight, drinking plenty of water and avoiding heavy alcohol consumption. Seek medical care immediately if you have a fever and your joint is hot and inflamed. For more information, see page 162.

■ Shoulder Pain

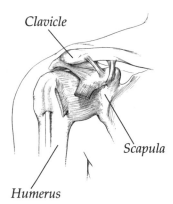

Clavicle

Scapula

Humerus

Treatment of shoulder pain depends on its cause. Bursitis and tendinitis are common causes of shoulder pain (see page 90), as are acute injury and rotator cuff tears (see page 93). Take note of how the pain began and what makes the pain worse. This information can be helpful if you need medical care.

Most shoulder pain is not life-threatening. Occasionally, however, shoulder pain signals a heart attack. Call 911 or your local rescue system right away if your pain:

- Starts as chest pain or pressure. The pain may occur suddenly or gradually. It may radiate to your shoulder, back, arms, jaw and neck.
- Is accompanied by excessive sweating, shortness of breath, faintness or nausea and vomiting.
- Is new and you have a known heart condition.

■ Acute Painful Shoulder

Acute shoulder pain centers on your upper arm and neck. Pain may suddenly limit arm movement. Possible causes include overuse or trauma. Your shoulder may become inflamed and swollen at the tip. It may be very painful to put on a coat or extend your arm straight out from your side.

Self-Care
- Use over-the-counter pain medications (see page 265).
- If the bone isn't broken or dislocated, it's important to move the joint through its full range four times a day to avoid stiffening or a permanent condition called "frozen shoulder." If necessary, ask a friend to help you move your arm gently through its full range.
- Once pain has resolved, exercise your arm daily.

Medical Help

Seek medical care if:
- Your shoulders appear uneven or you cannot raise the affected arm
- You have extreme tenderness at the end of your collarbone
- An injury causes you to wonder if a bone is broken
- You have redness, swelling or fever
- Your shoulder is not improving after a week of self-care

Mayo Clinic Guide to Self-Care

■ Rotator Cuff Injury

The rotator cuff is formed by the attachment of several tendons to the shoulder. Because of the shoulder's complexity, many problems are simply diagnosed as rotator cuff injuries. The tendons in your shoulder may have tiny tears, be irritated or pinched between your bones (called impingement). Pain may be more severe at night. This type of injury usually results from repetitive overhead motions (such as painting a ceiling, swimming, playing a racket sport or throwing a baseball or softball) or from trauma, such as falling on your shoulder.

Self-Care
- Follow the instructions for P.R.I.C.E. (see page 87).
- Take anti-inflammatory medicines (see page 265).
- Do stretching exercises and put the shoulder through its full range of motion four times daily.
- Wait until the pain is gone before gradually returning to the activity that caused the injury. You may have to wait 3 to 6 weeks.
- Alter your technique in racket sports, pitching or golf.

Medical Help
Seek medical care if the area is hot and inflamed and you have a fever, if your shoulders are uneven or if you can't move your arm at all.

  If the pain hasn't diminished in 1 week despite the use of self-care measures, see your doctor.

■ Elbow and Forearm Pain

Bursitis and tendinitis are common sources of pain in your elbow (see page 90). Bursitis may produce a small, egg-shaped, fluid-filled sac at the tip of your elbow. If the pain hasn't improved after a few days of treatment and the area is still very sensitive to pressure, seek medical care. You may need an X-ray to determine whether a bone is broken.

  A **dislocated elbow** may occur in a child if an adult suddenly pulls or jerks the child's arm. The elbow of a child—especially if younger than 6 years—cannot withstand this stress. Dislocation is very painful and limits movement. Seek medical treatment immediately. Your health care provider will return the bones to their proper position, which usually relieves the pain. An X-ray can rule out other problems. Use a sling for 2 weeks or as directed to stabilize the joint.

  A **hyperextended elbow** occurs when your elbow is pushed beyond its normal range of motion, often as a result of a fall or misplay during a tennis swing. Pain and swelling occur in your elbow and in the tissues beneath your elbow. Try P.R.I.C.E. (see page 87) and support your elbow with a splint or sling until the pain stops. If the pain has not improved in a week, see your health care provider.

Medical Help
Seek medical care immediately if:
- Your elbow seems deformed
- Your elbow is very stiff and has limited range of motion after a fall
- The pain in your arm is severe

■ Tennis Elbow or Little League Elbow

This recurrent pain is actually a form of tendinitis (called epicondylitis). It affects the outside or inside of your forearm, just below your elbow. Pain may extend down toward your wrist. It's caused by repeated tiny tears in tendons that attach muscles of your lower arm to your elbow. Common causes include swinging a racket, baseball pitching, painting a house, using a screwdriver or hammer or any movement requiring twisting arm motions.

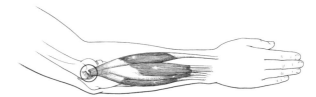

Tennis elbow produces pain on the outside or inside of your forearm near your elbow (see circle) when you exercise the joint. Tiny tears or inflammation causes the discomfort.

Self-Care

- Follow the instructions for P.R.I.C.E. (see page 87).
- Massage may speed healing by improving circulation in the area.
- Splinting your elbow and forearm at night may reduce pain.
- Take an anti-inflammatory medication (see page 265).
- It may take 6 to 12 weeks of treatment for the pain to disappear.

Prevention

- Prepare for any sport season with appropriate preseason conditioning. Do strengthening exercises with a hand weight by flexing and extending the wrists.
- Wear forearm support bands just below your elbow.
- Warm up properly. Gently stretch the forearm muscles before and after use.
- Try applying a warm pack for 5 minutes before activity and an ice pack after heavy use.

Medical Help

Seek medical care immediately if:
- Your elbow is hot and inflamed and you have a fever
- You can't bend your elbow at all or it looks deformed
- A fall or injury causes you to wonder if a bone is broken
    If the pain doesn't improve in a week or so, see your doctor to rule out other complications.

Wrist, Hand and Finger Pain

Think of all the things you do each day with your wrists, hands and fingers. You may not consider the many nerves, blood vessels, muscles and small bones that work together as you turn a key in the door—until the movement becomes painful.

Pain and swelling in your wrists, hands and fingers can result from injury or overuse. They can begin gradually or rapidly. They may be due to the following:

- A strain or sprain (see pages 87 and 88)
- Fracture, bursitis, tendinitis or gout (see pages 89, 90 and 92)
- Arthritis or fibromyalgia (see page 161 and page 91).

Self-Care

- Follow the instructions for P.R.I.C.E. (see page 87).
- Take over-the-counter pain medicines (see page 265).
- If an initial X-ray doesn't show a fracture and it's still quite painful a week later, ask your health care provider to check again. Some fractures may require special X-ray views or be invisible in the first few days.
- If pain continues, you may need further testing, rest in a splint or cast or physical therapy.

Prevention

- Remove your rings before manual labor. If you injure your hand, remove your rings before your fingers become swollen.
- Take frequent breaks to rest muscles you've used steadily. Vary your activities.
- Use flexibility and strengthening exercises.

Medical Help

Seek medical care immediately if:

- You suspect a fracture
- A fall or accident has caused rapid swelling and moving the area is painful
- The area is hot and inflamed and you have a fever
- Your fingers suddenly become blue and numb

Common Problems

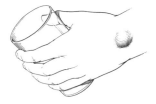

A ganglion is a swelling beneath the skin. It's a fluid-filled cyst lined with tissue bulging from a joint or tendon sheath.

Ganglions are fluid-filled lumps that usually appear on the back of the wrist, but they may be in the front, in the palm or over finger joints. They're filled with jelly-like material leaking from a joint or tendon, although they feel firm or solid. Ganglions are sometimes painful and, if bothersome, may require treatment. Seek medical care immediately if the lump becomes painful and inflamed or if the cyst breaks through the skin and drains (usually at the end of the fingers).

A **jammed finger** commonly occurs during sports activities. Pain may be caused by a sprain (stretched ligaments) or a fracture involving the joint surface. Follow the P.R.I.C.E. guidelines on page 87. To protect it during use, "buddy tape" the injured finger to an adjacent finger. Seek medical care immediately if:

- Your finger appears deformed
- You cannot straighten your finger
- The area becomes hot and inflamed and you have a fever
- Swelling and pain are significant or persistent

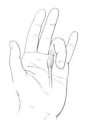

A **trigger finger** is a condition that causes the finger to lock or catch in a bent position. It will straighten with a visible sudden "snap," and if it is severe, the finger may not fully straighten. Triggering is more pronounced in the morning and after firmly grasping an object. It is caused by a binding "knot" in the palm which prevents smooth tendon motion. Change your habits to avoid overuse. Seek medical care immediately if your finger is hot and inflamed and you have a fever.

■ Carpal Tunnel Syndrome

A narrow tunnel through your wrist (the carpal tunnel) protects your median nerve, which provides sensation to your fingers. When swelling occurs in the tunnel, the median nerve can become compressed, and pain is produced.

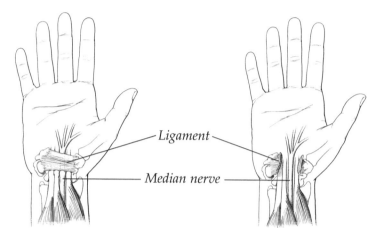

Ligament

Median nerve

Finger-bending (flexor) tendons and an important nerve pass through a tight space (the carpal tunnel) as they enter the hand. Swelling in the tunnel may squeeze the nerve. Most problems occur without a clear cause. Swelling is more common in women than in men. If occurs more frequently in people who are pregnant or overweight. Smoking, medical conditions such as diabetes, thyroid disease or arthritis also seem to play a role, as do occupations or hobbies that involve awkward wrist postures along with heavy, repetitive lifting or grasping actions.

Symptoms include the following:
- Tingling or numbness in your thumb, index and middle fingers (but not your little finger). This tingling may occur at night, and wake you from sleep, and may also occur while you are driving or holding the phone or a newspaper.
- Pain radiating or extending from your wrist into your forearm or down into your palm or fingers.
- A sense of weakness or clumsiness; dropping objects.
- If the condition is advanced, a constant loss of feeling in the affected fingers.

Self-Care

- Take regular breaks from heavy or repetitive activity, at least 5 minutes every hour.
- Vary your activities. Stretch your wrists and hands at least once every hour.
- Keep fit; watch your weight and don't smoke.
- If you have tingling in your hand or fingers that wakes you at night, or if you note numbness in your hand when you wake up in the morning, try wearing a wrist splint that holds your wrist straight at night. The splint should be snug but not tight.
- If the symptoms continue or worsen, see your health care provider.

Thumb Pain

Pain at the base of your thumb may be the first sign of osteoarthritis in your hands (see page 161). You may notice pain and swelling at the base of your thumb when you write, open jars, turn your key in the door or ignition or try to hold small objects. It may be limited to one joint or extend to many. It's most common in women older than 55. The pain can be the result of a previous injury, repetitive activity (such as screwing bolts) or heredity.

Self-Care

- Avoid activities that cause pain.
- Rest your thumb. Use a splint to stabilize the wrist and thumb. Remove the splint at least four times a day to move and stretch the joints to maintain flexibility.
- Use over-the-counter pain medications (see page 265).
- Exercise your thumb daily while your hands are warm. Move your thumb in wide circles. Bend it to touch each of the other fingers on your hand.
- Use tools specially designed for people with arthritis.

Medical Help

Seek medical care immediately if pain limits activities or is too severe to tolerate most days. Cortisone injections, arthritis medicine and, occasionally, an operation are effective in alleviating pain.

Hip Pain

Hip pain frequently follows a fall or accident. It also may occur after vigorous speed walking or aerobics. Common causes include bursitis, tendinitis and osteoarthritis (see pages 90 and 161, respectively) or strains and sprains (see pages 87 and 88). Only rarely is hip pain caused by having one leg shorter than the other, and differences in leg length of half an inch or more (1 to 2 cm) are common and normal.

Self-Care

- Follow the instructions for P.R.I.C.E. (see page 87).
- Avoid activities that aggravate the pain.
- Take over-the-counter pain medicines (see page 265).
- Strengthen the hip group muscles (especially the hip abductors, which move the leg out from the body) to relieve pain and improve function in an arthritic hip.

Medical Help

Seek medical care immediately if:

- You have fallen or had an accident and wonder if your hip may be broken
- You have followed the self-care instructions above after an accident or fall and your hip is more painful the following day
- You have osteoporosis and have injured your hip in a fall

Common Problems

Many leg difficulties result from a combination of overuse, deconditioning (poor strength and flexibility), being overweight, trauma and poor circulation. Lifestyle changes may improve your legs' comfort.

Use the following exercises to strengthen your muscles and avoid injuries:
● Walk. Begin with short strides. Lengthen your stride as your muscles loosen.
● Bike. Gradually increase your distance and speed over weeks.
● Swim. Stretch and tone your muscles.
● Work paired muscles equally. For example, exercise the quadriceps (the muscles on the front of the thigh) equally with the hamstrings (muscles on the back of the thigh).

■ Pulled Hamstring Muscle

Athletes often bruise or strain hamstring muscles, especially during sports such as soccer or track-and-field activities. You may suspect such an injury if you experience pain after a slip or rigorous activity.

Self-Care

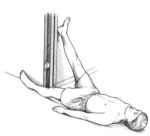

● Follow the instructions for P.R.I.C.E. (see page 87). If symptoms don't begin to improve after a week of P.R.I.C.E. treatment, see your health care provider.

To avoid hamstring injury, do this simple exercise called the "doorframe stretch":
● Lie on the floor in front of a doorway and extend your left leg straight ahead across the threshold. Slide into the doorframe with the leg to be stretched up against the wall and straighten the leg. Hold for 30 seconds. Repeat, reversing leg positions. Do not lock your knee.
● As you get better, strive to bring your leg position perpendicular to your body.

■ Pain, Cramps and Charley Horses

A cramp, sometimes called a charley horse, is actually a muscle spasm. Cramps commonly occur in an athlete who is overfatigued and dehydrated during sports, especially in warm weather. However, almost everyone experiences a muscle cramp at some time. For most people, cramps are only an occasional inconvenience.

Self-Care

● Gently stretch and massage a cramping muscle.
● For lower leg (calf) cramps, put your weight on the leg and bend your knee slightly, or do the calf stretch outlined on page 106.
● For upper leg (hamstring) cramps, straighten your legs and lean forward at your waist. Steady yourself with a chair. Or do the hamstring stretch described above.
● Apply heat to relax tense, tight muscles.
● Apply cold to sore or tender muscles.
● Drink plenty of water. Fluid helps your muscles function normally.
● If you have troublesome leg cramps, ask your health care provider about possible medication options.

Self-Care

Prevention

Stretch your leg muscles daily, using the following stretch for the Achilles tendon and calf (see the illustration on page 106):

- Stand an arm's length from a wall. Lean forward, resting your hands and forearms on the wall.
- Bend one leg at the knee and bring it toward the wall. Keep the other leg stiff. Keep both heels on the floor. Keep your back straight and move your hips toward the wall. Hold for 30 seconds.
- Repeat with the other leg. Repeat five times per leg.
- Stretch your muscles carefully and warm up before exercising vigorously.
- Stop exercising if a cramp begins.

◼ Shin Splint

When pain occurs on the front, inside portion of the large bone of your lower leg (the tibia), it may be the result of a shin splint. Shin splints occur when tiny fibers of the membrane that attaches muscle to the tibia are irritated and inflamed, producing pain and sometimes swelling. Shin splints commonly occur in runners, basketball and tennis players and army recruits.

Self-Care

- Follow the instructions for P.R.I.C.E. (see page 87).
- Apply ice massage to the painful area.
- Try over-the-counter pain relievers (see page 265).
- Wait until the pain leaves before resuming the activity that caused it. The pain may last several weeks or even months. Meanwhile, bike or swim to maintain flexibility and strength.

Prevention

- Use stretching exercises before running to loosen the muscles in your legs and feet. Tap your foot up and down and side to side.
- A soft shoe insert may help cushion your leg.
- You may need a specially made insert (orthotic) to wear in your shoes, especially if you have flatfeet.
- A trainer can help evaluate and adjust your running style.

Medical Help

Seek medical care immediately if:

- Pain in your shin follows a fall or accident and is severe
- Your shin is hot and inflamed
- You have pain in your shin at rest or at night

Special X-rays may be used to look for a stress fracture.

◼ Swollen Legs

Occasional swelling in your legs is a common problem and has many causes, including being overweight, sitting or standing for a long time, retaining fluids (common in pregnant or menstruating women), varicose veins, an allergic reaction and too much sun exposure.

Common Problems

Serious and ongoing swelling can be caused by the following medical conditions, which require medical attention:

- An *inflamed vein (phlebitis)*: Phlebitis can be dangerous if a blood clot develops and breaks loose. It usually occurs in the lower portion of one leg. The leg becomes sore, red and swollen. It often follows a period of inactivity—a long car or plane ride or after an operation, for example. See your health care provider immediately.
- *Poor circulation (claudication)*: A cramping pain occurs at about the same point each time you walk. It goes away when you stop and rest. It's caused by a narrowed or blocked area in your leg arteries. See your health care provider.
- *Heart failure*: If your heart is unable to keep up with the demands on it, you may retain fluid in your legs. This condition affects both legs at the same time and is not painful. See your health care provider.
- Liver or kidney disease. See your health care provider.

Self-Care

For Occasional Swelling
- Lose weight and limit salt intake.
- Elevate your legs to a level above your heart for 15 to 20 minutes every few hours to let gravity help move fluid toward your heart.
- For prolonged sitting and travel, walk around frequently and stretch your legs.

For Conditions That Cause Swelling
Although you cannot treat these conditions yourself, you can lower your risk if you do the following:
- Stop smoking.
- Control blood pressure.
- Exercise moderately and regularly.
- Attain a desirable weight.

Medical Help

Seek medical care immediately if you have unexplained, painful swelling in your legs or if a swollen leg becomes hot and inflamed.

◼ Knee Pain

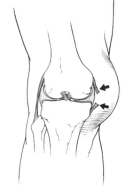

Arrows point to a torn ligament, a common form of knee injury. Swelling occurs and the joint becomes unstable.

Your knee is the largest joint in your body and is quite complex. The parts of your knee work together to support you each day as you bend, straighten and twist.

Your knee is very susceptible to injury because of its exposed location. It's not designed to handle sideways stress, and it carries a lot of weight.

Knee injuries are often complex. Many are sports-related or result from trauma. Sometimes pain is simply a matter of wear and tear. You cannot accurately tell how severe a knee injury is by the extent of pain and swelling. It's more important that your knee can bear weight, feels stable and has its full range of motion.

Pain can be due to the following:
- Strains and sprains (see pages 87 and 88) from sudden twists or blows to your knee. A sprain will be on the opposite side of your knee from the side that took the blow. It may take days for swelling to develop fully.
- Tendinitis (see page 90), possibly as a result of intense bicycling or stair climbing. Runner's knee is a form of tendinitis. This overuse injury produces pain at the front of your knee. Your tendons become inflamed and it hurts to move your knee.

- Bursitis (see page 90).
- Osteoarthritis (see page 161). Arthritis often causes pain when you move or put weight on your knees.
- Torn cartilage or ligaments in your knee caused by twisting or impact. These are common injuries for skiers and basketball players who trip or fall.
- Loose pieces of your kneecap or cartilage floating around your joint. They may become pinched in your knee joint. This condition is painful and can cause your joint to lock.
- A tender, bulging cyst behind your knee (popliteal or Baker's cyst). It hurts to bend, squat or kneel.

Self-Care

- Follow the instructions for P.R.I.C.E. (see page 87).
- Take an anti-inflammatory medicine (see page 265). Remember that you may not feel injury-alerting pain after you take pain medicine.
- Flex and straighten your leg gently every day. If it's difficult for you to move your knee, someone can help move it for you at first. Try to straighten it and keep it straight.
- If you use a cane, carry it on the side that's not injured.
- Avoid strenuous activity until your knee heals. Start non-impact exercises slowly.
- Avoid squatting, kneeling or walking up and down hills.

Prevention

- Exercise regularly to strengthen your knee muscles. Bend your knee only to 90° during exercise. Don't do deep knee bends.

Medical Help

Seek medical care immediately if:
- The injury produces intense, immediate pain and your knee doesn't function properly.
- Your knee is very painful, even when you're not putting weight on it.
- The pain follows a popping sound or snapping sensation. Torn knee ligaments may need surgical repair. Delay reduces the likelihood of success.
- Your knee locks rigidly in one position, or your kneecap is visibly deformed (dislocated).
- Your knee seems unusually loose or unstable.
- You have rapid, unexplained swelling or a fever.
   If pain is not improving after 1 week of home treatment, see your health care provider.

Knee Supports and Braces

If your knees are unstable, try a brace or support bandage such as:
- A rubbery, neoprene sleeve. This slips over your knee and has a hole over your kneecap.
- An inexpensive, nonprescription knee brace. This may be hinged on the outer side or on both sides of your knee.

Caution: These devices appear to offer more support than they actually do. Although they don't protect your knee from injury, they may make it feel warm and secure and will protect it from scrapes. Use braces or supports under the direction of your doctor or therapist.

■ Ankle and Foot Pain

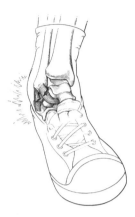

An ankle sprain occurs when ligaments that support your ankle are stretched or torn.

Your ankle is one of the most commonly injured joints. The ankle, where three bones meet, allows a wide-ranging foot movement and bears your full body weight. Common causes of foot or ankle pain include the following:

- Strains or sprains (see pages 87 and 88).
- Fractures (see page 89). High-impact activities such as basketball or aerobics can cause stress fractures. Stress fractures are really hairline cracks. They're often invisible on an X-ray for up to 6 weeks after the injury.
- Bursitis or tendinitis (see page 90).
- Achilles tendinitis occurs when the tendon that links your leg muscles to the bone at the back of your heel becomes inflamed. The tiny tears in the tendon may follow strenuous exercise. You'll feel a dull ache or pain, especially when you run or jump. The tendon also may be mildly swollen or tender.
- Bunion. Ill-fitting footwear is often the cause of this condition. Your big toe bends toward or overlaps the next toe. The base of your big toe extends beyond your foot's normal profile. That bump is called a bunion. The rubbing of shoes may cause corns, calluses and joint pain.

Self-Care

- Follow the instructions for P.R.I.C.E. (see page 87).
- Walking on an unstable joint may increase the damage, unless you stabilize it with an ankle brace, air splint or high, laced boots.

If you suspect a **fracture,** see your health care provider. If you have a stress fracture:
- Allow at least 1 month for healing. You usually won't need a cast.
- Avoid high-impact activities for 3 to 6 weeks.

If you have **Achilles tendinitis:**
- Wear soft-soled running shoes, and avoid running or walking up or down hills.
- Avoid any impact on your heel for several days.
- Use gentle calf stretches daily (see pages 99 and 106).

If you have **bunions:**
- Wear shoes with adequate toe width. Wear sandals or go barefoot in the summer. Larger deformities may require special shoes.

Prevention

- Choose well-fitting, good-quality footwear. Shoes with a wider toe box will eliminate pressure on your toes. Avoid tight, thin-soled, high-heeled shoes.
- Stretch your Achilles tendon. Before exercise, follow the calf stretches outlined on pages 99 and 106.

Medical Help

Seek medical care immediately if:
- Your foot pain is severe and the area is swollen after an accident or injury
- Your foot is hot and inflamed or you have a fever
- Your foot or ankle is deformed or bent in an abnormal position
- The pain is so severe that you can't move your foot
- You can't bear weight 72 hours after any injury

▪ Flatfeet

All babies appear to have flatfeet. By the time we're teens, most of us develop arched feet. Arches go both from side to side and lengthwise and help distribute weight evenly across our feet.

Some people never develop arches. Others become flatfooted after they put many miles on their feet. But that isn't necessarily a problem. People with flatfeet sometimes have fewer lower back, leg or foot injuries.

Flatfeet can be a problem when:
- They place pressure on your foot's nerves and blood vessels
- They cause imbalance and joint problems in your ankles, knees, hips or lower back
- You carry excess body weight

Self-Care

- Arch supports in well-fitting shoes may give you a better weight-bearing position.
- See your health care provider if your flatfeet are continually painful.

Kids' Care

Baby fat may make your infant's feet look flat. At about age 5 years, your child may begin to develop an arch. One in seven children never develops well-formed arches.

There are two kinds of flatfeet:
- *Flexible flatfeet* look flat only when your child stands up. Arches reappear if your child stands on tiptoe or takes weight off the foot. Flatfeet are painless and tend to run in families. There's usually no need to treat them. Some health care providers recommend arch supports in firm shoes for increased comfort.
- *Fixed flatfeet* can be more difficult. If your child's feet are painful, stiff or extremely flat, special footwear or an operation may help.

Flatfeet are feet that have little or no arch. Above at left (top and bottom) is a normal foot and footprint. If your child's foot and footprint more nearly resemble the illustrations at right, then he or she has flatfeet.

■ Burning Feet

Pain may be mild or severe burning or stinging. It may be constant or temporary. This condition is especially common in people older than 65 years. The cause may be difficult to pinpoint and may include the following:

- Irritating fabrics
- Poorly fitting shoes
- Athlete's foot (a fungal infection) (see page 122)
- Exposure to a toxic substance like poison ivy

Suspect a nerve or blood vessel disorder if you have:

- Burning with prickling, weakness or a change of sensation in your legs
- Burning with nausea, diarrhea, loss of urine or bowel control or impotence
- Other family members with the problem
- A persistent condition
- Diabetes mellitus

Self-Care

- Wear nonirritating cotton or cotton-synthetic blend socks and shoes of natural materials that breathe. A specially fitted insole may help, if it's in good condition.
- Eliminate activities that aggravate your condition.
- Soak your feet in cool tap water for 15 minutes twice each day.
- Reduce your stress and get adequate sleep.
- Use over-the-counter pain medications (see page 265).

■ Hammertoe and Mallet Toe

Unlike a bunion, which affects the big toe, hammertoe may occur in any toe (most commonly the second toe). The toe becomes bent and painful. Generally, both joints in a toe are affected, giving it a clawlike appearance. Hammertoe can result from wearing shoes that are too short, but the deformity also occurs in persons with long-term diabetes who have muscle and nerve damage as a result of the disease. A mallet toe is deformed at the end of the toe.

Self-Care

- A specially designed insert (orthotic) that fits into your shoe may help.
- Be sure your shoes fit well (that is, they accommodate your foot length and width).

Tips for Proper Shoe Fit

You can avoid many foot, heel and ankle problems with shoes that fit properly. Here's what to look for:

- Adequate toe room. Avoid shoes with pointed toes.
- Low heels will help you avoid back problems.
- Laced shoes are roomier and adjustable.
- Select comfortable athletic shoes, strapped sandals or soft, roomy pumps with cushioned insoles.

- Avoid vinyl and plastic shoes. They don't breathe when your feet perspire.
- Buy shoes at midday. Your feet are smaller in the morning and swell throughout the day. Measure both feet.
- As you age, your shoe size may change (especially the width).
- Have your shoe store stretch shoes in tight spots.

■ Swelling

Most people have swollen feet occasionally. Causes include all of those noted in Swollen Legs on page 99.

Self-Care
- Reduce your salt intake.
- Exercise your legs. Elevate your legs above your heart.
- Lie down for 30 minutes in mid day with your feet elevated higher than your heart.

Prevention
- Wear support stockings. They apply constant pressure and reduce foot and ankle swelling. Poorly fitting stockings (too tight in the calf) can cause swelling.
- Maintain a regular exercise program.

Medical Help
Seek medical care immediately if one foot becomes swollen rapidly, your foot is inflamed and you have a fever.

■ Morton's Neuroma

Morton's neuroma causes a sharp, burning pain in the ball of your foot. It may feel like you're walking on stones. Your toes may sting, burn or feel numb. Soft tissue grows around a nerve in your foot (called a neuroma), often between your third and fourth toes. It may not hurt early in the day, but only after you stand or walk in tight shoes.

Self-Care
- Wear well-fitting shoes with enough room in the toe box, or wear sandals.
- Shoe supports (orthotics) or a foot pad may help.
- Reduce high-impact activities for a few weeks.

Medical Help
- A cortisone injection may reduce pain.
- The growth may be surgically removed if pain is chronic and severe.

■ Heel Pain

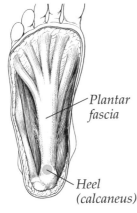

Plantar fascia

Heel (calcaneus)

Heel pain often results from stress on the plantar fascia.

Heel pain is irritating, but rarely serious. Although it can result from a pinched nerve or a chronic condition, such as arthritis or bursitis, the most common cause is plantar fasciitis. This is an inflammation of the plantar fascia, the fibrous tissue along the bottom of your foot which connects to your heel bone (calcaneus) and toes.

The pain usually develops gradually, but it can come on suddenly and severely. It tends to be worse when you are getting out of bed in the morning, when the fascia is stiff. Although both feet can be affected, it usually occurs in only one foot.

The pain generally goes away once your foot limbers up. It can recur if you stand or sit for a long time. Climbing stairs or standing on tiptoes also can produce pain. A bone spur (usually painless) may form from tension on your heel bone.

Plantar fasciitis can affect people of all ages. Factors increasing your risk include excess weight, improperly fitting shoes, foot abnormalities and activities that place added pressure on your feet. Treatment involves steps to relieve the pain and inflammation. Don't expect a quick cure. Relief may take 6 months or longer.

- Cut back on jogging or walking. Substitute exercises that put less weight on your heel, such as swimming or bicycling.
- Apply ice to the painful area for up to 20 minutes after activity.
- Stretching increases flexibility in your plantar fascia, Achilles' tendon and calf muscles. Stretching in the morning before you get out of bed helps reverse the tightening of the plantar fascia which occurs overnight.
- Strengthening muscles in your foot can help support your arch.
- Buy shoes with a low to moderate heel (1 to 2 inches) and good arch support and shock absorbency.
- Over-the-counter medications may ease the pain (see page 265).
- If you're overweight, shed excess pounds.
- Try heel pads or cups. They help cushion and support your heel.

These exercises stretch or strengthen your plantar fascia, Achilles' tendon and calf muscles. Hold each for 20 or 30 seconds, and do one or two repetitions two or three times a day.

Toe curls with towel

Toe extension

Calf/heel stretch on stairs

Standing calf/heel stretch

Medical Help

If the self-care measures aren't effective, or if you believe your condition is due to a foot abnormality, see your doctor. Treatment options include the following:

- Custom orthotics.
- Night splints to keep tension on the tissue so it heals in a stretched position.
- Deep heat, which increases blood flow and promotes healing.
- A cortisone injection in your heel often can help relieve the inflammation when other steps aren't successful. But multiple injections aren't recommended because they can weaken and rupture your plantar fascia, as well as shrink the fat pad covering your heel bone.
- Doctors can detach your plantar fascia from your heel bone, but this is recommended only when all other treatments have failed.

Lungs, Chest and Breathing

Breathing is one of our most basic reflexes. We do it thousands of times a day. When we breathe in (inhale), we draw fresh oxygen into our lungs and bloodstream. When we breathe out (exhale), we remove the air from our lungs which contains carbon dioxide, a waste product of our bodies' activities. Breathing is something that most of us take for granted—until we have trouble with it.

◼ Coughing: A Natural Reflex

A cough is a reflex—just like breathing. It's actually a way of protecting your lungs against irritants. When your breathing passages, called bronchi, have secretions in them, you cough to clear the passages so you can breathe more easily. A small amount of coughing is ordinary and even healthy as a way to maintain clear breathing passages.

However, strong or persistent coughing can be an irritant to your breathing passages. Repeated coughing causes your bronchi to constrict. This change can irritate the membranes (the interior "walls" of your breathing passages).

What Causes Coughing? Coughing is frequently a symptom of a viral upper respiratory tract infection, which is an infection of your nose, sinuses and airways. A cold and influenza are common examples. Your voice box may become inflamed (a condition called laryngitis), causing hoarseness, which could affect your ability to speak. Coughing also may result from throat irritation caused by the drainage of mucus down the back of your throat (a condition called postnasal drainage).

The Cough

A cough begins when an irritant reaches one of the cough receptors in your nose, throat or chest (see dots). The receptor sends a message to the cough center in your brain, signaling your body to cough. After you inhale, your epiglottis and vocal cords close tightly, trapping air within your lungs. Your abdominal and chest muscles contract forcefully, pushing against your diaphragm. Finally, your vocal cords and epiglottis open suddenly, allowing trapped air to explode outward.

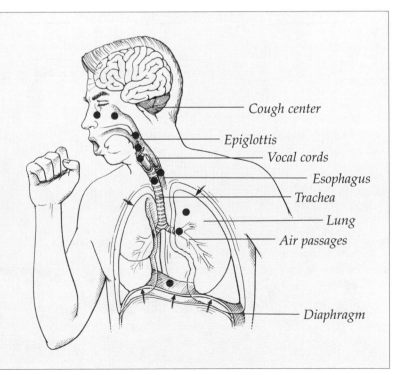

Cough center

Epiglottis

Vocal cords

Esophagus

Trachea

Lung

Air passages

Diaphragm

Coughing also occurs with chronic disorders. People with allergies and asthma have bouts of involuntary coughing, as do people who smoke. Irritants in the environment such as smog, dust, secondhand smoke and cold or dry air can cause coughing.

Sometimes coughing is caused by stomach acid that backs up into your esophagus or, in rare cases, your lungs. This condition is called gastroesophageal reflux (see page 64). Some people also develop a "habit" cough.

Self-Care

- **Drink plenty of fluids.** They help keep your throat clear. Drink water or fruit juices—not soda or coffee.
- **Use a humidifier.** The air in your home can get very dry, especially during the winter. Dry air irritates your throat when you have a cold. Using a humidifier to moisturize the air will make breathing easier (see below).
- **Honey, hard candy or medicated throat lozenges** may help to soothe a simple throat irritation and may help prevent coughing if your throat is dry or sore. Try drinking a cup of tea sweetened with honey.
- **Try expectorants,** medications that help you to clear your throat of mucus. ("To expectorate" means "to spit.") Expectorants may increase the flow of normal fluids in your throat and help relieve some of the pain.
- **Use cough suppressants,** available in both liquid and solid form. They act on the portion of your brain that controls your cough reflex. Mild over-the-counter versions are available. Stronger versions are available only by prescription.
- If your cough is caused by a backup of stomach acids, try sleeping with the head of your bed elevated 4 to 6 inches. Also avoid food and drink within 2 to 3 hours of bedtime.

Medical Help

Contact a doctor if your cough lasts more than 2 or 3 weeks, or if it is accompanied by fever, increased shortness of breath or bloody phlegm. Managing a chronic cough requires careful evaluation.

Home Humidifiers—Help or Hazard?

When breathing dry indoor air makes you cough, increase the humidity. But don't let the remedy to one problem create another. Dirty humidifiers can be a source of bacteria and fungi. To minimize growth, the U.S. Consumer Product Safety Commission suggests the following:

- **Change the water every day.** Empty the tank and dry the surfaces with a soft towel. Then refill with clean water.
- **Some products recommend use of distilled water.** Tap water contains minerals that can create bacteria-friendly deposits. When released into the air, these minerals often appear as white dust on your furniture.

- **Sanitize the humidifier every 1 to 2 weeks.** Empty the tank. Fill it with a solution of 1 teaspoon bleach to 1 gallon water. Let the solution soak for 20 minutes and then empty the tank. Rinse the tank until you can no longer smell bleach.
- **Keep the humidity between 30 and 50 percent.** Levels higher than 60 percent may create a buildup of moisture. When moisture condenses on surfaces, bacteria and fungi can grow. Periodically check the humidity with a hygrometer, available at your local hardware store.
- **Follow the manufacturer's instructions** for regularly cleaning the humidifier to avoid a buildup of bacteria.

◾ Bronchitis

Bronchitis is a common condition, much like the common cold. It usually is caused by a viral infection that spreads to the bronchi, producing a deep cough that, in turn, brings up yellowish gray matter from your lungs. The bronchi are the main air passages of your lungs. When the walls that line the bronchi become inflamed, this condition is called bronchitis.

Self-Care

- Get plenty of rest. Drink lots of fluids. Use a humidifier in your room.
- Take a nonprescription cough medicine (see page 266). Adults can take aspirin, NSAIDS or acetaminophen for a fever. Children should take only acetaminophen or ibuprofen.
- Avoid irritants to your airways, such as tobacco smoke.

Medical Help

Acute bronchitis usually disappears in a matter of days. Contact a doctor if you experience shortness of breath or a high temperature for more than 3 days. If your cough lasts for more than 10 days and your sputum (the matter you spit up from your lungs) becomes yellow, gray or green, the doctor may prescribe an antibiotic.

◾ Croup

Croup is caused by a virus that infects the voice box (larynx), windpipe (trachea) and bronchial tubes. Croup occurs most often in children between the ages of 3 months and 5 years, and it more often affects boys than girls. Because of a narrowing of the airway, a child with croup has a tight, brassy cough that may resemble the barking of a seal. The child's voice becomes hoarse, and it is difficult for the child to breathe. The child may become agitated and begin crying, actions that make breathing even more difficult. Croup typically lasts 5 or 6 days. During this period, it may go from mild to severe several times. The symptoms are usually worse at night.

Self-Care

- Reassure your child. Cuddle, read a book or play a game for distraction.
- Give clear, warm fluids to help loosen thickened secretions.
- Keep the child away from smoke (it aggravates the symptoms).
- Expose the child to warm, humid air. Try one of the following methods:
  - Lay a wet washcloth loosely over your child's nose and mouth so that air moves easily in and out. (Do not do this if your child is in respiratory distress.)
  - Fill a humidifier with warm water and have your child put his or her face in or near the mist and breathe deeply through the mouth.
  - Have your child sit in a steamy bathroom for at least 10 minutes. Return as often as needed. (Try one trip outside if the weather is cool or cold.)
- Sleep in the same room as your child so you will be alert to any worsening of the condition.

Medical Help

Occasionally, croup may cause nearly complete blockage of the airway. Get emergency help if you notice any of the following symptoms: drooling or difficulty swallowing, difficulty bending the neck forward, blue or dusky lips, worsening cough and more difficulty with breathing and high-pitched noises when inhaling.

Common Problems

Wheezing

Wheezing occurs when you hear a high-pitched whistling sound coming from your chest as you breathe out. It is caused by a narrowing of the airways in the lungs and indicates breathing difficulty. Also, your chest may feel tight.

Wheezing is a common symptom of asthma, bronchitis, smoking, allergies, pneumonia, emphysema, lung cancer and heart failure. It also can be caused by environmental factors, such as chemicals or air pollution. Wheezing requires medical attention. See a doctor if you have difficulty breathing and are wheezing.

Shortness of Breath

In general, unexpected shortness of breath is a symptom that needs medical attention. Shortness of breath can be caused by illnesses ranging from heart attacks to blood clots in the lung to pneumonia. It also can be caused by pregnancy.

In its chronic form, shortness of breath is a symptom of illnesses such as asthma, emphysema, other lung diseases and heart disease. All of these chronic conditions also require medical attention. There are, however, some exercises you can do to help relieve shortness of breath if you have chronic lung disease (see below).

Simple Exercises Can Improve Your Breathing

Some simple breathing exercises may help you if you have emphysema or another chronic lung disorder. They help you control the emptying of your lungs by using your abdominal muscles. You also can increase the efficiency of your lungs. Ask your physician about them. Do them two to four times daily.

Diaphragmatic Breathing
Lie on your back with your head and knees supported by pillows. Begin by breathing in and out slowly and smoothly in a rhythmic pattern. Relax.

Place your fingertips on your abdomen, just below the base of your rib cage. As you inhale slowly, you should feel your diaphragm lifting your hand.

Practice pushing your abdomen against your hand as your chest becomes filled with air. Make sure your chest remains motionless. Try this while inhaling through your mouth and counting slowly to 3. Then purse your lips and exhale through your mouth while counting slowly to 6.

Practice diaphragmatic breathing on your back until you can take 10 to 15 consecutive breaths in one session without tiring. Then practice it on one side and then on the other. Progress to doing the exercise while sitting erect in a chair, standing up, walking and, finally, climbing stairs.

Pursed-Lip Breathing
Try the diaphragmatic breathing exercises with your lips pursed as you exhale, that is, with your lips puckered (the flow of air should make a soft "sssss" sound). Inhale deeply through your mouth and exhale. Repeat 10 times at each session.

Deep-Breathing Exercise
While sitting or standing, pull your elbows firmly backward as you inhale deeply. Hold the breath in, with your chest arched, for a count to 5 and then force the air out by contracting your abdominal muscles. Repeat the exercise 10 times.

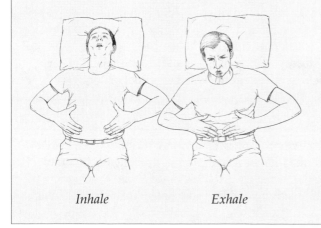

Inhale   *Exhale*

■ Chest Pain

Pain in your chest can be severe. It also can be difficult to interpret. The pain could be caused by something as simple as indigestion or by a serious medical situation.

Emergency Care

If pain in your chest persists, contact a health care provider immediately!
   Heart attack: In addition to pain or pressure in your chest, you could experience pain in your face, arms, neck or back. Other symptoms of a heart attack may include shortness of breath, sweating, dizziness, nausea and vomiting. If you think you are having a heart attack, seek medical help or call 911 immediately. If you go to a hospital, *do not drive yourself!*

Other Causes of Chest Pain

Here are common forms of chest pain that don't require immediate medical attention:
   Chest wall pain: This is one of the most common forms of harmless chest pain. If probing the tender area with your finger causes the pain to return, then serious conditions, such as heart attack, are less likely. Chest wall pain usually lasts only a few days, and it can be treated with aspirin in adults. For children, treat with ibuprofen or acetaminophen. Apply low and intermittent heat to the area to help reduce the pain.
   Heartburn: Symptoms are a warm or burning discomfort in the upper part of your abdomen and under your breastbone. You also may have an acid or sour taste in your mouth. Heartburn sometimes can be so painful that the symptoms are confused with the onset of a heart attack. Chest pain from heartburn usually can be relieved by belching or by taking an antacid.
   Precordial catch: This is a condition that occurs most often in young adults. The symptom is a brief, sharp pain under the left breast which makes breathing difficult. There are no self-care measures. The condition goes away momentarily. The cause of this common condition is unknown, although it is apparently harmless.
   Angina: Angina is the term used for chest pain, or pressure, associated with heart disease. It is caused by a lack of oxygen reaching the heart muscle. It usually develops with physical exertion or when you're under emotional stress. When you've been diagnosed as having heart disease, develop a treatment plan with your doctor.

- Don't try to "work through" an episode of angina. Stop and treat it.
- It is usually treated with rest and a medication such as nitroglycerin.
- If you have a change in your pattern of angina, such as increased frequency or nighttime attacks, see your doctor immediately.
- If you've tried measures to stop an angina attack but it lasts longer than 15 minutes or you're also having light-headedness or palpitations, seek emergency medical help.

■ Palpitations

A palpitation is the feeling you have in your chest when it feels as if your heart "skips a beat." Many people experience heart palpitations from time to time. Usually they are not dangerous, but check with your doctor to be sure. Palpitations can be caused by stress or by external factors such as consumption of caffeine and alcohol. Frequently, changes in lifestyle relieve the symptoms.

Common Problems

Nose and Sinuses

Your nose is the main gateway to your respiratory system. Normally, your nose filters, humidifies and warms the air you breathe as it moves from your nasal passage into your throat and lungs, 12 to 15 times a minute.

Occasionally, your nose is the site of conditions such as a nosebleed, cold, hay fever or a sinus infection. Luckily, most disorders of the nose and sinuses are temporary and easy to cure.

The following pages address the common disorders of the nose and its adjacent cavities, the sinuses. For information on respiratory allergies, see page 158.

◼ Foreign Objects in the Nose

If a foreign object becomes lodged in the nose, follow these steps:
- Do not probe at the foreign object with a cotton swab or other tool. Do not try to inhale the object by forcefully breathing in; breathe through the mouth until the object is removed.
- Blow your nose gently to try to free the object, but do not blow hard or repeatedly.
- If the object protrudes from the nose and can be easily grasped with tweezers, gently remove it.

If these methods fail, seek emergency medical assistance.

◼ Loss of Sense of Smell

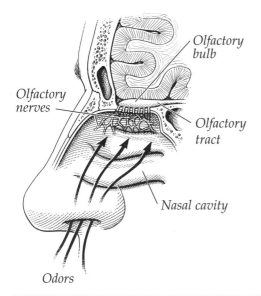

Olfactory bulb

Olfactory nerves

Olfactory tract

Nasal cavity

Odors

Your sense of smell and, to a large degree, your sense of taste begin with the olfactory nerve endings, which are found in the upper portion of your nose. The olfactory nerves contain very fine and sensitive fibers that transmit signals from the olfactory bulb to your brain.

Most people temporarily lose their sense of smell when they have a head cold. Usually, the sense of smell returns once the infection is gone.

However, when the sense of smell is lost without an apparent cause, the condition is called anosmia. Anosmia occurs from either an obstruction in your nose or nerve damage. An obstruction prevents odors from reaching the delicate nerve fibers in your nose. These nerves carry messages or signals to your brain. Nasal polyps, tumors, neurologic conditions or swelling of the mucous membrane can cause obstruction. Viral infections, chronic nasal infections or allergies also can damage the nerves that allow you to smell.

Medical Help

If you lose your sense of smell and you do not have a cold, consult your physician. Your physician will check for polyps or tumors of the nasal passages. When the problem is caused by a virus, the sense of smell usually returns when the tissues of the olfactory area heal.

Nosebleeds

Nosebleeds are common. Most often they are a nuisance and not a true medical problem. But they can be both. Why do they start, and how can they be stopped?

Among children and young adults, nosebleeds usually begin on the septum, just inside the nose. The septum separates your nasal chambers.

In middle age and older, nosebleeds can begin on the septum, but they also may begin deeper in the nose's interior. This form of nosebleed is much less common. It may be caused by hardened arteries or high blood pressure. These nosebleeds begin spontaneously and are often difficult to stop. They require a specialist's help.

Self-Care

Use your thumb and index finger to squeeze together the soft portion of your nose, located between the end of your nose and the hard, bony ridge.

- **Sit or stand up.** By remaining upright, you reduce blood pressure in the veins of your nose. This action will discourage further bleeding.
- **Pinch your nose** with your thumb and index finger and breathe through your mouth. Continue the pinch for 5 or 10 minutes. This maneuver sends pressure to the bleeding point on the nasal septum and often stops the flow of blood.
- **Don't apply ice to the nose.** This is of little or no benefit. The cold only tightens blood vessels on the surface of the nose and does not penetrate deeply enough to help.
- **To prevent bleeding,** increase the humidity of the air you breathe in your home. A humidifier or vaporizer can help keep your nasal membranes moist. Lubricating your nose with Vaseline or other lubricants is often helpful.
- **To prevent rebleeding after bleeding has stopped,** do not pick or blow your nose until several hours after the bleeding episode, and do not bend down. Keep your head higher than the level of your heart.
- **If rebleeding occurs,** sniff in forcefully to clear your nose of blood clots, spray both sides of your nose with a decongestant nasal spray such as Afrin, Dristan or Neosynephrine. Pinch your nose again in the technique described above and call your doctor.

Medical Help

Seek medical care immediately if:
- The bleeding lasts for more than 15 to 30 minutes
- You feel weak or faint, which can result from the blood loss
- The bleeding is rapid or if the amount of blood loss is great
- Bleeding begins by trickling down the back of your throat

If you experience frequent nosebleeds, make an appointment with your physician. You may need to have the blood vessel that is causing your problem cauterized. Cautery is a technique in which the blood vessel is burned with electric current, silver nitrate or a laser.

Kids' Care

Frequent nosebleeds in children can be a sign of a benign tumor. It occurs at puberty in boys and rarely in girls. It may shrink on its own after puberty, but it can grow rapidly, produce obstruction of nasal passages and sinuses and cause frequent and often severe nosebleeds. If the tumor does not shrink, the physician may suggest a procedure to remove it surgically.

■ Stuffy Nose

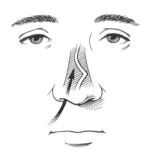

Your nasal septum separates your nasal chambers. A deviated septum may cause nasal obstruction.

Stuffy nose is a common medical complaint. A stuffy nose usually means nasal congestion or an obstruction that causes difficulty breathing. In most cases, a stuffy nose is a mere nuisance. Other causes of nasal obstruction are nasal polyps, tumors, enlarged adenoids and foreign objects in the nose.

Four causes of nasal obstruction and congestion are outlined below.

Common cold: See Aaachoo! Is It a Cold or the Flu? on page 115.

Deformities of the nose and nasal septum (the cartilage and bony partition separating your two nasal chambers) are usually due to an injury. The injury may have occurred years earlier, even in childhood. Deformities of the nose such as a deviated septum are fairly common problems. The deviation also can cause nosebleeds or sinusitis. For many people, a deviated septum poses few problems. However, if the condition makes breathing difficult, a surgical procedure may be the answer. The surgery, called septoplasty, realigns your septum.

Allergies: Allergic rhinitis (which means nasal inflammation from allergies) is the medical term for hay fever, rose fever, grass fever and other seasonal allergies. The allergic reaction is an inflammatory response to specific foreign substances that enter the nose, such as pollen, mold or house dust.

Vasomotor rhinitis: This form of inflammation is often episodic and associated with triggers such as smoke, air conditioning or vigorous exercise.

Self-Care

- For colds, see Aaachoo! Is It a Cold or the Flu? on page 115.
- Regularly and gently blow your nose if mucus or debris is present.
- Breathing steam can loosen the mucus and clear your head.
- Take a warm shower or sit in the bathroom with the shower running.
- Drink plenty of liquids.
- Use nonprescription nasal sprays or nose drops for no more than 3 or 4 days. Nonprescription oral decongestants (liquid and pills) may be helpful.
- Try saline drops.

Medical Help

If nose congestion persists for more than 1 to 2 weeks, consult your physician, who will examine your nose for the cause of the obstruction, such as polyps or tumors. If the physician determines you have an allergy, he or she may prescribe a course of therapy that may include antihistamines and inhaled anti-inflammatory medications.

Beware of Nose Drop Addiction

Frequent use of decongestant drops and sprays can result in a condition called nose drop addiction. This is a vicious cycle requiring more frequent use of nose spray to keep your nasal passages clear.

Prolonged use of nasal sprays and drops can cause irritation of your mucous membrane, a stinging or burning in your nose and a chronic inflammation.

The only way to treat the problem is to stop using nose drops. You may want to take an oral decongestant instead. Your condition may become worse for a while, but over a period of weeks your breathing should become nearly normal as the ill effects of the nose drops wear off.

Remember, use decongestant drops or sprays for no more than 3 or 4 days.

Mayo Clinic Guide to Self-Care

■ Runny Nose

Runny nose commonly occurs early in a cold and in allergic irritation. Gently blowing your nose may be all the self-care you need. If the discharge is persistent and watery, an over-the-counter antihistamine may be helpful. If the discharge is thick, follow the recommendations for stuffy nose on page 114.

Aaachoo! Is It a Cold or the Flu?
Both are viral, upper respiratory tract infections

	Cold	Flu, Influenza
Usual symptoms	• Runny nose, sneezing, nasal congestion • Sore throat (usually scratchy) • Cough • No fever or low fever • Mild fatigue	• Runny nose and sneezing • Sore throat and headache • Cough • Fever (usually more than 101 F) and chills • Moderate to severe fatigue and weakness • Achy muscles
Cause	One of more than 200 viruses typically causes 2 to 4 colds a year in adults and 4 to 8 a year in kids	One of a few viruses from the influenza A or influenza B family. On average, adults have less than one infection a year
Seriousness	Usually not serious except in people with lung disease or other serious illness	Can be serious. A special concern in elderly people and those with chronic health conditions
Can I work?	Often. Use care to avoid spreading a cold to others. Wash hands frequently	No, not until fever, fatigue and all but the mild symptoms have resolved
Preventable?	Possibly, through careful handwashing, not sharing food, towels or handkerchiefs and getting good nutrition and enough rest	Usually, through vaccination. You need to be immunized every fall (see page 223)
Do antibiotics help?	No, not unless you also have a bacterial infection	Sometimes. Antiviral antibiotics are available, but work only it taken at the onset of the illness.
Self-care	• Drink plenty of warm liquids. Homemade chicken soup can help clear mucus • Increase sleep and rest • Use cold remedies cautiously, see page 266 • Try zinc gluconate lozenges (13.3 mg, one every 2 hours while awake). For adult use only during a cold. Don't use if you are pregnant or immunocompromised (have cancer, AIDS or a chronic disease)	• Drink plenty of fluids to avoid dehydration • Increase sleep and rest • Use over-the-counter pain relievers cautiously, as needed (see page 265)
Seek medical help	• If you have difficulty breathing, faintness, change in alertness, severe sore throat, cough producing a lot of sputum or mucus (especially if green or yellow), pain in the face or a chronic health condition • If symptoms have not resolved in 10 days	

A word about pneumonia
Pneumonia can occur after a cold or flu or on its own. Pneumonia can be caused by viruses, bacteria or other organisms. Typically, you will have a prominent cough that brings up a lot of phlegm. A fever is common. You may experience a sharp pain when you breathe deeply, called pleurisy. If you are concerned about pneumonia, see your health care provider. You may need a chest X-ray and antibiotics.

Common Problems

■ Sinusitis

Signs of sinusitis include pain about your eyes or cheeks, fever and difficulty breathing through your nose. Occasionally, tooth pain occurs with the condition, or it may mimic a migraine headache.

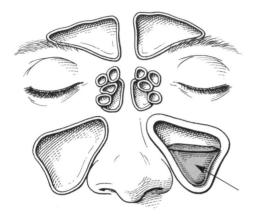

An infected maxillary sinus (arrow) is the most common site of sinusitis.

Your sinuses are cavities in the bones around your nose. They are connected to your nasal cavities by small openings. Normally, air passes in and out of your sinuses and mucus drains through these openings into your nose.

Sinusitis is an infection of the lining of one or more of these cavities. Usually, when your sinus is infected, the membranes of your nose also swell and cause a nasal obstruction. Swelling of the membranes of your nose may close off the opening of your sinus and thus prevent draining of pus or mucus. Pain in your sinus may result from inflammation itself or from the pressure as secretions build up in your sinus.

The infection can be bacterial, viral or fungal. A common cold is the most frequent cause. Allergies also can cause sinusitis.

Self-Care

- Stay indoors in an even temperature.
- Refrain from bending over with your head down—this movement usually increases the pain.
- Try applying warm facial packs, or cautiously inhale steam from a basin of boiling water.
- Drink plenty of liquids to help dilute the secretions.
- Gently and regularly blow your nose.
- Take pain relievers for discomfort.
- Use over-the-counter (OTC) decongestants and short-term decongestant sprays.
- Try OTC saltwater nose drops.
- If you are using OTC antihistamines, take care. They can do more harm than good by drying out your nose too much and thickening secretions. Use them only on the recommendation of your physician, and follow instructions carefully.

Medical Help

See your physician if you have a fever of more than 101 F, if the pain does not resolve in 24 hours or if the pain occurs repeatedly. X-rays and other examinations may be performed to discover the seriousness of the infection. If the infection is bacterial, your physician may prescribe a course of oral antibiotics to be taken for 7 to 14 days.

Skin, Hair and Nails

Because your skin, hair and nails are an integral part of your appearance, changes and problems involving them are often distressing. External irritants, infections, aging and even emotional stress can affect your skin, hair and nails in many ways. Rarely, underlying medical conditions and allergies to foods or medications trigger abnormalities.

Fortunately, many of these problems are not serious and respond well to self-care measures. The following pages explain some of the more common disorders and offer some self-care tips to help you find relief. But first, here are some general guidelines for proper skin care.

■ Proper Skin Care

Regardless of your skin color or type or your age, monitoring your exposure to the sun—and its ultraviolet rays—can help prevent unnecessary damage and, eventually, skin cancer.

Dark skin can tolerate more sun than fair skin. However, any skin can become blotchy, leathery and wrinkled from continued overexposure to the sun. Protective clothing, sunscreen preparations and daily lubrication or moisturizing can help.

Proper cleansing is another important strategy in protecting your skin. The best procedures and cleansing ingredients vary according to the type of skin you have—oily, dry, balanced or a combination of these.

Self-Care

- When washing your face, use tepid (never hot) water and a facecloth or sponge to remove dead cells. Use a mild soap. A superfatted soap, such as Basis or Dove, may be better for dry skin. You may need to clean oily skin two or three times each day.
- In general, avoid washing your body with very hot water or strong soaps. Bathing dries your skin. If you have dry skin, use soap only on your face, underarms, genital areas, hands and feet. After bathing, pat (rather than wipe) your skin dry, then immediately lubricate it with an oil or cream. Use a heavy, water-in-oil moisturizer rather than a light "disappearing" cream that contains mostly water, and avoid creams or lotions that contain alcohol. Keep the air in your home somewhat cool and humid.
- Shaving can be hard on a man's skin. If you shave with a blade razor, always use a sharp blade. Soften your beard by applying a warm facecloth for a few seconds; then use plenty of shaving cream. Pass the blade over your beard only once, in the direction of hair growth. Reversing the stroke to obtain a close shave can cause a skin irritation. Electric razors also may irritate your skin. Skin preparations are available to treat skin irritation.
- Match cosmetics to your skin type: an oil base is suitable for dry skin, and a water base is suitable for oily skin.
- For women, remove eye makeup before facial cleansing. Use cotton balls to avoid damaging the delicate tissue around your eyes.

Common Problems

■ Acne

It's a fear and frustration for teens, but acne can affect adults too. Acne is caused by plugged pores and bacteria in the skin. Oil from glands combines with dead skin to plug the pores, also called follicles. Follicles bulge, producing pimples and other types of blemishes:

- Whiteheads: clogged pores that have no opening
- Blackheads: pores that are open and have a dark surface
- Pimples: reddish spots that signal an infection by bacteria in plugged pores
- Cysts: thick lumps beneath the surface of your skin, formed by the buildup of secretions

Three of four teenagers have some acne. It is most prevalent in adolescence because hormonal changes stimulate the sebaceous glands during these years. The sebaceous glands secrete a fatty oil called sebum, which lubricates your hair and skin. Menstrual periods, the use of birth control pills or cortisone medications and stress may aggravate acne in later life.

Although a chronic problem for many people from puberty through early adulthood, acne eventually clears in most cases.

Self-Care

- Identify factors that aggravate your acne. Avoid oily or greasy cosmetics, sunscreens, hair styling products or acne coverups. Use products labeled "water-based" or "noncomedogenic."
- Wash problem areas daily with a cleanser that gently dries your skin and causes follicles to flake.
- Try over-the-counter acne lotion (containing benzoyl peroxide, resorcinol or salicylic acid as the active ingredient) to dry excess oil and promote peeling.
- Moderate exposure to the sun or careful use of a sun lamp may help. However, too much sun may cause wrinkles and skin cancer later in life.
- Keep your hair clean and off the face.
- Watch for signs of spreading infection beyond the edges of a pimple.
- Unless a food is clearly aggravating your acne, you don't need to eliminate it. Foods like chocolate, once thought to be a cause of acne, generally aren't the culprit.
- Don't pick or squeeze blemishes. These actions can cause infection or scarring.

Medical Help

Persistent pimples or inflamed cysts may need medical attention and treatment with prescription drugs. In rare cases, a sudden onset of severe acne in an older adult may signal an underlying disease requiring medical attention.

Physicians may use cosmetic surgery to diminish scars left by acne. The main procedures are dermabrasion or peeling by freezing or chemicals. However, if your skin tends to form scar tissue, these procedures can make your complexion much worse.

Peeling procedures eliminate superficial scars. Dermabrasion, usually reserved for more severe scarring, consists of abrading the skin with a rapidly rotating wire brush. Your physician will use a local anesthetic or topical freezing of your skin during the procedure. General anesthesia and hospitalization ordinarily are not required.

Boils

Boils are pink or red, very tender bumps under your skin which occur when bacteria infect one or more of your hair follicles. The bumps are usually larger than 1/2 inch in diameter. They typically grow rapidly, fill with pus and then burst, drain and heal. Although some boils resolve a few days after they appear, most burst and heal within about 2 weeks.

Boils can occur anywhere on your skin, but most often on the face, neck, armpits, buttocks or thighs. Poor health, clothing that binds or chafes and disorders such as acne, dermatitis, diabetes and anemia can increase your risk of infection.

Self-Care

To avoid spreading this infection and to minimize discomfort, follow these measures:
- Soak the area with a warm washcloth or compress for about 30 minutes every few hours. Doing so may help the boil burst and drain much sooner. Use warm saltwater. (Add 1 teaspoon of salt to 1 quart of boiling water and let it cool.)
- Gently wash the sore twice a day with antibacterial soap. Cover the sore with a bandage to prevent spreading.
- Apply an over-the-counter antibiotic ointment such as bacitracin.
- Never squeeze or lance a boil, because you might spread the infection.
- Launder towels, compresses or clothing that has touched the infected area.

Medical Help

Contact your health care provider if the infection is located on your spine or on your face, worsens rapidly or causes severe pain, has not disappeared within 2 weeks or is accompanied by fever or reddish lines radiating from the boil. In some cases, antibiotics or surgical drainage may be necessary to clear your infection.

Cellulitis

Cellulitis may appear gradually over a couple of days or rapidly over a few hours. It begins as a localized area of red, painful, warm skin. It may be accompanied by fever and swelling. This fairly common infection occurs when bacteria or fungus enters your body through a break in the skin and infects the deeper layers of your skin.

Good hygiene and proper wound care can help prevent this type of infection. However, bacteria can enter your skin through even tiny cuts or abrasions, such as a crack around your nostrils or a simple puncture wound.

Self-Care

To prevent cellulitis and other wound infections, follow these measures:
- Keep skin wounds clean.
- Apply an antibiotic cream or ointment. If a rash develops, stop using the ointment and talk to your doctor or pharmacist. Ingredients in these ointments can cause a mild rash in some people.
- Cover the area with a bandage to help keep it clean and keep harmful bacteria out. Keep draining blisters covered until a scab forms.
- Change the bandage daily or whenever it becomes wet or dirty.

Medical Help

Contact your doctor if you suspect you have cellulitis. Antibiotics are usually necessary to prevent this infection from spreading and causing severe damage.

Common Problems

■ Corns and Calluses

These thickened, hardened layers of skin commonly appear on your hands and feet. Corns often appear as raised bumps of hardened skin less than ¼-inch long. Calluses vary in size and shape. Corns and calluses are your skin's attempt to protect itself. Although they can be unsightly, treatment may be necessary only if they cause discomfort. For most people, eliminating the source of friction or pressure will help corns and calluses disappear.

Self-Care

- Wear properly fitted shoes, with adequate toe room. Have your shoe shop stretch your shoes at any point that rubs or pinches. Place pads under your heels if your shoes rub. Try over-the-counter remedies to cushion or soften the corn while wearing shoes.
- Wear padded gloves when using hand tools, or try padding your tool handles with cloth tape or covers.
- Rub your skin with a pumice stone or washcloth during or after bathing to gradually thin some of the thickened skin. This advice is not recommended if you have diabetes or poor circulation.
- Try over-the-counter corn dissolvers containing salicylic acid (available in plaster-pad disks or solutions containing a thickener called collodion).
- Do not cut or shave corns or calluses with a sharp edge.

Medical Help

If a corn or callus becomes very painful or inflamed, contact your health care provider.

■ Dandruff

New studies suggest a yeastlike organism may cause dandruff. The *Malassezia ovalis (Pityrosporum ovale)* fungus causes irritation and increased sloughing of the top layer of skin cells on your scalp.

Self-Care

- Shampoo regularly. Start with a mild, nonmedicated shampoo. Gently massage your scalp to loosen flakes. Rinse thoroughly.
- Use medicated shampoo for stubborn cases. Look for shampoos containing zinc pyrithione, salicylic acid, coal tar or selenium sulfide in brands such as Head & Shoulders, Neutrogena T/Sal or T/Gel, Tegrin, Denorex or Selsun Blue. Use a dandruff shampoo each time you shampoo, if necessary, to control flaking. Rotating different types of shampoo may help.
- Kill dandruff-causing fungi that live on your scalp by using the new antifungal shampoo, Nizoral A-D. This shampoo is available over-the-counter or by prescription.
- If you use tar-based shampoos, use them carefully. They can leave a brownish stain on light-colored or gray hair and make your scalp more sensitive to sunlight.
- Use a conditioner regularly. For mild dandruff, alternate dandruff shampoo with your regular shampoo.

Medical Help

If dandruff persists or your scalp becomes irritated or severely itchy, you may need a prescription shampoo. Dandruff is not contagious and is rarely serious, but your skin may be more susceptible to infection. If your dandruff persists, you may have some other skin condition. See your doctor.

◼ Dryness

This is by far the most common cause of itching, flaking skin. Although dryness can be a problem any time of the year, cold air and low humidity can be especially tough on your skin. Dry skin due to the weather depends on where you live (for example, the Minnesota "winter itch" and the Arizona "summer itch").

Self-Care

- Take fewer baths or showers. Keep them short and use lukewarm water and minimal amounts of soap. Mild superfatted soaps such as Basis or Dove will dry skin less. Add Aveno oatmeal powder or other bath oils to your bath.
- Pat (rather than wipe) your skin dry after bathing.
- Apply an oil or cream to your skin immediately after drying. Use a heavy, water-in-oil moisturizer, not a light "disappearing" cream that contains mostly water.
- Avoid creams or lotions containing alcohol.
- Use a humidifier and keep room temperatures cool.

◼ Eczema (Dermatitis)

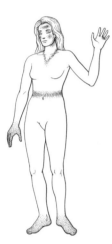

Frequent locations of irritation from contact dermatitis, the most common form of dermatitis.

The terms eczema and dermatitis are both used to describe irritated and inflamed (swollen or reddened) skin. Patches of dry, reddened and itchy skin are the major symptoms. Patches can thicken and develop blisters or weeping sores in severe cases.

Contact dermatitis results from direct contact with one of many irritants that can trigger this reaction. Common culprits include poison ivy (see Poisonous Plants, page 29), laundry and cleaning products, rubber, metals, jewelry, perfume or cosmetics.

Neurodermatitis can occur when something such as a tight garment rubs or scratches (or causes you to rub or scratch) your skin.

Seborrheic dermatitis (cradle cap in infants, see Baby Rashes, page 124) can appear as a stubborn, itchy dandruff. You may notice greasy, scaling areas at the sides of your nose, between your eyebrows, behind your ears or over your breastbone.

Stasis dermatitis may cause the skin at your ankles to become discolored (red or brown), thickened and itchy. It can occur when fluid accumulates in the tissues just beneath your skin.

Atopic dermatitis causes itchy, thickened, fissured skin, most often in the folds of the elbows or backs of the knees. It frequently runs in families and is often associated with allergies.

Self-Care

- Try to identify and avoid direct contact with irritants.
- Follow the self-care tips to prevent dry skin (see above).
- Soak in water for 20 to 30 minutes per day.
- After moisturizing, apply a cream containing 0.5 to 1 percent hydrocortisone.
- Avoid scratching whenever possible. Cover the itchy area with a dressing if you can't keep from scratching it. Trim nails and wear gloves at night.
- Shampoo with an antidandruff product if your scalp is affected.
- Support hose may help relieve stasis dermatitis.
- Dress appropriate to conditions to help avoid excessive sweating.
- Wear smooth-textured cotton clothing.
- Avoid wool carpeting, bedding and clothes and harsh soaps and detergents.
- Occasional use of over-the-counter antihistamines can reduce itching.

Common Problems

■ Fungal Infections

Fungal infections are caused by microscopic organisms that become parasites on your body. Mold-like fungi called dermatophytes cause athlete's foot, jock itch and ringworm of the skin or scalp. These fungi live on dead tissues of your hair, nails and the outer layer of your skin. Poor hygiene, continually moist skin and minor skin or nail injuries increase your susceptibility to fungal infections.

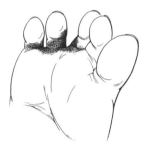

Typical pattern of athlete's foot.

Athlete's foot usually begins between your toes, causing your skin to itch, burn and crack. Sometimes the sole and sides of the foot are affected, becoming thickened and leathery in texture. Although locker rooms and public showers are often blamed for spreading athlete's foot, the environment *inside* your shoes is probably more important. It is also more common with age.

Jock itch causes an itching or burning sensation around your groin. In addition to the itching, you will usually notice a red rash that may spread to the inner thighs, anal area and buttocks. This infection is mildly contagious. It can be spread by contact or sharing towels.

Ringworm often affects children. Symptoms are itchy, red, scaly, slightly raised, expanding rings on the trunk, face or groin and thigh fold. The rings grow outward as the infection spreads, and the central area begins to look like normal skin. This infection is passed from shared clothing, combs and barber tools. Pets also can transmit the fungus to humans.

Self-Care

General
- Practice good personal hygiene to prevent all forms of fungal infections.
- Use antifungal creams or drying powder two or three times a day until the rash disappears. Use medications that contain miconazole (Zeasorb-AF, Micatin), clotrimazole (Lotrimin AF, Mycelex OTC) or undecylenic acid (Desenex, Cruex).

For Athlete's Foot
- Keep your feet dry, particularly the area between your toes.
- Wear well-ventilated shoes. Avoid shoes made of synthetic materials.
- Don't wear the same shoes every day, and don't store them in plastic.
- Change socks (cotton or polypropylene) twice a day if your feet sweat a lot.
- Wear waterproof sandals or shoes around public pools, showers and locker rooms.

For Jock Itch
- Keep your groin clean and dry.
- Shower and change clothes after exercise.
- Avoid clothes that chafe, and launder athletic supporters frequently.

For Ringworm
- Thoroughly clean brushes, combs or headgear that may have been infected.
- Wash hands before and after examining your child.
- Keep your child's linens separate from the rest of the family's.

Medical Help

See your health care provider if symptoms last longer than 4 weeks or if you notice increased redness, drainage or fever. You may require treatment with prescription medications.

Mayo Clinic Guide to Self-Care

■ Hives

Hives are raised, red, often itchy welts of various sizes that appear and disappear on the skin. They are more common on areas of the body where clothes rub your skin. Hives tend to occur in batches and last anywhere from a few minutes to several days.

Angioedema, a similar swelling, causes large welts below your skin, especially near your eyes and lips but also on your hands and feet and inside your throat.

Hives and angioedema result when your body releases a natural chemical called histamine in your skin. Allergies to foods, drugs, pollen, insect bites, infections, illness, cold and heat and emotional distress can trigger a reaction. In most cases, hives and angioedema are harmless and leave no lasting marks. However, serious angioedema can cause your throat or tongue to block your airway and cause loss of consciousness.

Self-Care

- Avoid substances that have triggered past attacks.
- Take cool showers. Apply cool compresses. Wear light clothing. Minimize vigorous activity.
- Use calamine lotion or over-the-counter antihistamines such as diphenhydramine hydrochloride (Benadryl) or chlorpheniramine maleate (Chlor-Trimeton) to help relieve the itching.
- If foods are suspected of causing the problem, keep a food diary.

Medical Help

Seek emergency care if you feel light-headed or have difficulty breathing or if hives continue to appear for more than a couple days.

■ Impetigo

Impetigo is a common skin infection that usually appears on the face. The infection begins when bacteria (streptococci) penetrate your skin through a cut, scratch or insect bite. Impetigo is highly contagious and easily spread by contact.

The infection starts as a red sore that blisters briefly, oozes for a few days and forms a sticky crust. Scratching or touching the sores can spread this contagious infection to other people and other parts of your body.

Impetigo is more common among young children. In adults, it appears mostly as a complication of other skin problems such as dermatitis.

Self-Care

Good hygiene is essential for preventing impetigo and limiting its spread. For limited or minor infections that have not spread to other areas, try the following:

- Keep the sores and skin surrounding them clean.
- Soak the area of the rash with a solution of 1 tablespoon of liquid bleach to 1 quart of water for 20 minutes. This will make it easier to remove the scabs.
- After washing with the bleach solution, apply an antibiotic ointment three or four times daily. Wash the skin before each application, and pat the skin dry.
- Avoid scratching or touching the sores unnecessarily until they heal. Wash your hands after any contact with them. Children's fingernails should be trimmed.
- Do not share towels, clothing or razors with others. Replace linens often.

Medical Help

If the infection spreads, your health care provider may prescribe oral antibiotics such as penicillin or erythromycin or an ointment of mupirocin (Bactroban).

Common Problems

■ Itching and Rashes

Because so many things can cause itching and rashes, pinpointing the source of the problem can be difficult. For information about specific problems that cause itching and rashes, see the following segments in this book: Allergic Reactions, page 12; Lice, page 126; Insect Bites and Stings, page 15; Baby Rashes, see below; Common Childhood Rashes, page 125; Hives, page 123; Dryness, page 121; and Eczema (Dermatitis), page 121.

■ Baby Rashes

Cradle cap: crusty, scaly skin on your baby's scalp. Wash your baby's hair only once a week with a mild shampoo and lukewarm water. Apply baby oil to the crusty areas and gently scrape off the scales with a soft brush after bathing. If the rash is red and irritated, apply a 0.5 percent hydrocortisone cream once a week.

Heat rash: fine red spots or bumps, usually on the neck or the upper back, chest or arms. This harmless rash often develops during hot, humid weather, especially if your baby is dressed too warmly. It also can occur if your baby has a fever.

Milia: tiny (pinpoint) white spots on the nose and cheeks. It is usually present at birth. The spots eventually disappear without treatment.

Infant acne: red bumps that can appear during the first few months after birth. Gently wash your baby's face daily with plain water and once or twice weekly with a mild soap. Do not use acne creams or lotions on an infant or young child.

Drool rash: a red rash on the cheeks and chin that comes and goes. This rash is caused by contact with food and sputum. Cleaning your baby's skin after feeding or spitting up usually helps clear this rash.

Diaper rash: reddish, puffy skin in the diaper area, especially in the folds of the skin. This irritation usually is caused by moisture, the acid in urine or stool and chafing of diapers. Some babies also get a rash from detergent used to wash cloth diapers, plastic pants, elastic or certain types of disposable diapers and diaper wipes. Sometimes a yeast infection is the cause.

Self-Care for Recurrent Diaper Rash

- Change your baby's diapers frequently, placing the diaper loosely around the child, and expose the skin to air whenever possible. Avoid using plastic pants.
- Use cloth diapers or disposable diapers without gathers. Wash cloth diapers in mild soap (Dreft or Ivory), and 1 cup of white vinegar should be added to the rinse cycle to help rid the diapers of bacteria. Avoid fabric softeners.
- Wash and pat dry the area at each diaper change, using plain water or a mild soap and water.
- Apply a thin layer of protective cream or ointment such as Desitin or A & D Ointment.
- Try switching to a different brand of diapers if you use disposable diapers.
- Avoid diaper wipes because many contain perfume and alcohol.
- If the rash is particularly difficult to cleanse, place the baby in a sink of warm water with 2 ounces of white vinegar mixed in.
- Do not apply cornstarch or talcum powder; they could worsen the condition.

Medical Help

See your health care provider if the above tips don't help; if the rash is purple or bruised-looking, crusty, blistered or weepy; or if the baby has a fever.

Mayo Clinic Guide to Self-Care

Common Childhood Rashes

Symptoms	Self-Care	Seek Medical Help

Chickenpox

Itchy, red spots on the face or chest which spread to the arms and legs. Spots quickly fill with a clear fluid to form blisters, rupture and turn crusty. New spots generally continue appearing over 4 to 5 days. Fever, a runny nose or cough often accompanies chickenpox. Chickenpox seldom lasts for more than 2 weeks after the first spot appears. Symptoms usually appear 14 to 21 days after exposure. The child is contagious until the rash crusts

- Give the child cool baths every 3 or 4 hours to reduce the itching. Sprinkle baking soda in the bath water for added relief
- Apply calamine lotion to the rash
- Switch to a bland diet of soft foods, and avoid citrus fruits if blisters are present in the mouth
- Trim fingernails. Put gloves on the child at night to prevent scratching

- If the rash involves the eyes, or if you develop a cough or shortness of breath
- If you are an older adult, have an impaired immune system or are pregnant and have not been previously exposed
- Doctors may prescribe a antiviral antibiotic medication in severe cases. A vaccine is available for children ages 12 months or older and adults who have not yet had the virus

Roseola

Often begins with a high fever lasting about 3 days. When it subsides, a rash appears on the trunk and neck and lasts a few hours to a few days. Virus typically affects children, especially between ages 6 months and 3 years

The rash causes little discomfort and disappears on its own without treatment. Acetaminophen and tepid sponge baths may help relieve the discomfort caused by the fever

- If the rash lasts longer than 3 days. Young children may experience convulsions triggered by the high fever

Measles

Typically begins with fever, often as high as 104 to 105 F, and a cough, sneezing, sore throat and inflamed, watery eyes. Two to 4 days later, a rash appears. It often begins as fine red spots on the face and spreads to the trunk, arms and legs. Spots may become larger and usually last about a week. Small white spots may appear on inside lining of the cheek

- Bed rest, acetaminophen and an over-the-counter cough medication may help relieve the discomfort
- Lukewarm baths, calamine lotion or Benadryl solution will relieve itching

- If you suspect that you or a family member has measles. Measles has uncommon but potentially serious complications, such as pneumonia, encephalitis or a bacterial infection
- A vaccine to prevent measles is given to children between 12 and 15 months and between 4 and 12 years of age

Fifth disease

Bright red, raised patches appear on both cheeks. During the next few days, a pink, lacy, slightly raised rash develops on the arms, trunk, thighs and buttocks. Rash may come and go for up to 3 weeks. Often, there are no symptoms, or only mild, cold-like symptoms

No specific treatment. Use acetaminophen to relieve the fever and any discomfort

- If you aren't sure whether a rash is fifth disease or if you are pregnant and suspect that you've been exposed

Common Problems

Lice

Louse

Lice are tiny parasitic insects. _Head lice_ often are spread among children by contact, clothing or hairbrushes. _Body lice_ are generally spread through clothing or bedding. _Pubic lice_ (commonly called "crabs") can be spread by sexual contact, clothing, bedding or even toilet seats.

The first sign of lice is intense itching. With body lice, some people have hives and others have abrasions from scratching. Head lice are found on the scalp and are easiest to see at the nape of the neck and over the ears. Small nits (eggs) that resemble tiny pussy willow buds can be found on the hair shafts. Body lice are difficult to find on the body because they burrow into the skin, but they usually can be detected in the seams of underwear. Pubic lice are found on the skin and hair of the pubic areas. Lice live only 3 days off the body; eggs hatch in about 1 week.

Self-Care

- Several lotions and shampoos, both prescription and over-the-counter, are available. Apply the product to all infected and hair parts of the body. Any remaining nits can be removed with tweezers or a fine comb. Repeat treatment with the lotion or shampoo in 7 to 10 days.
- Your sexual partner should be examined and treated if infected.
- Keep infected children home until you complete this first treatment.
- Wash sheets, clothing and hats with hot, soapy water and dry them at high heat. Soak combs and brushes in very hot, soapy water for at least 5 minutes.
- Vacuum carpets, mattresses, pillows, upholstered furniture and car seats.

Medical Help

Consult your physician before using products in a child younger than 2 months or if you are pregnant.

Scabies

Almost impossible to see without a magnifying glass, scabies mites cause itching by burrowing under the skin. Itching is usually worse at night. The burrowing leaves tiny bumps and thin, irregular, pencil-like marks or tracks on your skin. They appear most often in the following areas: between your fingers, in your armpits, around your waist, along the insides of your wrists, on the back of your elbows, on your ankles and soles of your feet, around your breasts and genitals and on your buttocks. However, almost any part of the skin may be involved.

Close physical contact and, less often, sharing clothing or bedding with an infected person can spread these tiny mites. Often an entire family or members of a day-care group or school class will experience scabies.

Self-Care

Bathing and over-the-counter preparations will not eliminate scabies. Talk to your health care provider if you have symptoms or if you believe you had contact with someone who has scabies.

Medical Help

Your doctor may prescribe a cream or lotion that you must apply all over your body and leave on overnight. All family members and sexual partners may require treatment. Also, all clothing and bedding that you used before treatment must be washed with hot, soapy water and dried with high heat.

Mayo Clinic Guide to Self-Care

■ Psoriasis

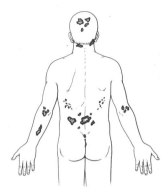

Some of the most common locations of psoriasis.

For some, psoriasis brings little more than recurrent bouts of mild itching, but for others, it's a lifetime of discomfort and unsightly skin changes.

Most often, psoriasis causes dry, red patches covered with thick, silvery scales. You may see a few spots of scaling or large areas of damaged skin. Knees, elbows, trunk and scalp are the most common locations. Patches on your scalp can shed large quantities of silvery-white scales resembling severe dandruff.

In more severe cases, pustules, cracked skin, itching, minor bleeding or aching joints also may develop. In addition, your fingernails and toenails may lose their normal luster and develop pits or ridges.

These skin eruptions are due to overly rapid growth of cells in your skin's outer layer. Many people also inherit a tendency toward psoriasis. Dry skin, skin injuries, infections, certain drugs, obesity, stress and lack of sunlight can all aggravate your symptoms. This condition is not contagious. You cannot spread it to other parts of your own body, or to other people, simply by touching it. Psoriasis typically goes through cycles. The symptoms can persist for weeks or months, followed by a break.

Self-Care

- Maintain good general health: a balanced diet, adequate rest and exercise.
- Maintain a normal weight. Psoriasis occurs often in skin creases or folds.
- Avoid scratching, rubbing or picking at the patches of psoriasis.
- Bathe daily to soak off the scales. Avoid hot water or harsh soap.
- Keep your skin moist (see Dryness, page 121).
- Use soaps, shampoos, cleansers or ointments containing coal tar or salicylic acid.
- Expose your skin to moderate sunlight, but avoid sunburn.
- Apply over-the-counter cortisone creams, 0.5 or 1 percent, for a few weeks when symptoms are especially bad.

Medical Help

If self-care remedies don't help, stronger cortisone-type creams or various forms of phototherapy may be prescribed. Phototherapy involves a combination of medications and ultraviolet light. Skin ointments containing a form of vitamin D (Dovenex) also may offer some relief. In severe cases, an anticancer drug called methotrexate or a drug used to prevent rejection in organ transplant recipients (cyclosporine) is sometimes prescribed.

■ Moles

Sometimes called "beauty marks," moles are usually harmless collections of pigment cells. They may contain hairs, stay smooth, become raised or wrinkled and even fall off in old age.

In rare cases, a mole can become cancerous. Talk to your health care provider if pain, bleeding or inflammation occurs or if you notice a change in a mole (see Signs of Skin Cancer, page 129). Keep an eye on moles located around your nails or genitals, and those that have been present since birth. Giant moles, present at birth, are a special problem, and they may need to be removed to avoid the risk of cancer.

Self-Care

Healthy moles usually don't require special care unless they become cut or irritated. Your normal skin care routine will suffice.

■ Shingles

Shingles (also known as herpes zoster) emerges when the virus that causes chickenpox (varicella zoster) reactivates after lying dormant within your nerve cells.

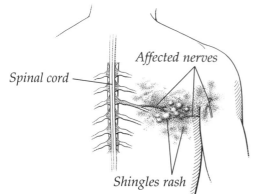

Spinal cord

Affected nerves

Shingles rash

The shingles rash is associated with an inflammation of nerves beneath the skin.

As this virus reactivates, you may notice pain or tingling in a limited area, usually on one side of your body or face. This pain occurs as the virus spreads along one of the nerves that spread outward on your face or from your spine. This pain or tingling can continue for several days or longer.

Subsequently, a rash with small blisters may appear. The rash may continue to spread over the next 3 to 5 days, often forming a band-like pattern on one side of your body. The blisters usually dry up in a few days, forming crusts that fall off over the next 2 to 3 weeks. The blisters contain a virus that is contagious, so avoid physical contact with others, especially pregnant women. Chickenpox in a newborn can be deadly.

Self-Care

You can relieve some of the discomfort by doing the following:
- Soak your blisters with cool, wet compresses (aluminum acetate solution).
- Wash blisters gently, and don't bandage them.
- Apply a soothing lotion such as calamine (Caladryl) lotion.
- Take over-the-counter pain relievers to alleviate pain.
- Over-the-counter analgesic creams also may alleviate your pain.

Medical Help

Contact your health care provider promptly in the following situations:
- If the pain and rash occur near your eyes. If left untreated, this infection can lead to permanent eye damage.
- If you or someone in your family has a weakened immune system (due to cancer, medications or a chronic medical condition).
- If the rash is widespread and painful.
- If you are older than 60 years.

Acyclovir (Zovirax) and famciclovir (Famvir) can hasten healing and reduce the severity of some complications caused by shingles.

When the Pain Persists After Shingles

Pain persisting for months or even years after a bout with shingles is called postherpetic neuralgia (PHN). It occurs in 50 percent of people older than 60 who have had shingles.

PHN is as individual as you are, and effective treatment for you may be useless for someone else. But new treatments show promise, and new findings support the benefit of early treatment of the acute viral infection that precedes PHN.

Because the pain of PHN tends to lessen as time passes, it's difficult to tell whether a medication is effective or the pain is subsiding on its own.

Several treatments may provide relief. They include analgesic medications, electrical stimulation, antidepressants, certain anticonvulsant medications and neurosurgery in severe cases.

Most people are free of pain after 5 years.

■ Signs of Skin Cancer

Each year, skin cancer is diagnosed in approximately 1 million people, and about 10,000 people die each year of the disease. More than 90 percent of skin cancers occur on areas regularly exposed to ultraviolet radiation (from sunlight or tanning lights), and this exposure is considered to be the chief cause. Other factors include a genetic tendency, chemical pollution and X-ray radiation.

Here are the signs of the three most common types of skin cancer:

Basal cell cancer, by far the most common skin cancer, usually appears as a smooth, waxy or pearly bump that grows slowly and rarely spreads and causes death.

Squamous cell cancer causes a firm, nodular or flat growth with a crusted, ulcerated or scaly surface on the face, ears, neck, hands or arms.

Melanoma is the most serious but least common skin cancer.

The ABCD rule (see below) can help you tell a normal mole from one that could be melanoma. In addition, rapid growth, bleeding and nonhealing sores could be symptoms.

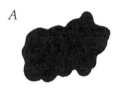

A

Asymmetry. Half of the lesion is unlike the other half.

B

Border irregular (ragged, notched or blurred).

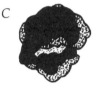

C

Color varies from one area to another. Different shades of tan and brown, black, red, white or blue.

D

Diameter is larger than the head of a pencil, about 1/4 of an inch.

Self-Care	• Avoid exposure to the sun to the point of a sunburn or a dark suntan. Both result in skin damage. Skin damage accumulates over time. Minimize your time in the sun and wear tightly woven clothing and a broad-brimmed hat. Remember, snow, water and ice reflect the sun's harmful rays. • Use sunscreen as part of your daily outdoor routine. Apply a broad-spectrum sunscreen with a sun protection factor (SPF) of at least 15. (Broad-spectrum means it provides protection against ultraviolet A and B radiation.) Use sunscreen on all exposed skin, including your lips. Apply sunscreen 30 minutes before sun exposure. • Avoid tanning salons. • Check your skin at least every 3 months for the development of new skin growths or changes in existing moles, freckles, bumps and birthmarks.
Medical Help	If you notice a new growth, change in skin or sore that doesn't heal in 2 weeks, see your physician. Don't wait for pain; skin cancers are usually not painful. The cure rate for skin cancer is high if you receive treatment early. If you have a family history of melanoma and many moles on your body (especially on the trunk), regular examination by a dermatologist may be appropriate.
Kids' Care	Getting severe, blistering sunburns as a child increases one's risk for the development of melanoma as an adult. Set time limits for your child when at the pool or beach. Remember, ultraviolet rays are strongest between 10 a.m. and 3 p.m. Clouds block only a small portion of ultraviolet rays.

Common Problems

▧ Warts

Warts are skin growths caused by a common virus, but they can be painful and disfiguring and can spread to others.

There are more than 50 types of warts. They can appear on any part of your body, but they are most common on the hands or feet. Warts found on the feet, called plantar warts, can be painful because they press inward as you stand on them.

You can acquire warts through direct contact with an infected person or surface, such as a shower floor. The virus that causes them stimulates the rapid growth of cells on the outer layer of your skin.

Each person's immune system responds to warts differently. Most warts are not a serious health hazard and disappear without treatment. Because warts are more common among children than adults, some believe that many adults develop immunity to them. In many adults, warts eventually disappear within 2 years.

Certain warts trigger or signal more serious medical problems. Genital warts (see page 184) require treatment to avoid spreading them through sexual contact. Some strains of the papilloma virus increase a woman's risk for cervical cancer. Women also can pass this virus to their babies during birth, causing some complications.

Self-Care

- Over-the-counter topical medications may remove warts. Look for products containing salicylic acid, which peels off the infected skin. They require daily use, often for a few weeks. **Caution:** The acid can irritate or damage normal skin.
- To avoid spreading warts to other parts of your body, avoid brushing, combing or shaving over areas where there are warts.

Medical Help

You may want to see your health care provider if your warts are tender or a cosmetic nuisance or interfere with your activities. Common treatments for warts include freezing with liquid nitrogen or dry ice, electrical burning, laser surgery or minor surgery.

▧ Wrinkled Skin

Skin wrinkles.

As much as people sometimes try to hide the fact that they're aging, wrinkles ("character lines") are an inevitable part of the aging process. As you grow older, your skin gets thinner, drier and less elastic. Sagging and wrinkling begin because connective tissue in your skin deteriorates. Some people don't seem to age as quickly as others. This difference is typically due to heredity. Cosmetic products that promise a fountain of youth are often expensive and fail to deliver real improvements.

Self-Care

There is no cure for wrinkled skin. These measures may help slow the process:
- Maintain good general health.
- Don't smoke cigarettes.
- Avoid prolonged exposure to the sun. Use sunscreens when you are outdoors.
- Avoid harsh soaps and hot water when bathing.

Medical Help

Prescription medical treatments such as retinoic acid creams may work if used for a long time. Cosmetic procedures such as chemical peels, dermabrasion or lasers can alter your skin's appearance if it disturbs you.

Hair Loss

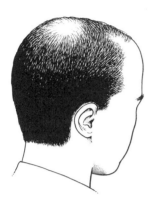

Male-pattern baldness typically appears first at the hairline or crown.

Healthy, lustrous hair has long been a symbol of youth and beauty. As a result, many people cringe at the first signs of hair thinning or baldness.

If your hair seems to be thinning, take comfort in the fact that it's normal to lose between 50 and 100 strands a day. Like your nails and skin, your hair goes through a cycle of growth and rest. Gradual thinning occurs as a normal part of the aging process.

Common baldness accounts for 99 percent of hair loss in both men and women and is genetic. Male-pattern baldness usually begins with thinning at your hairline, followed by moderate to extensive hair loss on the crown of your head. Bald patches rarely develop in women with common baldness. Instead, their hair becomes thinner all over the head. Heredity, hormones and age all play important roles in common baldness, so the best way to know what you will look like later in life is to look at your parents' families.

Gradual hair loss also can occur any time your hair's delicate growth cycle is upset. Diet, medications, hormones, pregnancy, improper hair care, poor nutrition, underlying diseases and other factors can cause too many follicles to rest at once, producing bald patches or diffuse thinning.

Sudden hair loss is usually due to a condition called alopecia areata. This fairly rare condition causes smooth, circular bald patches, up to 3 inches across, that may overlap. Stress and heredity may play a role in this disorder. About 90 percent of the time, the hair grows back within 6 to 24 months with no treatment.

Self-Care

There is no "magic bullet" to prevent hair loss or encourage new growth. However, the following tips can help keep your hair healthy.
- Eat a nutritionally balanced diet.
- Handle your hair gently. When possible, allow your hair to dry naturally in the air.
- Avoid tight hairstyles such as braids, buns or ponytails.
- Avoid compulsively twisting, rubbing or pulling your hair.
- Check with hair care experts about hairpieces or styling techniques that help minimize the effects of common baldness.
- An over-the-counter medication called minoxidil can promote new hair growth in a small percentage of people, but the drug eventually loses its effectiveness and can be costly. Other hair growth products for baldness are of no proven benefit.

Medical Help

Although there is no cure for common genetic baldness, you may want to ask your health care provider about medical treatments or hair replacement surgery. Because sudden hair loss can signal an underlying medical condition that may require treatment, contact your physician for evaluation.

Kids' Care

If your child has patches of broken hairs on the scalp or eyebrows, he or she may be rubbing or pulling out the hair. This signals a behavioral disorder called trichotillomania. Contact your health care provider for evaluation.

Common Problems

Nail Fungal Infections

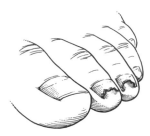

Typical fungal infection.

This stubborn, but harmless, problem often begins as a tiny white or yellow spot on your nail. Fungal infections can develop on your nails or under their outer edges if you continually expose them to a warm, moist environment. Depending on the type of fungus, your nails may discolor, thicken and develop crumbling edges or cracks.

Fungal infections usually affect your toenails more frequently than your fingernails and are more common among the elderly. Your risk for a toenail fungal infection is greater if your feet perspire heavily, and if you wear socks and shoes that hinder ventilation and don't absorb perspiration. You also can contract this infection by walking barefoot in public places and as a complication of other infections.

Fingernail fungal infections often result from overexposure to water and detergents. Moisture caught under artificial nails also can encourage fungus growth.

Self-Care

To help prevent fungal infections, try the following:
- Keep your nails dry and clean. Dry your feet thoroughly after bathing.
- Change your socks often and wear leather-soled shoes.
- Use an antifungal spray or powder on your feet and inside your shoes.
- Don't pick at or trim the skin around your nails.
- Avoid walking barefoot around public pools, showers and locker rooms.

Medical Help

Self-care measures usually fail to prevent the infection. Topical antifungal creams or oral antifungal medications such as griseofulvin, itraconazole, terbinafine hydrochloride and fluconazole are effective. In severe cases, surgical removal may be required.

Ingrown Toenails

Pain and tenderness in your toe often signal that you have an ingrown toenail. This common condition occurs when the sharp end or side of your toenail grows into the flesh of your toe. It affects your big toe most often, especially if you have curved toenails, if your shoes fit poorly or if you cut your nails improperly.

Self-Care

- Trim your toenails straight across and not too short.
- Wear socks and shoes that fit properly, and don't place excessive pressure on your toes. Wear open-toe shoes, if necessary, or try sandals.
- Soak your feet in warm salt water (1 tablespoon per quart) for 30 minutes four times a day to reduce swelling and relieve tenderness.
- After soaking, put tiny bits of sterile cotton under the ingrown edge. This will help the nail eventually grow above the skin edge. Change the cotton daily until the pain and redness subside.
- Apply an antibiotic ointment to the tender area.
- If there is severe pain, apply cotton saturated with an over-the-counter ingrown toenail reliever to the area. It will provide temporary relief.

Medical Help

If you experience severe discomfort or pus or redness that seems to be spreading, seek medical attention. Your doctor may need to remove the ingrown portion of the nail and prescribe antibiotics.

Mayo Clinic Guide to Self-Care

Throat and Mouth

■ Sore Throat

The tight, scratchy feeling in our throats is a familiar sign that a cold or flu is on the way. Most sore throats run their course in a few days, sometimes needing over-the-counter lozenges or gargles.

Most sore throats are caused by two types of infections—*viral* and *bacterial*—but they also can be caused by allergies and dry air. When a sore throat involves enlarged, tender tonsils, it's sometimes called tonsillitis.

Viral infections usually are the source of common colds and the flu and the sore throat that accompanies them. Colds usually go away on their own in about a week, once your system has built up antibodies that destroy the virus. Antibiotic medications are *not* effective in treating viral infections. The common symptoms are as follows:

- Sore or scratchy, dry feeling
- Coughing and sneezing
- Mild fever or no fever
- Hoarseness
- Runny nose and postnasal dripping

Bacterial infections are not as common as viral infections, but they can be more serious. "Strep throat" is the most common bacterial infection. Often a person with strep was exposed to someone else with strep throat in the past 2 to 7 days. Children ages 5 to 15 who are in a classroom or other group setting are most likely to get strep throat. It generally is spread by nose or throat secretions. Less commonly, infection may be transmitted through food, milk or water contaminated with streptococci, the bacterial agent. Strep throats require medical treatment. Common symptoms are:

- Swollen tonsils and neck glands
- Back of throat is bright red with white patches
- Fever, often more than 101 F, and often accompanied by chills
- Pain when swallowing

Most sore throat "bugs" are passed by direct contact. Mucus and saliva from one person's hands are transferred to objects, doorknobs and other surfaces, then to your hands and eventually to your mouth or nose.

Mononucleosis: A Tiresome Illness

Infectious mononucleosis. You've probably heard it called the "kissing disease." It's also known as mono, and it can be spread by kissing or, more commonly, through exposure resulting from coughing, sneezing or sharing a glass or cup.

Mono is caused by the Epstein-Barr virus. Anyone can get mono. By some estimates, 50 percent of the population has had mono by age 5. Most people older than 35 already have been exposed to the Epstein-Barr virus and have built up antibodies. They're immune and won't get it again. Full-blown mono is common in people age 7 to 35, especially teenagers.

Most people with mono experience fatigue and weakness. Other symptoms include a sore throat, fever, swollen lymph nodes in the neck and armpits, swollen tonsils, headache, rash and loss of appetite. Most symptoms abate within 10 days, but you shouldn't expect to return to your normal activities or contact sports for 3 weeks (your liver or spleen may be enlarged and at risk of injury). It may be 2 to 3 months before you feel completely normal. Rest and a healthful diet are the only treatments.

If symptoms linger more than a week or two or if they recur, see a doctor.

Common Problems

Self-Care

- Double your fluid intake. Fluids help keep your mucus thin and easy to clear.
- Gargle with warm salt water. Mix about a teaspoon of salt with a glass of warm water to gargle and spit. This will soothe and help clear your throat of mucus.
- Suck on a lozenge or hard candy, or chew sugarless gum. Chewing and sucking stimulate saliva production, which bathes and cleanses your throat.
- Take pain relievers. Over-the-counter medications, such as acetaminophen, ibuprofen and aspirin, relieve sore throat pain for 4 to 6 hours. Don't give aspirin to children or teenagers (see page 265).
- Rest your voice. If your sore throat has inflamed your larynx (voice box), talking may lead to more irritation and temporary loss of your voice, called laryngitis.
- Humidify the air. Adding moisture to the air prevents your mucous membranes from drying out (which causes irritation and makes it harder to sleep). Saline nasal sprays are also helpful.
- Avoid smoke and other air pollutants. Smoke irritates a sore throat. Stop smoking, and avoid all smoke and fumes from household cleaners or paint. Keep children away from secondhand smoke exposure.

Prevention

- Wash your hands frequently, especially during the cold and flu season.
- Keep your hands away from your face to avoid getting bacteria and viruses into your mouth or nose.

Medical Help

Serious throat infections, such as epiglottitis, can cause swelling that closes your airway. Seek emergency care if your sore throat is accompanied by any of the following symptoms:

- Drooling or difficulty swallowing or breathing
- A stiff, rigid neck and severe headache
- A fever of more than 102 F (103 F for children) or a fever that lasts for more than 48 hours
- A rash
- Persistent hoarseness or mouth ulcers lasting 2 weeks or more
- Recent exposure to strep throat

If the doctor suspects strep throat, a test will be ordered. You may learn the results before leaving the doctor's office, usually within 1 hour. Because this test misses about 20 percent of strep throats, many clinics do both the rapid test and a 24-hour throat culture. The rapid strep test also gives inaccurate results if you have recently been taking antibiotics. If the test result is positive, your doctor will prescribe an antibiotic, usually penicillin or a related medication.

Tonsils are rarely removed, except when recurrent infections cause serious problems.

Caution

If your doctor does prescribe a medication, take it for the full time indicated. Stopping use of the medication early can allow some bacteria to remain in the throat, potentially leading to a recurrence and complications such as rheumatic fever or a blood infection.

If your child has been taking antibiotics for at least 24 hours, has no fever and feels better, it is usually OK for him or her to return to school or day care.

Lump in Your Throat

The expressions "all choked up" and "the words stuck in my throat" are a reflection of the relationship between your throat and your emotional system. That "lump" in your throat that you feel is muscle tension.

When you are anxious, depressed or under stress, the small muscular opening in the lower part of your throat (the pharynx) begins to tense. This muscle may tighten without your being aware of it. When the muscle tightens, it sends a signal to your brain saying that something is in your throat, even when nothing is there.

This condition is so common it has its own name (globus syndrome), and although it is unpleasant, it usually resolves in a matter of days.

Other causes of a lump in your throat include side effects of medications, such as antihistamines or medications for high blood pressure and depression; recent cold or cough; hiatal hernia; being overweight; and acid indigestion (especially if you overeat at night).

Self-Care

- Drink plenty of fluids.
- Chew gum or suck on lozenges to stimulate saliva, which will soothe your throat.
- Avoid heartburn (stomach acid may be slipping up your food pipe and into your throat). Take antacids at bedtime, and don't go to bed on a full stomach.
- Avoid chocolate, fatty meals, alcohol and overeating.

Medical Help

If the lump in your throat does not go away after a few days, see your health care provider. Your doctor will perform tests to determine the exact cause of the lump and may adjust your medications to see if that will solve the problem.

Bad Breath

Everyone would like to have breath that always is "kissing sweet." Because fresh breath is important to us, makers of mints and mouthwashes sell millions of dollars worth of products every year. However, these products are only temporarily helpful for controlling bad breath. They actually may be less effective than simply rinsing your mouth with water and brushing and flossing your teeth.

There are many causes of bad breath. First, your mouth itself may be the source. Bacterial breakdown of food particles and other debris in and around your teeth can cause a foul odor. A dry mouth, such as occurs during sleep or as the result of some drugs or smoking, enables dead cells to accumulate on your tongue, gums and cheeks. As a result, they decompose and cause odor.

Eating foods containing oils with a strong odor causes bad breath. Onions and garlic are the best examples, but other vegetables and spices also may cause bad breath.

Lung disease can cause bad breath. Chronic infections in the lungs can produce very foul-smelling breath. Usually, much sputum (the mucus you cough up) is produced by these conditions. Several illnesses can cause a distinctive breath odor. Kidney failure can cause a urine-like odor, and liver failure may cause an odor described as "fishy." People with diabetes often have a fruity breath odor. This smell is also common in ill children who have eaten poorly for a few days. Bad breath in these situations can be corrected by treatment of the underlying condition.

For most people, bad breath can be improved by following a few simple steps:
- Brush your teeth after every meal.
- Brush your tongue to remove dead cells.
- Floss once a day to remove food particles from between your teeth.
- Drink plenty of water (not coffee, pop or alcohol) to keep your mouth moist.
- Avoid strong foods that cause bad breath. Toothbrushing or use of mouthwashes only partially disguises odors of garlic or onion which come from your lungs.
- Change your toothbrush every 2 to 3 months.
- Rinse your mouth after using inhaler medications.

■ Hoarseness or Loss of Voice

Loss of voice (laryngitis) or hoarseness occurs when your vocal cords become swollen or inflamed and no longer vibrate normally. They produce an unnatural sound, or they may not produce any sound at all.

Your speaking voice is formed when your diaphragm (the muscle above your stomach) pushes air from your lungs through your vocal cords. Air pressure forces your vocal cords to open and close, and the controlled escape of air vibrates the vocal cords, producing the sound that is your voice.

In addition to hoarseness, you may feel pain when speaking or have a raw and scratchy throat. Sometimes, your voice sounds higher or lower than normal.

The common causes of hoarseness or loss of voice are infections (as a result, you frequently lose your voice when you have a cold or flu), allergies, vocal strain (talking too loudly for too long or yelling), smoking and chronic esophageal reflux. Reflux, the backwash of acidic stomach contents into the food pipe, can sometimes spill over into the voice box.

Self-Care

- Limit your talking and whispering. (Whispering strains your vocal cords as much as talking.)
- Drink lots of warm, noncaffeinated fluids to keep your throat moist.
- Avoid clearing your throat.
- Stop smoking, and avoid exposure to smoke. Smoke dries your throat and irritates your vocal cords.
- Stop drinking alcohol, which also dries your throat and irritates your vocal cords.
- Use a humidifier to moisturize the air you breathe. (Follow the manufacturer's instructions to clean the humidifier and prevent bacterial buildup.)

Medical Help

If hoarseness lasts for more than 2 weeks, seek medical help. Your doctor may prescribe medications for infection or allergy. Take them just as prescribed. Hoarseness is rarely caused by cancer.

Mouth Sores

Irritating, painful and repetitive. That's how many people describe canker sores and cold sores. But the terminology can be confusing. Cold sores have nothing to do with the common cold. What's more, the cause, appearance, symptoms and treatments of canker sores and cold sores are very different. There are other mouth sores and conditions that are often mistaken for canker sores and cold sores.

Canker Sores

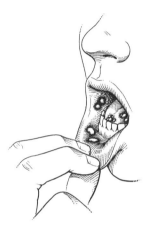

A canker sore is an ulcer on the soft tissue inside your mouth—on the tongue, soft palate and inside the cheeks. Typically, you notice a burning sensation and a round whitish spot with a red edge or halo. Pain lessens in a few days.

Despite a great deal of research into the problem, the cause of canker sores remains a mystery. Current thinking suggests that stress or tissue injury may cause the eruption of common canker sores. Some researchers think certain foods (for example, citrus fruits, tomatoes and some nuts) may complicate the problem. A minor injury, such as biting the inside of your mouth, may trigger a canker sore.

There are two types of canker sores: simple and complex. The simple type of canker sore may appear three or four times a year and last 4 to 7 days. The first occurrence is usually between the ages of 10 and 20, but it can occur in younger children. As a person reaches adulthood, the sores occur less frequently and may stop developing altogether. Women seem to get them more often than men, and they seem to run in families.

Complex canker sores are less common but much more of a problem. People with this condition may have sores 50 percent of the time—as old sores heal, new ones appear.

Self-Care

There is no cure for either simple or complex canker sores, and effective treatments are limited. However, the following practices may provide temporary relief:
- Avoid abrasive, acidic or spicy foods, which may increase the pain.
- Apply ice to the canker sore.
- Brush your teeth carefully to avoid irritating the sore.
- Use a topical ointment containing phenol.
- Rinse your mouth with over-the-counter preparations: try diluted hydrogen peroxide or elixir of Benadryl.
- Use an over-the-counter pain reliever.

Medical Help

For severe attacks of canker sores, your dentist or physician may recommend a prescription mouthwash, a corticosteroid salve or an anesthetic solution called viscous lidocaine.

Contact your physician in any of the following situations:
- New high fever with canker sores
- Spreading sores or signs of spreading infection
- Pain that is not controlled with the measures listed above
- Sores that do not heal completely within a week

See your dentist if you have sharp tooth surfaces or dental appliances that are causing the sores.

Common Problems

■ Cold Sores (Fever Blisters)

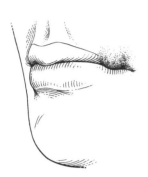

Also known as fever blisters, cold sores are very common. They may appear on your mouth, lips, nose, cheeks or fingers.

The herpes simplex virus causes cold sores. Herpes simplex virus type 1 usually causes cold sores. Herpes simplex virus type 2 is usually responsible for genital herpes. However, either form of the virus can cause sores in the facial area or on the genitals. You get cold sores from another person who has an active condition. Eating utensils, razors, towels or direct skin contact are common means of spreading this infection.

Symptoms may not start for as long as 20 days after you were exposed to the virus. Small, fluid-filled blisters develop on a raised, red, painful area of skin. Pain or tingling often precedes blisters by 1 to 2 days. Symptoms usually last 7 to 10 days.

After the first infection, the virus periodically reemerges at or near the original site. Fever, menstruation and exposure to the sun may trigger a recurrence.

The herpes simplex virus can be transmitted even when blisters aren't present. But the greatest risk of infection is from the time the blister appears until it has completely crusted over. Cold sores occur most often in adolescents and young adults, but they can occur at any age. Outbreaks decrease after age 35.

Self-Care

Cold sores generally clear up without treatment. The following steps may provide relief:

- Rest, take over-the-counter pain relievers (if you have a fever) or use over-the-counter creams for comfort (they won't speed healing). Children should avoid aspirin use.
- Do not squeeze, pinch or pick at any blister.
- Avoid kissing and skin contact with people while blisters are present.
- Wash your hands carefully before touching another person.
- Use sunblock on your lips and face before prolonged exposure to the sun—during both the winter and the summer to prevent cold sores.

Medical Help

If you experience frequent bouts of cold sores, an antiviral antibiotic may be the answer. (The drug acyclovir is commonly prescribed.) These drugs inhibit the growth of the herpes virus. Studies of skiers who use sunscreen with and without acyclovir indicate that the drug offers significant additional protection.

You may feel a tingling sensation before the outbreak of a cold sore. This is called the prodrome. Many physicians recommend using acyclovir as soon as the prodrome begins.

Caution

- If you have a cold sore, take special care to avoid contact with infants or anyone who has a skin condition known as eczema (see page 121). They're more susceptible to infection. Also, avoid people who are taking medications for cancer and organ transplantation because they have decreased immunity. The virus can cause a life-threatening condition in them.
- Pregnant women and nursing mothers should avoid using acyclovir for treatment of cold sores unless specifically advised by their doctor to use it.
- Herpes simplex virus infections have potentially serious complications. The virus can spread to your eye. This is the most frequent cause of corneal blindness in the United States. If you have a burning pain in the eye or a rash near the eye or on the tip of your nose, see your doctor immediately.

■ Other Oral Infections and Disorders

Gingivostomatitis (also called trenchmouth): This is an oral infection that is common among children. It's caused by a virus and often accompanies a cold or flu. The infection generally lasts about 2 weeks and ranges from mild to severe. If your child has sores on the gums or on the inside of the cheeks, has bad breath, has a fever and feels generally unwell, consult your dentist or physician. Treatment of any underlying infection will help clear the mouth infection. A medicated oral rinse may help relieve the pain and promote healing. Practice good oral hygiene and eat a nutritious diet of soft foods and drink plenty of fluids. Use a mouthwash made of half a teaspoon of salt dissolved in 8 ounces of water, or use an over-the-counter mouthwash.

Oral thrush: This is caused by a fungus. There will be creamy-white soft patches in the mouth or throat. It often occurs when your body has been weakened by illness or when your mouth's natural balance of microbes has been upset by medications. Many people will experience an outbreak of oral thrush at some point in their lives. It is most common among babies, young children and the elderly. Although painful, oral thrush is not a serious disorder. However, it can interfere with eating and impair your nutrition. There is no self-care for this condition, but a dentist or physician can prescribe an oral medication that is taken for 7 to 10 days. Thrush tends to recur.

Leukoplakia: Thickened, white patches on a cheek or the tongue are often signs of leukoplakia. Leukoplakia is the mouth's reaction to chronic irritation. It may be caused by ill-fitting dentures or a rough tooth rubbing against the cheek or gum. When white patches develop in the mouths of smokers, the condition is called "smoker's keratosis." Snuff and chewing tobacco also produce chronic irritation. You can have leukoplakia at any time during your life, but it is most common among the elderly. Treatment involves removing the source of irritation. Once the source of irritation has been removed, the patch may clear up, usually within weeks or months. A doctor or dentist should evaluate white patches in the mouth. Tobacco use can lead to cancer of the lip, tongue or lungs.

Oral cancer: Cancer of the mouth usually occurs along the side or the bottom of the tongue or on the floor of the mouth. The tumors often are painless at first and frequently are visible or can be felt with a finger. Regular examination of the soft tissues of the mouth is essential for early diagnosis. If you notice any persistent change from the usual appearance or feel of the soft tissues in your mouth, consult your dentist or physician. Early detection is important for successful treatment. Almost 25 percent of people with oral cancer die because of delayed discovery and treatment.

Common Problems

Routine self-examination of your mouth and tongue may enable you to see or feel an oral cancer when it is small and treatment may be most effective.

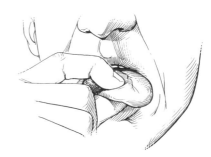

Men's Health

■ Testicular Pain

Any sharp and sudden pain in your testicles should be treated carefully, because it can be a symptom of a serious medical condition. Seek medical help if you have sudden pain in your testicles that does not go away in 10 or 15 minutes or if you have pain that recurs. Some causes of sudden testicular pain are discussed below.

Testicular torsion is caused when the *spermatic cord*, which carries blood to and from the testicle, gets twisted. This twisting cuts off the blood supply to the testicle, causing sharp and sudden pain. Testicular torsion sometimes occurs after strenuous physical activity, but it can happen with no apparent cause, even during sleep. This condition can occur at any age, but it usually occurs in boys. Symptoms include sudden and severe pain, which can cause fever, nausea and vomiting. You also may notice the elevation of one testicle within the scrotum.

Epididymitis occurs when the *epididymis*, a coiled tube that carries sperm from the testicles to the spermatic cord, becomes inflamed, usually by a bacterial infection. Symptoms include aching to moderately severe pain in the scrotum, which develops gradually over several hours or days; fever and swelling may occur. Epididymitis is occasionally caused by chlamydia, a sexually transmitted disease (see page 183). In these cases, your sexual partner may be infected and should also receive a medical examination.

Orchitis is an inflammation of the testicle, usually due to an infection. Orchitis frequently occurs with epididymitis (see above). Orchitis may occur when you have the mumps, or it may develop if you have a prostate infection. Orchitis is rare, but it could cause infertility if left untreated. Symptoms include pain in the scrotum, swelling (usually on one side of the scrotum only) and a feeling of weight in the scrotum.

Screening for Cancer of the Testicle

Testicular cancer is rare. It occurs most often in young men age 15 to 35. The major symptom is a lump, swelling or "heavy feeling" in a testicle.

A simple 2-minute self-examination each month could save the life of a man with early signs of testicular cancer. Perform the examination after a shower or warm bath, when the skin of your scrotum is loose and relaxed. Examine one testicle at a time. Roll it gently between your thumbs and forefingers, feeling for any lump on the surface of the testicle. You also should notice whether the testicle is enlarged, hardened or otherwise in a different condition than during the last examination. If you notice anything unusual, it may not necessarily mean cancer, but you should contact your physician.

Do not be alarmed if you feel a small, firm area near the rear of the testicle and a tube leading up from the testicle. This is normal. These are the *epididymis* and the *spermatic cord*, which store and transport sperm.

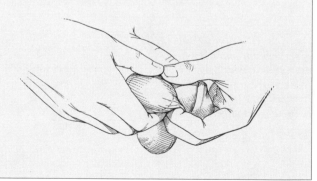

Mayo Clinic Guide to Self-Care

Enlarged Prostate

The *prostate* is a walnut-sized gland that is located just below the bladder and is present only in males. The prostate produces most of the fluids in the semen. Testosterone, the male sex hormone, causes the prostate to slowly enlarge with age. As the prostate enlarges, it can restrict the flow of urine through the *urethra* (the tube that passes urine from your bladder), causing slow or difficult urination. The symptoms can be mild and cause little difficulty with urinating, or they can be very painful if complete blockage occurs. Other symptoms may include more frequent nighttime voiding, dribbling after voiding or voiding twice in a row within 10 to 15 minutes.

Prostate enlargement can start as men reach their late 40s. Four of five men experience prostate enlargement by the time they reach age 80. From 25 to 30 percent of men will have some kind of procedure performed on their prostates to correct symptoms during their lifetime.

An enlarged prostate can produce difficulty with urination because the flow of urine is restricted.

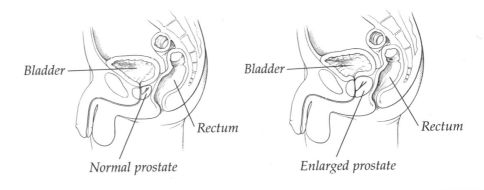

Bladder —   Bladder —

Rectum   Rectum

Normal prostate   Enlarged prostate

Medical Help

Your health care provider will ask you detailed questions about your symptoms and may do tests on urine and blood samples. Using a gloved, lubricated finger, your health care provider may examine your prostate for enlargement and lumps. Called the "digital rectal examination," this procedure causes only mild discomfort.

Initial treatment for an enlarged prostate may be medications that reduce the size of the prostate gland or improve urine flow by relaxing the tissues in the area of the prostate gland. Surgery can reduce the size of the prostate or remove it completely.

Screening for Prostate Cancer

Cancer of the prostate is the second leading cause of cancer death in American men. Prostate cancer occurs most frequently in men older than 60.

Screening for prostate cancer is controversial. Some doctors believe that many men will have unnecessary surgery or radiation because of screening. Others believe that screening is essential. The American Cancer Society recommends yearly screening for prostate cancer for men 50 or older, for men who have at least a 10-year life expectancy and for younger men who are at high risk. This involves digital rectal examination and a blood test for PSA (prostate-specific antigen). Ultrasound examination is another way to detect cancer. If detected early, prostate cancer often can be cured. Symptoms are the same as those for prostate enlargement unless cancer has spread to the bone.

■ Painful Urination

Painful urination is usually caused by a *urinary tract infection* (UTI). UTIs are more common in women, but they also occur in men. Other symptoms include frequent or urgent urination, an inability to release more than a small amount of urine (followed by an urgent need to urinate again) and a burning sensation while urinating.

If your kidney also is infected, you may experience pain in your abdomen or back, chills, a fever or vomiting. A kidney infection is a serious condition that requires immediate medical attention.

Common Causes

E. coli bacteria: E. coli bacteria are common in the bowel. If E. coli bacteria enter the urethra (the tube through which urine passes), and then enter your urine or bladder, a UTI can result.

Chlamydia: One of several sexually transmitted organisms that can infect the urethra, causing penile drainage and painful urination.

Prostate problems: An enlarged prostate gland can restrict the flow of urine, causing urine retention and UTIs. Also, if your prostate gland produces fewer proteins as you age, the absence of these proteins may make you more susceptible to UTIs. (See Enlarged Prostate, page 141.)

Medical procedures: A urinary catheter or medical instruments can introduce bacteria into your urethra and bladder, causing a UTI.

Narrowed urethra: Injury to or frequent inflammation of the urethra can cause a narrowing (called a stricture) of the urethra. Strictures restrict urine flow and can cause UTIs.

Dehydration: Lack of fluids can lead to stagnant urine, which can cause a UTI.

Medical Help

See your health care provider, who will take a urine sample and perform tests to determine whether you have a UTI. Do not force fluids just before you give a urine sample because your urine may be diluted and the results may be inaccurate. In most instances, UTIs can be treated with medications. Be sure to take all the medication, even if your symptoms go away after a few days. Failure to take all the medication can lead to a recurrence of the UTI.

■ Impotence

Occasional episodes of impotence are common in men. When impotence is a recurring problem, however, it can harm a man's self-image and affect his relationships. Fortunately, impotence often can be treated successfully. Impotence is defined as an inability to achieve or maintain an erection adequate for sexual intercourse.

The causes of impotence can be psychological or physical. Stress, anxiety or depression can lead to impotence. Impotence also can be a side effect of alcohol use and some medications (such as some drugs used to treat high blood pressure). Impotence can be caused by diseases such as diabetes or multiple sclerosis or other chronic diseases. Impotence may be the result of a direct injury to the genitals or an injury that affects the spinal cord or nervous system. Radiation treatments or major pelvic surgeries, such as those performed for cancer of the prostate, bladder or rectum, also may result in impotence.

Self-Care	If you can still get an erection at certain times of the day, such as the morning, you may benefit from the following advice: • Limit alcohol consumption, especially before sexual activity. • Quit smoking. • Exercise regularly. • Reduce stress. • Work with your partner to create an atmosphere conducive to lovemaking.
Medical Help	**Psychological treatment:** If stress, anxiety or depression is the cause of impotence, you may want to seek counseling with a mental health professional or a sex therapist (either alone or with your partner). **Medications:** Pills or male hormone shots may be prescribed by your doctor. **Penile injections:** If impotence is caused by a decreased blood supply to the penis, medications that increase blood flow are prescribed. They are injected into the penis, and the injections can be performed at home after training by your physician. **Vacuum constriction device:** A tube is placed over the penis, and air is withdrawn; as a result, blood flows to the penis and causes an erection. A rubber constricting band is placed around the base of the penis to prolong the erection. This low-cost device is available at most drugstores with a doctor's prescription. **Surgery:** Surgery can be performed to increase blood flow to the penis or to implant devices to assist in achieving an erection. **Intraurethral medication:** A small suppository (half the size of a grain of rice) is slid into the opening of the penis.

■ Male Birth Control

Vasectomy involves cutting and sealing the *vas deferens*, the tube that carries sperm. The procedure does not interfere with a man's ability to maintain an erection or reach orgasm, nor does it stop the production of male hormones or of sperm in the testicles. The only change is that the sperm's link to the outside is severed permanently. After a vasectomy, you continue to ejaculate about the same amount of semen because sperm account for only a small part of the ejaculate.

Before your vasectomy, you will be given an injection of anesthetic in the scrotum to numb the area so you will not feel pain. After your physician has located the vas deferens, a pair of small cuts are made in the skin of the scrotum. Each vas deferens is then pulled through the opening until it forms a loop. Approximately a half inch is cut out of each vas deferens and removed. The two ends of each vas deferens are closed by stitches or cauterization (or both) and are placed back in the scrotum. The incisions are closed with stitches.

The operation takes about 20 minutes. After a vasectomy, refrain from any strenuous activity, including intercourse, for at least 2 weeks. The stitches are generally of a type that dissolves in 2 to 3 weeks. You may notice some swelling and minor discomfort in the scrotum for several weeks. However, if the pain becomes severe or if fever develops, call your physician.

The failure rate for a vasectomy is less than 1 percent. Until your physician has determined that your ejaculate does not contain sperm, you should continue to use alternative contraception. This typically takes several months and several ejaculations.

Women's Health

■ Lump in Your Breast

Most breast lumps are not cancerous. However, because of the risk of cancer, all lumps should be carefully assessed. Many breast lumps are fluid-filled cysts that enlarge near the end of your monthly cycle. The lumps may or may not be painful. Perform a breast self-examination each month after your period to check for lumps and any other changes in your breasts (see below).

Self-Care

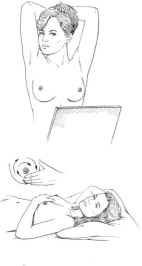

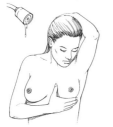

- Do a breast self-examination each month so you'll know whether a lump is new.
- Examine your breasts on the same day each month if you are past menopause. If you are still menstruating, the best time to examine your breasts is 7 to 10 days after your last period started. Breast cancer lumps usually aren't painful. Use your eyes and hands to search for lumps, thickened areas or swelling in your breasts. Notify your health care provider of any changes.
- Refer to the illustrations at left.
  - Look into a mirror with your arms at your sides. Elevate your arms and thoroughly examine the skin on your breasts for puckering, dimples or changes in their size or shape. Look for changes in the natural symmetry of both breasts. Check to see whether your nipples are pulled in (inverted). Also note any unusual discharge from your nipples. Check for the same signs while you rest your hands on your hips and again with your hands behind your head.
  - Examine your breasts while standing in the shower and while lying on your back. Hold one hand behind your head and use a circular massaging motion with the other hand to check the tissue over the entire opposite breast, including the nipple and the tissue under your armpit. Repeat the procedure on the other side. Soap and water during a shower can make the procedure easier.
  - Check for lumps that don't disappear or change. Abnormal lumps may seem to appear suddenly and remain. They vary in size and firmness and often feel hard with irregular edges. Sometimes they just feel like thickened areas without distinct outlines. Cancerous lumps usually aren't painful.
- If the lump causes discomfort, take a mild pain medication (see page 265) or eliminate caffeine from your diet.

Medical Help

See your doctor if a lump in your breast doesn't go away after your menstrual cycle. A fluid-filled cyst may be drained with a needle after an injection of a local anesthetic. If you have a breast infection, an antibiotic is typically prescribed. Lumps that are not filled with fluid may require a needle biopsy or surgical removal to determine whether they are cancerous.

Women beyond menopause should see their doctor if a lump lasts more than a week or becomes reddened, painful or enlarged.

Mayo Clinic Guide to Self-Care

Mammograms: Who Should Have Them?

A mammogram is a special breast X-ray that can detect tumors so small that your physician cannot even feel them. Mammography saves lives by identifying breast cancer at a stage when it is potentially curable. However, the test is not perfect. Occasionally it fails to show a tumor, and at other times it indicates a problem when there is not one. Screening by mammography is best combined with regular breast examinations.

There is controversy within the medical profession about the age at which you should begin to have regular mammograms. The breasts of young women are often too dense to X-ray well. Fortunately, young women rarely develop breast cancer. Because every woman's risk of cancer, preferences and concerns are different, the final decision about screening needs to be made by you and your doctor. Here are some guidelines.

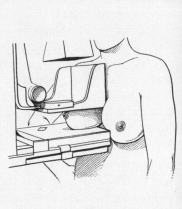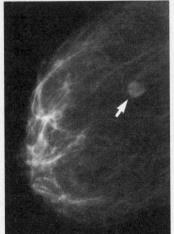

Mammograms are produced by a special X-ray device that can detect tumors before you or your physician can feel them.

Age	Expert Opinion	What to Do
Younger than 40	Experts agree generally	Monthly breast self-exam No mammogram
Younger than 40 at high risk (sister or mother with breast cancer at a young age)	Talk to your doctor for an individualized program	Monthly breast self-exam Annual physical exam Mammogram, often beginning 5-10 years before age at which mother or sister had cancer
40-49 not at high risk	Some disagreement	Monthly breast self-exam Physical exam every 1-2 years Mammogram, not at all to yearly
40-49 at high risk	Some disagreement	Monthly breast self-exam Annual physical exam Annual mammogram
50-74 at normal or high risk	General agreement	Monthly breast self-exam Annual physical exam Annual mammogram
75 or older	Some disagreement	Monthly breast self-exam Annual physical exam Annual mammogram

Note: Risk factors for breast cancer include prior breast cancer, breast cancer in mother or sister, never pregnant or first pregnancy when older than 35, early onset of menses or late menopause. Your doctor also may consider other risk factors.

Common Problems

■ Pain in Your Breast

The most common cause of pain in the breast is mastitis, which is caused by an infection or inflammation. It usually occurs in only one breast. Generalized tenderness in both breasts is common, especially during the week before a menstrual period, and it is also a symptom of premenstrual syndrome (see page 147). Exercises, such as jogging and aerobics, can cause breast tenderness. Tenderness also may be caused by an inflamed cyst. If fever and redness are present, infection is a concern. Infections, although not common, can occur with breast-feeding.

Self-Care

- Wear a comfortable and supportive bra.
- Take an over-the-counter pain reliever (see page 265).
- Reduce the salt in your diet before your period.
- Avoid caffeine.
- If pain is due to high-impact exercises, switch to a low-impact workout such as biking, walking or swimming and use an athletic bra.
- See other tips in the section on premenstrual syndrome (page 147).

Medical Help

If you have fever or redness along with the pain, see your doctor. You probably need an antibiotic. If pain is associated with a lump or a change in the texture of your breast, see your doctor.

■ Painful Menses

Most women are familiar with menstrual cramps. During menstruation, you may feel pain in the lower abdomen, possibly extending to the hips, lower back or thighs. Some women also have nausea, vomiting, diarrhea or general aching. It is normal to have mild abdominal cramps on the first day or two of your period (more than half of women do). However, about 10 percent of women experience pain so severe that they can't manage their normal routine unless they take medication.

If there is not an underlying gynecologic disorder, the pain is called primary dysmenorrhea. It is caused by high levels of prostaglandin (a substance that makes the muscles of the uterus contract and shed its lining). Although painful, primary dysmenorrhea is not harmful. It often disappears by your mid-20s or after you have a baby.

Pain that is caused by an underlying gynecologic disorder is called secondary dysmenorrhea. It may be due to a fibroid tumor (a benign tumor in the wall of your uterus), a sexually transmitted disease, endometriosis, pelvic inflammatory disease or an ovarian cyst or tumor.

Self-Care

- Nonsteroidal anti-inflammatory drugs or aspirin (see page 265) relieves pain in about 80 percent of women.
- Try soaking in a warm tub or exercising.

Medical Help

Treatment of the underlying cause should relieve the pain. If no cause for the pain is found, birth control pills may relieve the discomfort.

Talk to your health care provider if the menstrual pain is severe or is associated with fever; if you have unusual nausea, vomiting or abdominal pain; or if the pain lasts beyond the third day of menstrual flow.

■ Irregular Periods

It is common for women to experience unexplained irregularities in their periods. Irregular periods are due to changes in hormone levels, which can be affected by stress or other emotional experiences, significant changes in the amount of aerobic exercise or dramatic changes in weight. High levels of exercise in a woman with an excessively lean body may stop periods altogether.

Self-Care

- Keep a menstrual calendar for at least three cycles. Record the first day of flow, the day of maximal flow, the day that flow stops and times of intercourse to help evaluate menstrual changes.
- If your periods are irregular for more than three cycles, talk to your doctor.
- If you miss a period and have had intercourse, look for symptoms of pregnancy.

■ Bleeding Between Periods

Occasional bleeding between menstrual periods is common. It may occur spontaneously or with sexual intercourse. Usually it is not serious, and is caused by a variation of your usual hormone cycles. Stress, new contraceptive pills, polyps (benign growths of tissue) and many other conditions can affect your menstruation. Because abnormal bleeding also can be the first warning sign of cancer, it needs prompt evaluation by your doctor.

■ Premenstrual Syndrome

If you experience a predictable pattern of physical and emotional changes in the days before your period, you may have premenstrual syndrome (PMS). PMS is related to the normal hormone cycles and occurs with normal hormone levels. One clue to its cause may lie in a woman's response to serotonin. Serotonin is a substance in the brain which has been associated with clinical depression and other emotional disorders. Sometimes an underlying psychological condition such as depression is aggravated by the hormonal changes before a period.

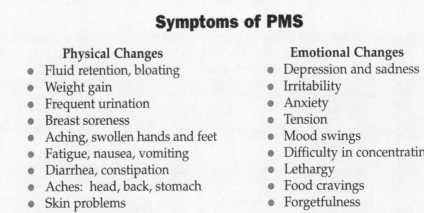

Symptoms of PMS

Physical Changes	Emotional Changes
• Fluid retention, bloating	• Depression and sadness
• Weight gain	• Irritability
• Frequent urination	• Anxiety
• Breast soreness	• Tension
• Aching, swollen hands and feet	• Mood swings
• Fatigue, nausea, vomiting	• Difficulty in concentrating
• Diarrhea, constipation	• Lethargy
• Aches: head, back, stomach	• Food cravings
• Skin problems	• Forgetfulness

Self-Care

You can usually manage PMS with a combination of education and lifestyle changes.

- Maintain your weight at a healthy level.
- Eat smaller, more frequent meals. Don't skip meals. Eat at the same time every day if possible.
- Limit salt and salty foods for 1 to 2 weeks before your period to reduce bloating and fluid retention.
- Avoid caffeine to reduce irritability, tension and breast soreness. See page 211 for information on caffeine.
- Avoid alcohol before your period to minimize depression and mood swings.
- Eat a well-balanced diet (see page 210).
- A diet that is adequate in calcium may help. Drink 2 to 3 cups of low-fat milk daily and choose other calcium-rich foods (see page 149). If you cannot tolerate foods with calcium or you're unsure about the adequacy of calcium in your diet, a daily calcium supplement (1,200 milligrams) may help.
- Reduce stress (see page 224). Stress can aggravate PMS.
- Walk, jog, bike, swim or perform some other aerobic exercise at least three times a week.
- Record your symptoms for a few months. You may find that PMS is more tolerable if you see that your symptoms are predictable and short-lived.

Medical Help

There are no physical findings or lab tests for diagnosing PMS. Instead, doctors rely on careful evaluation of your medical history. As part of the diagnostic process, women are asked to record the onset, duration, nature and severity of symptoms for at least two menstrual cycles.

If your PMS symptoms seriously affect your life and the suggestions listed above don't help, your doctor may recommend the following medications:

- Nonsteroidal anti-inflammatory drugs (NSAIDs) can ease cramps and breast discomfort (see page 265).
- Birth control pills often relieve symptoms by stopping ovulation.
- An injection of medroxyprogesterone acetate (Depo-Provera) can be used to temporarily stop ovulation and menstruation in severe cases.
- Antidepressants help about 60 percent of women who have severe emotional symptoms from PMS. Examples of these antidepressants are fluoxetine (Prozac), sertraline (Zoloft), paroxetine (Paxil), fluvoxamine (Luvox) and venlafaxine (Effexor). These drugs can be used in doses lower than those usually prescribed for depression and may be effective when taken only during the week or two before menstruation.
- If antidepressants are not effective, the antianxiety drug alprazolam (Xanax) may help, but it is a powerful and potentially addictive medication that should not be used long-term.

◼ Menopause

Menopause is a natural stage of life which begins in most women between ages 40 and 55 years. The average age at onset has been increasing over the years and is currently about 51 years.

During menopause, the ovaries gradually stop producing estrogen. Your periods become irregular. The process may last several months to several years. Eventually, your menstrual periods stop, and you can no longer become pregnant.

As your ovaries produce fewer hormones, various changes occur, although they vary a great deal from person to person. Your uterus atrophies (shrinks), and the lining of your vagina becomes thin. Your vagina also may become dry, making intercourse painful. Hot flashes cause flushing or sweating that may last from several minutes to more than an hour and may interrupt sleep and produce night sweats.

During and after menopause, your body fat typically is redistributed as metabolism changes. Your bones lose density and strength. Osteoporosis may occur (see below).

Mood changes are not uncommon during menopause. They may be related to sleep disruption due to "hot flashes," other hormonal changes, or the normal midlife issues that affect both men and women. Many women find that menopause can have a positive effect on their physical and emotional health.

Self-Care

- Accept the changes as normal and healthy.
- Eat a balanced diet, exercise regularly and dress in layers.
- Use a water-soluble lubricating jelly if intercourse is painful.

Medical Help

Your doctor may prescribe estrogen replacement therapy to relieve hot flashes, halt the thinning of vaginal tissue, prevent or delay the progression of osteoporosis and possibly prevent or delay heart disease.

Estrogen replacement therapy does not affect mood swings. However, estrogen replacement therapy may increase the risk of breast or endometrial cancer. Therefore, if you still have your uterus, you generally should be given progesterone as well as estrogen.

Another hormone, megestrol acetate, can reduce the frequency and severity of hot flashes in women who can't use estrogens. If hormones are prescribed, you may resume menstrual bleeding.

How to Prevent Osteoporosis

The loss of estrogen after menopause greatly increases the likelihood of osteoporosis, a disorder in which your bones become porous and brittle. The most effective way to manage osteoporosis is to prevent it by maximizing your bone density when you are young.

- Eat enough calcium (1,000 to 1,200 mg per day) throughout adulthood to help prevent osteoporosis. Foods rich in calcium include milk, yogurt, cheese, salmon and broccoli. Just 1 glass of milk is about 300 mg of calcium.
- If you are at an increased risk, your physician may suggest calcium tablets. Calcium, however, may be harmful for certain conditions. See your physician before taking a high-calcium supplement.
- Participate in weight-bearing exercises such as walking, dancing, and jogging.

Urination Problems

Urinary tract infections (UTIs) are common among women. With the beginning of sexual activity, women have a marked increase in the number of infections. Sexual intercourse, pregnancy and urinary obstruction all contribute to the likelihood of such an infection. Symptoms of UTI include pain or a burning sensation during urination, increased frequency of urination and a feeling of urgency every time you need to urinate. If you have an infection, your doctor will prescribe an antibiotic.

Urinary incontinence is involuntary loss of urine. The condition is often divided into "urge" and "stress" incontinence. If leakage occurs when you feel the need to void it is called "urge" incontinence. It is often caused by a mild UTI or by excessive use of bladder stimulants such as caffeine. "Stress" incontinence is loss of urine when pressure is put on your bladder by coughing, laughing, jumping or lifting something heavy. It usually is caused by weakening of the muscles that support your bladder. These muscles can weaken because of childbirth, being overweight or aging.

Self-Care for Urine Leakage

- Try Kegel exercises. Begin by contracting your pelvic muscle, as you would to prevent a bowel movement or to stop urine flow. Relax, and then repeat the contraction. Do this 20 or 30 times. Rest 10 seconds between contractions. Repeat the exercise several times a day. Don't do it in the bathroom while urinating.
- Empty your bladder more often.
- Lean forward when urinating to empty your bladder more completely.
- Decrease your intake of caffeine-containing foods and beverages (see page 211).
- Use a pad to protect against small leaks. Change it every couple of hours.
- Use tampons while exercising.

Vaginal Discharge

Vaginal discharge is one symptom of vaginitis. Vaginitis is an inflammation of your vagina. It usually is caused by an infection or an alteration in the normal vaginal bacteria. In addition to vaginal discharge, you may have itching, irritation, pain during intercourse, pain in your lower abdomen, vaginal bleeding and odor.

There are three common types of vaginitis: trichomoniasis, yeast infections and bacterial vaginosis. Trichomoniasis is caused by a parasite. It may cause a smelly, greenish yellow, sometimes frothy discharge. It usually develops as a result of sexual intercourse. Trichomonal vaginitis usually is treated with metronidazole tablets. Your partner also should be treated. Yeast infections are caused by a fungus. You are more susceptible to a yeast infection if you are pregnant or have diabetes; if you are taking antibiotics, cortisone or birth control pills; or if you have an iron deficiency. The main symptom is itching, but a white discharge also may be present. Bacterial vaginosis usually produces a gray, smelly discharge. This infection also can be treated with metronidazole tablets or another antibiotic.

Self-Care for Yeast Infection

- Use an over-the-counter antifungal cream or suppository for suspected yeast infections.
- Abstain from intercourse or have your partner use a condom for a week after beginning treatment.
- See your health care provider if symptoms persist after 1 week.

Mayo Clinic Guide to Self-Care

◼ Cancer Screening

See page 145 for breast cancer screening recommendations. Screening tests for cervical cancer include a Pap smear and a pelvic examination. The Pap smear detects more than 90 percent of cervical cancers at a curable stage.

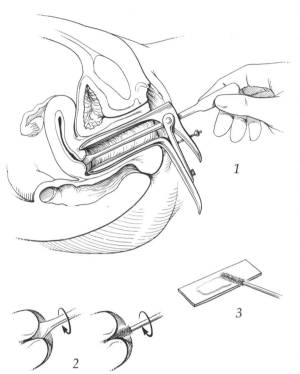

With speculum in place, your physician rotates a wooden spatula and then a brush to remove a sample of cells (1 and 2). The cells are smeared onto a glass slide (3) for examination under a microscope.

Cervical cancer develops slowly, often over 10 to 20 years. It begins with changes in cells on the surface of the cervix. Doctors refer to these abnormal cells as precancerous. They may become cancerous with time.

Early precancerous changes in surface cells are called dysplasia or squamous intraepithelial lesions. Some of these abnormalities go away on their own, but others progress. Precancerous conditions generally do not cause any symptoms, including pain.

Because doctors aren't in agreement about how often the Pap smear should be done, discuss with your physician what's best for you. Guidelines for a cost-effective screening strategy suggest the following:

- An initial Pap test at age 18 or with the beginning of sexual activity
- Subsequent Pap tests every 1 to 3 years
- After three consecutive Pap tests with normal results, a woman and her doctor may opt for less frequent testing
- For women who've had a total hysterectomy for a benign disease and no prior abnormal Pap tests, routine Pap tests are no longer necessary

Women at high risk should have more frequent testing. You are at high risk if:

- You began sexual activity as a teenager, especially if you had multiple sex partners
- You currently have more than one sex partner
- You have had a sexually transmitted disease, including genital warts
- You have had an abnormal Pap test or a prior cancer
- You use tobacco

The Reliability of Pap Tests

The Pap test is a screening test and is not perfect. It may miss abnormal cells, causing a false negative result. That's why it's important to get regular Pap smears. A result could be inaccurate for these reasons:

- The patient washes away abnormal cells

through sexual activity or douching before her examination.

- The doctor doesn't collect cells from the entire cervical area, missing abnormal cells; doesn't smear the sample onto the slide properly; or doesn't "fix" the cells immediately and correctly.

Contraception

Method	How It Works	Effectiveness*	Cautions
Natural family planning	Relies on a woman's menstrual cycle to determine which days are safe for intercourse	May be more than 90 percent	Works best in stable relationships. Requires special training
Oral contraceptives (birth control pills)	Synthetic hormones prevent ovulation and impair implantation. They are usually a combination of an estrogen and a progestin	More than 99 percent	Take pill at the same time every day. Do not smoke, especially after age 35. If you miss two periods in a row, consult your health care provider
Contraceptive implants	Match-sized hormone sticks that are implanted under the skin of your upper arm	More than 95 percent	Sometimes difficult to remove
Intrauterine device (IUD)	Inserted into the uterus. Inhibits sperm migration and fertilization. Two are in use: one with progesterone and one with copper	95 to 98 percent	Increased tubal pregnancy; increase in menstrual blood loss with copper device. Check the string regularly to be sure that the device is still in place
Diaphragm	A rubber cap is inserted into vagina to cover the cervix. It must be fitted	About 95 percent when used consistently and correctly with a spermicide	May cause cervical irritation and increased risk of urinary tract infections. Must be inserted before intercourse
Cervical cap	The plastic cervical cap must be fitted by your health care provider to cover your cervix	85 percent	May cause cervical irritation. Difficult to fit. Pap smear abnormalities. Must be inserted before intercourse
Female condom	Several different forms. Extends to the outside of the vagina	90 percent	Difficult to insert for some people
Depo-Provera shots	Shot in the arm or buttock every 2 to 3 months	More than 95 percent	May cause menstrual irregularities, headache, acne and weight gain
Tubal ligation (female sterilization)	Fallopian tubes are tied and cut or cauterized, thus preventing the egg from traveling down the tube and sperm from moving up the tube	More than 99 percent	Requires surgery, usually as an outpatient

*Effectiveness is defined as preventing pregnancy during 1 year of typical use.

■ Pregnancy

Although pregnancy is a natural state, you want to take especially good care of your health to help ensure that your baby will have the best possible start in life. It's a good idea to see your health care provider for a complete physical examination before you become pregnant. You will be checked for several conditions that may not cause symptoms but can complicate pregnancy. These include diabetes, high blood pressure, pelvic tumors and anemia. If there is a health problem, your health care provider will want to control the condition, ideally before you become pregnant. Your health care provider will also review your immunizations to be sure you're immune to rubella (a viral infection called German measles).

Self-Care

To Prepare for Pregnancy

- If you are overweight, reduce your weight before you become pregnant. Do not begin a diet if you are pregnant.
- If you smoke, stop. And, if possible, avoid secondhand smoke (see page 193).
- Don't drink alcohol if you are trying to become pregnant.
- Take a multivitamin daily. Make sure it contains folic acid, which decreases the risk of neural tube defects (birth defects of the spinal column).
- Check with your health care provider about taking over-the-counter or prescription medicines.

During Pregnancy

Once you are pregnant, the best ways to ensure a healthy baby are to:

- Obtain a book on pregnancy. Understand the changes your body is experiencing.
- Make regular visits to your health care provider.
- Eat a healthful diet. Allow for appropriate weight gain.
- Avoid harmful substances such as cigarettes, alcohol and some medications and chemicals.
- Take a prenatal vitamin with folic acid, as prescribed by your physician.
- **Caution:** Bleeding from your vagina during pregnancy may indicate that something is wrong. Call your health care provider immediately. Although some harmless spotting and bleeding occur in many women during early pregnancy, your health care provider will want to rule out miscarriage, ectopic (tubal) pregnancy or other conditions such as a cervical lesion.

Home Pregnancy Tests

Home pregnancy tests provide a private way to find out whether you are pregnant. Most tests use a wand or stick placed into a urine stream or a collected urine specimen to detect the hormone hCG (human chorionic gonadotropin). The placenta begins to produce this hormone soon after conception. When performed correctly, the tests are 95 percent accurate 10 days after a missed period.

Home pregnancy tests can help you get your pregnancy off to a good nutritional start by using prenatal vitamin supplements early. They also help you avoid things that could harm the fetus such as alcohol and smoking and also some medications or chemicals at home or work. Home pregnancy tests also provide early warning for women who have had tubal pregnancy or early miscarriage so they can see their health care provider as soon as possible.

Common Problems

Common Problems During Pregnancy

Common but bothersome concerns you may have during pregnancy are morning sickness, heartburn, backache and other problems. These may make you uncomfortable, but usually they do not threaten your health or the health of your developing baby. If they are severe or persist despite self-care measures, see your doctor.

Morning Sickness
About half of all pregnant women experience morning sickness during the first 12 weeks of pregnancy. Although it doesn't always happen during the morning, the term is used to describe nausea, queasiness or vomiting. It is usually harmless. If you have problems with morning sickness:
- Munch a few crackers before arising in the morning.
- Eat several small meals a day so that your stomach is never empty.
- Avoid smelling or eating foods that trigger the nausea, and avoid spicy, rich and fried foods if you are nauseated.
- Drink plenty of liquids, especially if you are vomiting. Try crushed ice, fruit juice or frozen ice pops if water upsets your stomach.
- Try using acupressure or motion-sickness bands to combat nausea.

Anemia
Some pregnant women develop anemia (an inadequate level of hemoglobin in the blood) because of an iron deficiency or an inadequate supply of folic acid. Symptoms of anemia include fatigue, breathlessness, fainting, palpitations and pale skin. This condition can be risky for both you and your baby. It is easily diagnosed with a blood test. If you are anemic:
- Eat a diet rich in iron (including meat, liver, eggs, dried fruit, whole grains and iron-fortified cereals).
- Eat plenty of leafy green vegetables, liver, lentils, black-eyed peas, kidney beans and other cooked dried beans, oranges and grapefruit.
- Follow your health care provider's recommendations.

Edema (Swelling)
When you are pregnant, your body tissues accumulate more fluid, and swelling is common. Warm weather may aggravate the condition. If you have problems with edema:
- Use cold-water compresses to help relieve swelling.
- Eat a low-salt diet.
- Lie down; elevate your legs for an hour in the middle of the day.
- If your face becomes swollen, especially around the eyes, it may be a sign of a serious condition called preeclampsia. See your doctor right away.

Varicose Veins
About 20 percent of all pregnant women have varicose veins. Pregnancy increases the volume of blood in your body and impairs the flow of blood from your legs to your pelvis. This change causes the veins in your legs to become swollen and sometimes painful. If you have problems with varicose veins:
- Stay off your feet as much as possible, and elevate them as often as you can.
- Wear loose clothing around your legs and waist.
- Wear support stockings from the time you awaken until you go to bed.

Constipation

Constipation may worsen during pregnancy. Bowel activity may be slowed because of the increased pressure on the bowels from the growing baby inside the uterus.

- Drink plenty of liquids—at least 8 to 10 glasses a day.
- Exercise moderately every day.
- Eat several servings of fresh fruits, vegetables and whole grains.
- Try taking a bulk-former that contains psyllium (available without a prescription). Do not take a laxative without discussing it with your health care provider.

Heartburn

Heartburn is a burning sensation in the middle of your chest, often with a bad taste in your mouth. It is caused by reflux—stomach acid flowing up into your food pipe (esophagus). It has nothing to do with your heart. During the later part of pregnancy, your expanding uterus pushes the stomach out of position, which slows the rate that food empties from the stomach.

- Eat smaller meals more often, but eat slowly.
- Avoid greasy foods.
- Don't drink coffee. Both regular and decaffeinated coffee may worsen heartburn.
- Don't eat for 2 to 3 hours before you go to bed, and raise the head of your bed 4 to 6 inches. Reflux is worse when you lie flat.
- If these steps don't work, consult your health care provider, who may recommend an antacid. (See page 64.)

Backache

Backache is common in pregnancy and may worsen if you bend, lift, walk too much or are fatigued. Pain may be in the lower back, or it may radiate down your legs. Your abdomen also may hurt because of the stretching of ligaments. During pregnancy your ligaments are more elastic and so your joints are more prone to strain and injury. Your center of balance also changes during pregnancy. This puts more strain on your back.

- Don't gain more weight than your health care provider recommends.
- Eliminate as much strain as possible. Try wearing a maternity girdle.
- Your health care provider may recommend exercises to relieve the pain.

Hemorrhoids

Hemorrhoids are enlarged veins at the anal opening. They become enlarged from increased pressure. They are often worse during pregnancy and often accompany constipation.

- Avoid becoming constipated.
- Don't strain during bowel movements.
- Take frequent warm-water baths.
- Apply a cotton pad soaked with cold witch hazel cream to the area.

Sleeping Problems

Your sleep may be disturbed during the later stages of pregnancy because of the frequent need to urinate, the movements of your baby or the many things on your mind.

- Avoid caffeine.
- Do not eat a large meal right before bedtime; take a warm bath before going to bed.
- Exercise more during the day.
- If you can't sleep, get out of bed and do something else.
- Do not take any medicines unless recommended by your health care provider.

■ Other Common Medical Conditions

Endometriosis

Endometriosis is a disorder of the reproductive system in which small pieces of the endometrium (the lining of the uterus) are thought to migrate out of the uterus through the fallopian tubes. The pieces implant on other pelvic organs, the pelvic walls and the outside of the ovaries or the fallopian tubes. During menstruation, blood from these patches is absorbed by the surrounding organs, which can cause inflammation. This process can create adhesions (scar tissue, which causes organs to stick together) on the ovaries and fallopian tubes, which can prevent pregnancy. Symptoms include painful periods, worsening of cramping during periods, pain deep in the pelvis during intercourse and pain during bowel movements or urination. The condition causes severe pain in some women, but others have no symptoms.

Endometriosis is diagnosed with laparoscopy (surgery in which a small viewing instrument is passed through a small incision near the navel). Treatment with hormones helps relieve the symptoms, stop the progression and prevent infertility. Sometimes more extensive surgery is needed.

Hysterectomy

Each year, half a million women have a hysterectomy (removal of all or a portion of the uterus). After a hysterectomy, you no longer menstruate, and you can no longer become pregnant.

A *vaginal hysterectomy* is removal of the uterus through an incision in the vagina. An *abdominal hysterectomy* is removal of the uterus through an incision in your abdomen. Abdominal hysterectomy is performed if you have suspected or confirmed uterine or ovarian cancer, extensive endometriosis or scarring in the pelvis, a history of pelvic infection or a uterus that's too large to remove vaginally.

Here's what you can expect during your recuperation:
- After a *vaginal hysterectomy*, you may feel pulling in your groin or have low back pain for a day or two. You may have a discharge for about 3 weeks as the stitches at the top of the vagina dissolve. An *abdominal hysterectomy* may cause more discomfort because the incision goes through the abdominal wall.

Toxic Shock Syndrome

Toxic shock syndrome (TSS) is a reaction to poisons produced by bacteria in the vagina. It typically occurs during menstruation and more frequently in tampon users. The symptoms of TSS develop suddenly, and the disease is serious. Your blood pressure can drop, and you may go into shock. Sometimes kidney failure results. TSS requires immediate medical attention.

Symptoms include a fever of 102 F or higher, vomiting, diarrhea, weakness, dizziness, fainting, disorientation and a rash resembling a sunburn, especially on your palms and soles.

If you use tampons, avoid superabsorbent brands. Change tampons at least every 8 hours. If you have ever had TSS, do not wear tampons at all.

Mayo Clinic Guide to Self-Care

Specific Conditions

- **Respiratory Allergies**
- **Arthritis**
- **Asthma**
- **Cancer**
- **Diabetes**
- **Heart Disease**
- **Hepatitis C**
- **High Blood Pressure**
- **Sexually Transmitted Diseases**

Asthma, arthritis, serious respiratory allergies, cancer, diabetes, high blood pressure, heart disease, hepatitis C and sexually transmitted diseases are common and costly medical conditions in which the normal rules of self-assessment and self-care may not apply. You should be examined by a physician for correct diagnosis and treatment of your condition.

In this section, we offer general guidelines on the prevention and management of these diseases. In some cases, we explain new developments that may be helpful to you. You should discuss new treatments with your doctor to determine their appropriateness to your condition.

Respiratory Allergies

Do you develop itchy, watery eyes or a stuffy, runny nose during the same season every year? Do you sneeze frequently when you're around animals or at work? If you answered "yes" to either of these questions, you may be 1 of 50 million Americans with an allergy (see Allergic Reactions, page 12, and Hives, page 123).

Allergic Reactions and Immune Response

An allergy is an overreaction by your immune system to an otherwise harmless substance, such as pollen or pet dander. Contact with this substance, called an allergen, triggers production of the antibody immunoglobulin E (IgE). IgE causes immune cells in the lining of your eyes and airways to release inflammatory substances, including histamine.

When these chemicals are released, they produce the familiar symptoms of allergy—itchy, red and swollen eyes, a stuffy or runny nose, frequent sneezing and cough, hives or bumps on the skin. This allergic reaction causes or aggravates some forms of asthma (see page 165).

Substances found outdoors, indoors and in the foods you eat can cause allergic reactions. The most common allergens are inhaled:

- **Pollen:** Spring, summer and autumn are the pollen-producing seasons in most climates. During these seasons, exposure to airborne pollen from trees, grasses and weeds is inevitable.
- **Dust mites:** House dust harbors all kinds of potential allergens, including pollen and molds. But the main allergy trigger is the dust mite. Thousands of these microscopic spider-like insects are contained in a pinch of house dust. House dust is a cause of year-round allergy symptoms.
- **Pet dander:** Dogs and especially cats are the most common animals to cause allergic reactions. The animal's dander (skin flakes), saliva, urine and sometimes hair are the main culprits.
- **Molds:** Many people are sensitive to airborne mold spores. Outdoor molds produce spores mostly in the summer and early autumn. Indoor molds shed spores all year long.

Discovering Causes

It's not clear why some people become sensitive to allergens such as pollen. But doctors know the tendency to develop allergies is inherited. If you're bothered by allergies, chances are someone in your immediate family also copes with allergic reactions.

Yet, you and your relatives won't necessarily be sensitive to the same allergens. You're less likely to inherit a sensitivity to a specific substance than you are to inherit the general tendency to develop allergies.

If your symptoms are mild, over-the-counter allergy medicines (usually a combination of an antihistamine and decongestant) may be all the treatment you need. But if your symptoms are persistent or bothersome, a trip to the doctor may bring you relief.

To diagnose allergies accurately, your doctor will need to know about your:

- Symptoms
- Past medical problems
- Past and current living conditions
- Possible exposure to allergens
- Family's medical history
- Diet, lifestyle and recreational habits

The next steps are typically a physical examination and skin tests. During a skin test, tiny, dilute drops of suspected allergens are applied to your skin. Then small pricks or punctures are made through the droplets. If your response to an allergen is positive, a skin reaction like a mosquito bite or small hive (called a wheal and flare) appears at the test site within about 20 minutes.

A positive result of a skin test means only that you might be allergic to a particular substance. To pinpoint the cause of your symptoms, your doctor considers the results of your skin test in addition to your history and physical examination.

The Difference Between Colds and Allergies

Because allergies often cause symptoms similar to those of a cold—congested head and chest, stuffy or runny nose, coughing and sneezing—many people mistake allergies for colds. With a cold, however, symptoms usually go away in a few days. If you have allergies, symptoms may flare under certain conditions or may seem never-ending.

Hay fever (medically referred to as allergic rhinitis) is a common respiratory allergy. The symptoms often appear during pollen season — spring, summer or autumn. Hay fever generally refers to seasonal allergic rhinitis due to pollen. It's not due to hay and there is no fever.

Some people have allergy symptoms mainly in the winter when their homes are closed to ventilation, allowing greater exposure to dust mites and molds. Others may experience symptoms when they enter a room with a cat. Still others find they have symptoms randomly occurring all year long.

Signs and symptoms of hay fever include the following:
- Stuffy or runny nose
- Itchy eyes, nose, throat or roof of your mouth
- Frequent sneezing
- Cough

Myths About Allergy

Allergies often seem vague in origin and unpredictable in response. So it's not surprising that several misconceptions about their causes and cure exist. Three common myths about allergies are described below.
- **Allergies are psychosomatic.** Although hay fever affects your eyes and nose, allergies aren't "all in your head." An allergy is a real medical condition involving your immune system. Stress or emotions may bring on or worsen symptoms, but emotions don't cause allergies.
- **Moving to Arizona will cure allergies.** Some people who are bothered by allergies to pollens and molds believe moving to the Southwest, where the foliage and climate are different, will cause their allergies to disappear. The desert may lack maple trees and ragweed, but it does have other plants that produce pollen such as sagebrush, cottonwood, ash and olive trees. People who are sensitive to some pollens and molds may become sensitive to the pollens and molds found in new environments.
- **Short-haired pets don't cause allergies.** An animal's fur (regardless of its length) isn't the culprit in allergies. The cause is the dander and sometimes saliva and urine. If you're allergic to furry pets, safer pets include fish and reptiles.

Self-Care

The best approach for managing allergies is to know and avoid your triggers:

Pollen
- Stay indoors when the pollen count is highest, between 5 a.m. and 10 a.m. Use an air conditioner with a good filter. Change it often.
- Wear a pollen mask when outdoors and for yard work.
- Vacation out of the region during the height of the pollen season.

Dust or Molds
- Limit your exposure by cleaning your home at least once a week. Wear a mask while cleaning, or have someone else clean for you.
- Encase mattresses, pillows and box springs in dustproof covers.
- Consider replacing upholstered furniture with leather or vinyl, carpeting with wood, vinyl or tile (particularly in the bedroom).
- Maintain indoor humidity between 30 and 50 percent. Use exhaust fans in your bathrooms and kitchen and a dehumidifier in your basement.
- Routinely change furnace filters according to the manufacturer's instructions. Also, consider installing a high-efficiency particulate-arresting (HEPA) filter in your heating system.
- Clean humidifiers frequently to prevent growth of molds and bacteria (see page 108).

Pets
- Avoid pets with fur or feathers. If you choose to keep a furry animal, wash it once a week with soap and water. Keep your animal outside as much as possible, and don't let it in your bedroom.

Medical Help

Antihistamines are widely used to control sneezing, runny nose and itchy eyes or throat. Antihistamines block the action of histamine, one of the irritating chemicals that are largely responsible for symptoms. **Caution:** Some antihistamines can cause drowsiness.

Decongestants relieve some allergy symptoms by reducing congestion or swelling in your nasal membranes. This allows you to breathe more easily. Many over-the-counter medications for allergies and colds combine decongestants with antihistamines.

Nasal sprays, available over-the-counter and by prescription, also can be part of your defense against allergies. The different forms are described here.
- *Corticosteroids:* Available by prescription, they relieve congestion when used daily but take at least a week to become fully effective.
- *Cromolyn sodium:* Nasal sprays containing cromolyn sodium prevent sneezing and an itchy, runny nose caused by mild to moderate allergies.
- *Saline:* Nonprescription nasal sprays containing a saltwater solution relieve mild congestion, loosen mucus and prevent crusting. You can use them safely as needed until symptoms improve.
- *Decongestants:* These sprays aren't intended for relief of chronic allergy symptoms. Avoid them or use sparingly for no more than 3 to 4 days.

Allergy shots (immunotherapy) involve injecting tiny amounts of known allergens into your system. After several injections, usually weekly, you may build up tolerance to the allergen. Then you may need monthly injections for up to several years.

Arthritis

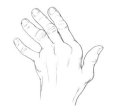

Rheumatoid arthritis can lead to a deformity in the large and middle knuckles.

Arthritis is one of the most common medical problems in the United States. It strikes one person in seven. There are more than 100 forms of arthritis, and they have varying causes, symptoms and treatments. Refer to the chart on page 162 for a summary of symptoms of the major forms of arthritis.

The warning signs of arthritis include the following:
- Swelling in one or more joints
- Prolonged early-morning stiffness
- Recurring pain or tenderness in any joint
- Inability to move a joint normally
- Obvious redness and warmth in a joint
- Unexplained fevers, weight loss or weakness associated with joint pain

Any of these signs, when new, that last for more than 2 weeks require prompt medical evaluation. Distinguishing arthritis from simple aches and pains (rheumatism) is important for treating the problem correctly.

Arthritis can result from the normal wear and tear of the joints (as with osteoarthritis) or from an injury, inflammation, infection or some unknown cause. Most joint ailments caused by inflammation are termed arthritis, from the Greek words *arthron*, for "joint," and *itis*, for "inflammation."

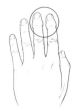

Heberden's nodes are bony lumps at the ends of fingers. They occur most often in women and are a sign of osteoarthritis.

The remainder of this chapter focuses on the management of osteoarthritis, which is the most common form of arthritis. Some of the self-care tips may apply to the other forms. Consult your physician regarding management of other forms of arthritis.

■ Exercise

Over time, exercise is probably the one therapy that will do the most good for managing your arthritis. Exercise must be done regularly to produce improvements. That's why you should check with your doctor and begin a regular exercise program for your specific needs.

Overall, you want to be in good general physical condition. This means maintaining flexibility, strength and endurance. Together, these will protect your joints against further damage, keep them aligned, reduce stiffness and minimize pain.

Different types of exercise achieve different goals. For flexibility, range-of-motion exercises (gentle stretching) move the joint from one end position to the other. In severe osteoarthritis, range-of-motion exercises may cause pain. Do not continue exercise beyond the point that is painful without the advice of your doctor or physical therapist.

Moving large muscle groups for 15 to 20 minutes is the primary way of exercising aerobically to strengthen muscles and build endurance. Walking, bicycling, swimming and dancing are good examples of aerobic-type exercises with low to moderate stress on the joint.

If you're carrying a lot of extra weight, moving around is more difficult. You're putting stress on your back, hips, knees and feet—all common places to have osteoarthritis. There's no positive evidence that excess weight causes osteoarthritis, but obesity clearly makes the symptoms worse.

Common Forms of Arthritis

Cause and Frequency	Key Symptoms	How Serious Is It?

Osteoarthritis

Associated with normal wear and tear on the joints. May be due to an imbalance of enzymes. Common in people older than 50; rare in young people unless a joint is injured	• Pain in a joint after use • Discomfort in a joint before or during a change in weather • Swelling and a loss of flexibility in a joint • Bony lumps at finger joints • Aching is common. Redness and warmth are less common	Usually not serious. It doesn't go away, although the pain may come and go. The effects are crippling in only rare cases. Joints such as the hip and knee may deteriorate to the point of needing replacement surgery. Age is the most significant factor.

Rheumatoid arthritis

The most common form of inflammatory arthritis.* Most often develops between ages 20 and 50. Probably caused by the body's immune system attacking joint-lining tissue	• Pain and swelling in the small joints of hands and feet • Overall aching or stiffness, especially first thing in the morning or after periods of rest • Affected joints are swollen, painful and warm during initial attack and flare-ups	It is the most debilitating form of arthritis. Disease frequently causes deformed joints. Some people experience sweats and fever along with the loss of strength in muscles attached to affected joints. Often chronic, although it can come and go

Infectious arthritis

Infectious agents include bacteria, fungus and viruses. Can be complication of sexually transmitted diseases. Can occur in anyone	• Pain and stiffness in one joint, typically a knee, shoulder, hip, ankle, elbow, finger or wrist • Surrounding tissues are warm and red • Chills, fever and weakness • May be associated with a rash	In most cases, prompt diagnosis and treatment of a joint infection result in rapid and complete recovery

Gout

Uric acid crystals form in joint. Most patients are men older than 40	• Severe pain that strikes suddenly in a single joint, often at the base of the big toe • Swelling and redness	An acute attack can be treated effectively. After an attack has run its course, the affected joint usually returns to normal. Attacks can recur and may require preventive treatment to lower uric acid levels in the blood

*Other types of inflammatory arthritis include *psoriatic arthritis,* which occurs in people with psoriasis, especially in the finger and foot joints; *Reiter's syndrome,* which often is transmitted by sexual contact and is characterized by pain in the joints, penile discharge, painful inflammation of the eye and a rash; *ankylosing spondylitis,* which affects the joints of the spine and, in advanced cases, causes a very stiff, inflexible backbone.

Medications Control Discomfort

The most common over-the-counter and prescription drugs used for osteoarthritis are described below. (See page 265 for more information on the use of these medications.)

- **Acetaminophen:** This nonprescription product relieves pain as well as aspirin and is less likely to upset your stomach. It doesn't help inflammation, but because joints often are not inflamed in osteoarthritis, it's a good choice most of the time.
- **NSAIDs:** The acronym stands for nonsteroidal anti-inflammatory drugs. NSAIDs include aspirin, ibuprofen, naproxen and ketoprofen. Dosage makes a difference, so your physician needs to specify the amount that's right for you. Aspirin may relieve pain with 2 tablets every 4 hours. You might need to take this dosage for a week or two for inflammation. Other NSAIDs may work as well as aspirin and may have fewer side effects, but they cost more. You may need to take fewer doses daily than you would aspirin.
- **Corticosteroids:** These are like a hormone made in the adrenal gland of your body. They decrease inflammation. About 20 types are available; the most common is prednisone. Doctors do not prescribe oral corticosteroids for osteoarthritis, but they may occasionally inject a cortisone drug into an acutely inflamed joint. Because frequent use of this drug may accelerate joint disease, injections may be limited to no more than two or three annually.

Caution

Many over-the-counter pain relievers and anti-inflammatory drugs can irritate the lining of your stomach and intestines and cause ulcers and even severe bleeding with long-term use. **Consult your physician if you are using NSAIDs or aspirin regularly for more than 2 weeks to treat joint pain.** A newer class of prescription medications, called cox-2 inhibitors, may be less damaging to the stomach.

Other Methods to Relieve Pain

Ask your doctor or your physical or occupational therapist about the therapies described below.

- **Heat** can relax muscles around a painful joint. You can apply heat superficially with warm water, a paraffin bath, electric pad, hot pack or heat lamp; but be careful to avoid a burn. For deep penetration, a physical therapist can use ultrasound or short-wave diathermy.
- **Cold** acts as a local anesthetic. It also decreases muscle spasms. Cold packs may help when you ache from holding muscles in the same position to avoid pain.
- **Splints** support and protect weak, painful joints during activity and provide proper positioning at night, which promotes restful sleep. Constant splinting, however, can weaken muscles and decrease flexibility.
- **Relaxation** techniques, including hypnosis, visualization, deep breathing, muscle relaxation, and other techniques may decrease pain.
- **Glucosamine supplements** are gaining in popularity. There is evidence that these over-the-counter dietary supplements can be helpful. But be careful when selecting one. Quality control often leaves much to be desired.
- **Other techniques,** such as low-impact exercise, weight management, orthotics (such as shoe inserts) and gait aids (canes and walking sticks), strengthen muscles and reduce pressure on joints and thus decrease pain.

■ Joint Protection

Correct "body mechanics" help you move with minimal strain. A physical or occupational therapist can suggest techniques and equipment that protect your joints while decreasing stress and conserving energy.

Modifications you can make include:

- Avoid grasping actions that strain your finger joints. For example, instead of a clutch-style purse, select one with a shoulder strap. Use hot water to loosen a jar lid and pressure from your palm to open it, or use a jar opener. Don't twist or use your joints forcefully.
- Spread the weight of an object over several joints. Use both hands, for example, to lift a heavy pan. Try using a walking stick or cane.
- Take a break periodically to relax and stretch.
- Poor posture causes uneven weight distribution and may strain ligaments and muscles.
- Throughout the day, use your strongest muscles, and favor large joints. Don't push open a heavy glass door. Lean into it. To pick up an object, bend your knees and squat while keeping your back straight.
- Special tools that make gripping easier are available for buttoning shirts and kitchen use. Contact your pharmacy or health care provider for information on ordering these items.

Don't Be Duped by Unproven Cures

One person in 10 who tries an unproven arthritis remedy reports harmful side effects. Here are some popular, but false, nutrition claims:

- **Cod liver oil "lubricates" stiff joints.** It may sound logical, but your body treats cod liver oil like any other fat; it provides no special help for joints. Large amounts of cod liver oil can lead to vitamin A and D toxicity.
- **Some foods cause "allergic arthritis."** There's no proof that food allergy causes arthritis. Also,

you can't relieve arthritis by avoiding tomatoes or other foods.

- **Fish oils reduce inflammation.** Research on rheumatoid arthritis suggests that omega-3 fatty acids in fish oils may give modest, temporary relief of inflammation. This finding is valid, but we don't advise fish oil supplements. You'd need about 15 capsules a day—and doctors don't know whether that's a safe amount. A lower dose won't help.

FOR MORE INFORMATION

- Arthritis Foundation, 1330 West Peachtree Street, Atlanta, GA 30309; (800) 283-7800; Internet address: http://www.arthritis.org.
- National Institute of Arthritis, Musculoskeletal and Skin Diseases Information Clearinghouse, National Institutes of Health, 1 AMS Circle, Bethesda, MD 20892-3675; (877) 226-4267; Internet address: http://www.nih.gov/niams.org.
- American College of Rheumatology, 1800 Century Place, Suite 250, Atlanta, GA 30345; (404) 633-3777; Internet address: http://www.rheumatology.org.

Asthma

Asthma occurs when the main air passages of your lungs, called the bronchial tubes, become inflamed. The muscles of bronchial walls tighten, and extra mucus is produced. Airflow out of your lungs is diminished, often causing wheezing.

Common symptoms are wheezing, difficulty breathing, "tightness" in the chest and coughing. In emergencies, the person will have extreme difficulty in breathing, bluish lips and nails, severe breathlessness, increased pulse rate, sweating and severe coughing.

Asthma is a serious medical condition, but with proper care and treatment you usually can control your symptoms and lead a normal life.

Approximately 10 percent of children and 5 percent of adults in the United States have asthma. About half of the children who have asthma develop the condition before age 10. Asthma is usually an inherited condition, and it is not contagious.

There are many causes, or "triggers," of asthma attacks. They can be triggered by an allergic reaction to dust mites, cockroaches, chemicals, pollen, mold or animal dander (dead skin cells that fall off animals). They can be triggered by exposure to substances in the home or workplace. Some people are more prone to suffer an asthma attack after exercise, especially if they exercise in cold air.

Respiratory infections caused by colds and the flu can aggravate the symptoms of asthma. (Adults with chronic asthma should get a yearly flu shot. Pregnant women and children, however, should check with their health care provider before receiving flu shots.) Some additional triggers of asthma include sulfites, which are sprayed on vegetables and fruits by restaurants and stores to keep them from turning brown. Other foods or beverages, such as wine, also may contain sulfites as a preservative. Aspirin and other nonsteroidal anti-inflammatory drugs (NSAIDs) may trigger an asthma attack in some people.

Asthma attacks can range from very mild to life-threatening (see below). Asthma attacks can last for just a few minutes, or they can go on for hours and even days. If you have asthma, you should be receiving treatment from a health care provider. Your health care provider will work with you to identify the triggers that cause your asthma attacks. Together, you will devise a strategy to limit your exposure to these triggers, help control your symptoms and make sure your breathing is not severely obstructed.

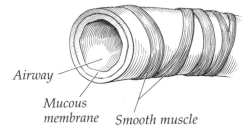

Airway
Mucous membrane
Smooth muscle

Normal airways in your lungs.

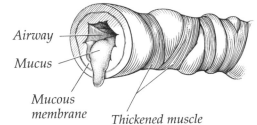

Airway
Mucus
Mucous membrane
Thickened muscle

In asthma, airways in your lungs are inflamed and swollen.

Recognizing a Life-Threatening Attack

Prevent fatal attacks by treating symptoms early. Don't wait for wheezing as a sign of severity; wheezing may disappear when airflow is severely restricted. Get emergency care if:

- Breathing becomes difficult and your neck, chest or ribs pull in with each breath
- Nostrils flare
- Walking or talking becomes difficult
- Fingernails or lips turn blue
- Peak airflow (measured with a handheld meter you can use at home) reading decreases 50 percent below your normal level or keeps decreasing even after you take your medication

The following tips help control symptoms by "trigger-proofing" your environment.

- Educate yourself about asthma. The more you know, the easier it is to control.
- Avoid allergens that might trigger your symptoms. If you are allergic to cats or dogs, remove these pets from your home and avoid contact with other people's pets. Avoid buying clothing, furniture or rugs made from animal hair.
- If you are allergic to airborne pollens and molds, use air-conditioning at home, at work and in your car. (If temperature changes irritate your symptoms, you may not be able to do this.) Keep doors and windows closed to limit exposure to airborne pollens and molds.
- Avoid activities that might contribute to your symptoms. For example, home improvement projects might expose you to triggers that lead to an asthma attack, such as paint vapors, wood dust or similar irritants.
- Check your furnace. If you have a forced-air heating system and you are allergic to dust, use a filter for dust control. Change or clean filters on heating and cooling units frequently. (The best filter is a high-efficiency particulate-arresting filter, referred to as a HEPA filter.) Wear a mask when you remove dirty filters.
- Install an electrostatic filter on your vacuum cleaner (or use a two-ply microfiltration bag).
- Avoid projects that raise dust. If you cannot, then use a dust mask, which is available at drugstores and hardware stores.
- Review exercise habits and consider adjusting your routine (see below). Consider exercising indoors, which may limit your exposure to asthma triggers.
- Avoid all types of smoke, even smoke from a fireplace or burning leaves. Smoke irritates the eyes, nose and bronchial tubes. If you have asthma, you should not smoke and people should never smoke in your presence.
- Reduce stress and fatigue.
- Read labels carefully.
- If sensitive to aspirin, avoid other nonsteroidal anti-inflammatory agents (ibuprofen such as Motrin, Advil, Nuprin; naproxen such as Naprosyn, Anaprox, Aleve; and piroxicam such as Feldene).

Staying Active With Well-Planned Workouts

Years ago if you had asthma, doctors told you not to exercise. Now they believe well-planned regular workouts are beneficial, especially if you have mild to moderate disease. If you're fit, your heart and lungs don't have to work as hard to expel air.

But, because vigorous exercise can trigger an attack, be sure to discuss an exercise program with your doctor. In addition, follow these guidelines:

- **Know when not to exercise.** Avoid exercise when you have a viral infection, when the pollen count is more than 100 or in below-zero or extremely hot and humid conditions. In cold temperatures, wear a face mask to warm the air you breathe.
- **Medicate first.** Use your inhaled short-acting beta agonist 15 to 60 minutes before exercise.
- **Start slowly.** Five to 10 minutes of warm-up exercises may relax your chest muscles and widen your airways to ease breathing. Gradually work up to your desired pace.
- **Choose the type of exercise wisely.** Cold-weather activities such as skiing and long-distance, nonstop activities such as running most often cause wheezing. Exercise that requires short bursts of energy, such as walking, golf and leisure bicycling, may be better tolerated.

Medical Help

Testing for allergies: Your health care provider may perform some tests to try to determine the triggers of your asthma attacks. A skin test or blood test may be performed. The blood test is more expensive and is less sensitive than skin tests, but it is sometimes preferable when the person being tested has a skin disease or is taking medications that might affect the test results.

Medications: Your doctor may prescribe some of the medications listed below to prevent or treat your asthma attacks. Take all the medications as prescribed, even if you are not experiencing any symptoms. Do not take more than the prescribed amount (excessive use of medications can be dangerous). These medications can be taken using an inhaler, or they may come in liquid, capsule or tablet form.

Preventers (anti-inflammatory medications) reduce the inflammation in your airways and also help reduce the production of mucus.
The result is a reduction of the spasms in your breathing passages. Take the daily dose of these medications as prescribed to prevent asthma attacks from occurring. Preventers include inhaled steroids, cromolyn sodium and nedocromil sodium.

Relievers (also called "bronchodilators"), unlike preventers, are taken once you are experiencing an asthma attack. Relievers help open narrow airways to allow you to breathe more easily during an attack. Relievers include beta agonists and theophylline.

Self-monitoring with peak flowmeter: You may be trained to use a peak flowmeter, a tube that measures how well you are breathing. The flowmeter acts like a gauge for your lungs, giving you a number that helps evaluate lung function. A low reading means your air passages are narrow and is an early warning that you may experience an asthma attack.

Inhalers: Risks of Misuse

Inhaling a bronchodilator (see Medical Help above) helps you breathe better immediately during an attack. But the drug doesn't correct inflammation.

Maximal daily use of a bronchodilator is two puffs every 4 to 6 hours. If you use one more frequently to control symptoms, you need a more effective medication.

Fast relief may make it difficult to recognize worsening symptoms. Once the medication wears off, asthma returns with more severe wheezing.

You're then tempted to take another dose of the medication, delaying adequate treatment with anti-inflammatory medications.

Overuse also risks toxic drug levels that may lead to an irregular heartbeat, especially if you have a heart condition.

Over-the-counter inhalers also can relieve symptoms quickly—but temporarily. Relying on inhalers can mask a worsening attack and delay treatment with anti-inflammatory medications.

FOR MORE INFORMATION

- Asthma and Allergy Foundation of America, 1233 20th St., Suite 402, Washington, D.C. 20036; (800) 727-8462.; Internet address: http://www.aafa.org.
- American Lung Association, 1740 Broadway, New York, NY 10019; (800) 586-4872; Internet address: http://www.lungusa.org.
- National Institute of Allergy and Infectious Disease (NIH), Building 31, Room 7A50, 31 Center Drive, MSC 2520, Bethesda, MD 20892-2520; (301) 496-5717; Internet address: http://www.niaid.nih.gov.

Cancer

The day your cancer is diagnosed becomes a major event in your life. You see everything that follows in the context of your cancer diagnosis and treatment. That's a normal reaction.

There are many different kinds of cancer. We're constantly finding new ways to detect and treat it. Recently, survival rates for some cancers have improved dramatically. Now, we talk of "living with cancer," rather than "dying of cancer" or becoming a "victim of cancer."

New cases of cancer by site and sex. The statistics are 2001 estimates by the American Cancer Society. Figures exclude basal and squamous cell skin cancers and superficial cancers (in situ carcinoma), except bladder. (By permission of the American Cancer Society.)

Male

Prostate
198,100 (31%)
Lung & bronchus
90,700 (14%)
Colon & rectum
67,300 (10%)
Urinary bladder
39,200 (6%)
Non-Hodgkin's lymphoma
31,100 (5%)
Melanoma of the skin
29,000 (5%)
Oral cavity
20,200 (3%)
Kidney
18,700 (3%)
Leukemia
17,700 (3%)
Pancreas
14,200 (2%)

All sites
643,000 (100%)

Female

Breast
192,200 (31%)
Lung & bronchus
78,800 (13%)
Colon & rectum
68,100 (11%)
Uterine corpus
38,300 (6%)
Non-Hodgkin's lymphoma
25,100 (4%)
Ovary
23,400 (4%)
Melanoma of the skin
22,400 (4%)
Urinary bladder
15,100 (2%)
Pancreas
15,000 (2%)
Thyroid
14,900 (2%)

All sites
625,000 (100%)

The diagram shows the estimated number of new cases of various kinds of cancer in 2001, according to the affected body part. The remainder of this chapter includes some advice for you or a family member with cancer.

For specific information on various types of cancer, refer to Index page 298.

■ Responding to the Cancer Diagnosis

As with any crisis or difficult time in life, you need healthful and effective coping strategies. Here are some suggestions:

1. **Get the facts.** Try to obtain as much basic, useful information as possible. Consider bringing a family member or friend with you to doctor appointments. Write down your questions and concerns beforehand. This approach helps you organize your thoughts, obtain accurate information, understand your cancer and treatment and participate in decision making. But remember, the answers are frequently educated guesses or statistics. Everyone is different. Questions often include the following:
   - Is my cancer curable?
   - What are my treatment options?

- What can I expect during treatment?
- Will my treatments be painful?
- When do I need to call my doctor?
- What can I do to prevent cancer from recurring?
- What are the risk factors for my family members (especially children)?

2. **Develop your own coping strategy.** Just as each person's cancer treatment is individualized, so is the coping strategy that you must follow. Here are some ideas:
   - Learn relaxation techniques (see page 225).
   - Share feelings honestly with family, friends, a pastor or counselor.
   - Keep a journal to help organize your thoughts.
   - When faced with a difficult decision, list pros and cons for each choice.
   - Find a source of strength in your faith.
   - Find time to be alone.
   - Remain involved with work and leisure activities.

3. **Keep communication open** between you and your loved ones, health care providers and others. You may feel particularly isolated if people try to protect you by keeping disappointing news from you or trying to put up a strong front. If you and others feel free to express your emotions, you can gain strength from each other.

4. **Your self-image is important.** Although some people may not notice physical changes, you will. Insurance will often help pay for wigs, prostheses and special adaptive devices.

5. **A healthful lifestyle** can improve your energy level and promote healthy cell growth. This includes adequate rest, good nutrition, exercise and fun activities.

6. **Let friends and family help you.** Often they can run errands, drive the carpool, prepare meals and help with household chores. Learn to accept help. Accepting help also gives those who care about you a sense of purpose at a difficult time.

7. **Review your goals and priorities.** Consider what's really important in your life. Reduce unnecessary activities. Find a new openness with loved ones. Share your thoughts and feelings with them. Cancer affects all of your relationships. Communication can help reduce the anxiety and fear that cancer can cause.

8. **Try to maintain your normal lifestyle.** Take each day one at a time. It's easy to overlook this simple strategy during stressful times. When the future is uncertain, organizing and planning for it can suddenly become overwhelming.

9. **Maintain a positive attitude.** Celebrate each day. If a day is difficult, let go of it and move on. Don't let cancer control your life.

10. **Fight stigmas.** Many of the old stigmas associated with cancer still exist. Your friends may wonder if cancer is contagious. Coworkers may doubt you're healthy enough to do your job and think you'll drain their health benefits. Reassure others that research shows cancer survivors are just as productive as other workers and don't miss work any more often. Remind friends that even if cancer has been a frightening part of your life, it shouldn't scare them to be near you.

11. **Look into insurance options.** If you're employed, you may feel "trapped," unable to change jobs for fear of not being eligible for new insurance. If you're retired, you may have difficulty purchasing supplemental insurance. Find out whether your state provides health insurance for people who are difficult to insure. Look into group insurance options through professional, fraternal or political organizations.

■ Nutrition: A Big "Plus"

There is no conclusive evidence that avoiding or overeating any specific food helps treat cancer. However, good nutrition is important to living with cancer. Your cancer treatment may reduce your appetite and change the flavor of foods. It also may interfere with absorption of nutrients in foods. Studies show that good nutrition can:

- Improve your chances of tolerating your treatment successfully
- Improve your sense of well-being
- Enhance your tissue and immune system functions
- Help meet demands for calories and proteins to rebuild damaged tissues

A new medicine, megestrol acetate (available in pill or liquid form), taken several times a day may help maintain or increase your weight.

Self-Care

Here are some specific tips for good nutrition:

- If the taste of meat bothers you, mild-tasting dairy products such as cottage cheese and yogurt are good alternative sources of protein. Try eating a peanut butter sandwich or peanut butter spread on fruit. Legumes such as kidney beans, chickpeas and black-eyed peas are good sources of protein, especially when combined with grains such as rice, corn or bread.
- Pack as many calories as possible into the foods you eat. Warm your bread, and spread it with butter, margarine, jam or honey. Sprinkle foods with chopped nuts.
- Lightly seasoned dishes made with milk products, eggs, poultry, fish and pasta often are well tolerated.
- If you have trouble eating an adequate amount of food at a single sitting, eat smaller amounts more frequently. Chew your food slowly.
- If the aroma of food being prepared makes you ill, use a microwave or choose foods that need little cooking or that can be warmed at a low temperature.
- Nourishing liquids can boost protein and calories. Cream soups, milk, cocoa, milk shakes or malts or commercially prepared nutritional beverages may help. Your physician or dietitian can help determine whether you need a supplement.

■ What About Pain?

Pain is a big fear among people with cancer, but it need not be. More than half of all people who have cancer don't have notable pain. In fact, patients with cancer often experience less pain than people with arthritis or nerve disorders. Pain is almost always controllable. Pain control medications include the following:

- **Nonnarcotic drugs:** Aspirin is highly effective, and it often provides relief equivalent to more powerful painkillers. Other nonsteroidal anti-inflammatory drugs and acetaminophen are equally effective and may require fewer doses per day than aspirin (see page 265). Antidepressants also are helpful pain relievers.
- **Narcotics** (morphine and codeine), used for severe pain, may be given by mouth (pills or liquid), injections, pumps you control or a slow-release skin patch.
- **Tranquilizers** may improve your comfort level when used with pain medications.

Nondrug pain control measures include radiation to shrink a tumor and lessen pain; injection or surgery to block pathways of nerves carrying pain messages to your brain; biofeedback, behavior modification, hypnosis, breathing and relaxation exercises, massage, transcutaneous electrical nerve stimulation or hot/cold packs.

Self-Care	• Don't wait for the pain to become severe before taking a pain medication. Take pain medicines on a schedule.
	• Don't be concerned about addiction. When used properly, the chance for addiction to narcotics is very small. Besides, if a narcotic is needed for a long time to relieve severe pain, the comfort it provides is often more important than any possibility of addiction.
	• Develop a strategy for dealing with emotions such as anxiety and depression. They can make the pain seem worse.

■ Cancer in Children

Cancer in children is uncommon, but when it happens parents face special issues and problems. Researchers have made great strides in finding effective treatments for childhood cancers. Today, more than 70 percent of American children with cancer survive.

Self-Care

If your child has cancer, it's important to:
- Carefully choose the person who will treat your child. Look for a medical center with the latest treatments for childhood cancers. It also should provide emotional support for your family.
- Try to maintain as normal a lifestyle as possible. Keeping schedules, rules and previous expectations in place will help your child cope and plant the idea of a long future.
- Talk to your child's teachers to establish behavioral and academic expectations.
- Do your best to deal with the possibility of death in an honest, straightforward manner. Children need to be told as much as they can understand. There is no single "right" way to tell children about death. Encourage them to ask questions. Give them simple answers. Their fears may keep them from asking questions, so start by asking how they feel. Never lie, make promises you may not be able to keep or be afraid to say, "I don't know."
- Promote activities that reduce anxiety (such as drawing) and express feelings (role-playing or puppets).
- Don't ignore the needs of your other children. Siblings can be very supportive to their ill brother or sister, but they must know that their special place in the family is secure.
- Read "Talking With Your Child About Cancer," from the National Institutes of Health (Pamphlet #91-2761, available from the National Cancer Institute) (see below).

FOR MORE INFORMATION
- The National Cancer Institute Information Service, (800) 4-CANCER; CancerFax (800) 624-2511 (24 hours); Internet address: http://cancernet.nci.nih.gov.
- The American Cancer Society, 1599 Clifton Road NE, Atlanta GA 30329-4251; (800) ACS-2345; Internet address: http://www.cancer.org.

Specific Conditions

Diabetes

Diabetes is a disorder of your metabolism—the way your body uses digested food for energy and growth. Normally, your digestive system converts a portion of the food you eat into a sugar called glucose. That sugar then enters your bloodstream, ready to fuel your cells.

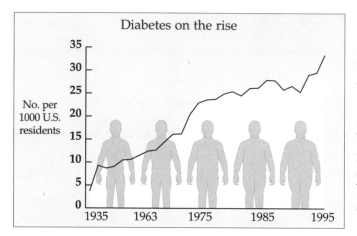

Diabetes on the rise

No. per 1000 U.S. residents

Diabetes has increased dramatically as obesity has become more common in the United States. The number of Americans diagnosed with any form of diabetes was just 3.7 per 1,000 U.S. residents in 1935. In 1995, it was 33.2 per 1,000 residents.

In order for your cells to receive the sugar, insulin, a hormone produced by your pancreas, must "escort" it in. Normally, your pancreas produces enough insulin to handle all the sugar that is present. There are two types of diabetes, both of which disrupt this process.

In type 1 diabetes, your pancreas produces reduced amounts of insulin. In type 2 diabetes, your body doesn't respond normally to the insulin that is made. In both types of diabetes, sugar enters body cells only in limited amounts. Some of the sugar then builds up in your blood, overflows into your urine and passes from your body unused.

Both types of diabetes can cause long-term complications such as heart disease, kidney failure, nerve damage, blindness and deterioration of blood vessels and nerves. Damage to your body's small and large blood vessels is at the root of most of these complications.

Type 1 and Type 2: What's the Difference?

Type 1 diabetes affects 1 in 10 people with diabetes. It is also known as insulin-dependent diabetes mellitus (IDDM) or juvenile-onset diabetes and usually develops before age 30. If you have type 1 diabetes, you must receive insulin daily for the rest of your life. The symptoms can develop abruptly and include the following:

- Excessive thirst
- Frequent urination
- Extreme hunger
- Unexplained weight loss
- Weakness and fatigue

Type 2 diabetes is the most common form of diabetes. It is also called non-insulin-dependent diabetes mellitus (NIDDM) or adult-onset diabetes. Type 2 most often occurs after age 40 in overweight people. Balanced diet, moderate weight loss and exercise often can control it. If diet and exercise aren't effective, you may need oral medication or insulin injections. Many people with type 2 diabetes have few or no symptoms. These symptoms can develop slowly and include the following:

- Excessive thirst
- Frequent urination
- Blurred vision
- Recurring bladder, vaginal and skin infections
- Slow-healing sores
- Irritability
- Tingling or loss of feeling in your hands or feet

Mayo Clinic Guide to Self-Care

Self-Care

Managing diabetes is a balancing act. Illness, eating too much or too little, a change in exercise, travel and stress all affect your blood sugar level. Here are some tips to help you gain tighter control of your blood sugar level.

Diet

A well-balanced diet is the cornerstone of diabetes management. Remember to:

- **Stick to a schedule.** Eat three meals a day. Be consistent in the amount of food you eat and the timing of eating. If you take insulin or an oral diabetes medication, you may need to eat a bedtime snack.
- **Focus on fiber.** Eat a variety of fresh fruits, vegetables, legumes and whole-grain foods. These are low-fat and rich sources of vitamins and minerals.
- **Limit foods that are high in fat** to less than 30 percent of your total calorie intake. Choose lean cuts of meats and use low-fat dairy products.
- **Don't push proteins.** Too much protein can take its toll on your kidneys. Limit meat to about 6 ounces a day. This will also help you limit cholesterol.
- **Avoid "empty" calories.** Candy, cookies and other sweets are not forbidden. But because they have little nutritional value, eat them in moderation and count them in your total carbohydrate intake.
- **Use alcohol in moderation.** If your doctor says it's safe, choose drinks that are low in sugar and alcohol, such as light beer and dry wines. Count alcoholic drinks in your total carbohydrate intake and do not drink on an empty stomach.
- **Watch your weight.** If you're overweight, losing even a few pounds can improve your blood sugar levels.

Exercise

Regular exercise helps maintain overall health, benefits your heart and blood vessels and may improve circulation. It helps control your blood sugar level and may help prevent type 2 diabetes. If you have type 2 diabetes, regular exercise and a healthful diet may reduce or even eliminate your need for injected insulin or an oral medication.

Exercise alone is not enough to achieve good control of your blood sugar level if you have type 1 diabetes. However, it may enhance the effects of insulin that you take. You may need to eat additional food just before or during exercise to prevent sudden changes in your blood sugar level. Follow your doctor's advice on exercise.

Monitoring Your Blood Sugar

Checking your blood sugar level regularly is essential for managing your diabetes. How often you need to perform this test depends on the type of diabetes you have, how stable your blood sugar levels are and other factors. Your health care team can help you determine reasonable goals for your blood sugar level. In addition to sticking with a proper diet and exercise, you also may need to learn how to adjust your medications, especially insulin, to keep your blood sugar level near normal.

Today, blood tests are the most accurate way to check your blood sugar level. To do so, you put a drop of fingertip blood onto a chemically treated test strip. The test strip reacts to the amount of glucose in your blood by changing color. You can read the blood glucose level by holding the test strip next to a color guide chart or by having an electronic glucose monitor read it. Reliable monitors cost between $40 and $120.

Self-Care

Medications

You may need medications to control your blood sugar level. But even with medication, exercise and diet are integral to managing your diabetes.

If you have type 1 diabetes, you must take insulin by injection. Insulin can't be taken by mouth because it breaks down in your digestive tract. The number of daily injections and type of insulin prescribed (short-, intermediate- or long-lasting) depend on your individual needs. If your blood sugar level is hard to control, your health care provider may prescribe frequent injections or an insulin pump.

If you have type 2 diabetes and have trouble controlling your blood sugar with diet and exercise alone, your doctor may prescribe one of several oral medications. These medications can help your pancreas produce more insulin or help insulin to work better in your body. If oral medications aren't working well, insulin injections are best. Good control of the blood sugar level is key to avoiding complications.

Caution

Diabetes can cause one or more of the following emergencies:

Insulin reaction: This is also called hypoglycemia (low blood sugar). It can occur when excess insulin, excess exercise or too little food causes a decreased blood sugar level. Symptoms usually appear several hours after eating and include trembling, weakness and drowsiness followed by confusion, dizziness and double vision. If untreated, a low blood sugar level may cause seizures or loss of consciousness.

If you are concerned that you are having an insulin reaction, try eating something containing sugar, such as fruit juices, candy or soft drinks containing sugar, and check your blood sugar level. If you are helping someone in this condition, seek emergency medical care if the person vomits or is unable to cooperate, or if symptoms persist beyond 30 minutes after treatment. Remain with the person for an hour after recovery to ensure that he or she is thinking clearly.

Diabetic coma: Also called diabetic ketoacidosis or DKA, this complication develops more slowly than an insulin reaction, often over hours or days. DKA occurs when the blood sugar level is too high (hyperglycemia). Nausea, vomiting, abdominal pain, weakness, thirst, sweet-smelling breath and deeper and more rapid breathing all can precede gradual confusion and loss of consciousness. This reaction is most likely to occur in persons with type 1 diabetes who are ill or skip an insulin dose. It can be the first symptom of previously undiagnosed diabetes.

Foot Care Reduces the Risk of Injury and Infection

Diabetes can impair the circulation and nerve supply to your feet. Foot care is essential:

- Inspect your feet daily. Look for sores, color changes or altered sensation. Get help or a mirror to view all surfaces.
- Bathe your feet daily. Use warm (not hot) soapy water. Dry them thoroughly.
- Trim nails straight across, file rough edges.

- Don't use wart removers or trim calluses and corns yourself. See your doctor or a podiatrist.
- Wear cushioned, well-fitted shoes. Check inside shoes daily for sharp edges. Don't walk barefoot.
- Avoid tight clothing around your legs or ankles. Don't smoke; smoking can make bad circulation worse.

FOR MORE INFORMATION

- The American Diabetes Association, 1701 N. Beauregard St., Alexandria, VA 22311; (800) DIABETES; Internet address: http://www.diabetes.org.

Mayo Clinic Guide to Self-Care

Heart Disease

Your heart pumps blood to every tissue in your body through a 60,000-mile network of blood vessels. Blood supplies the tissues with oxygen and nutrients that are essential for good health.

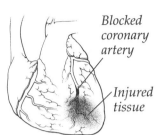

Blocked coronary artery

Injured tissue

A heart attack occurs when arteries supplying your heart with blood and oxygen become blocked.

Problems can arise in the heart muscle, the heart valves, the electrical conduction system, the pericardium (the sac that surrounds the heart) or the coronary arteries (the arteries that supply blood to the heart muscle itself). This chapter focuses on problems in the coronary arteries. Coronary artery problems cause "heart attacks," which kill 500,000 Americans annually.

As you age, fatty deposits may form in the coronary arteries in your heart, creating a condition called coronary artery disease. Atherosclerosis—"hardening of the arteries"—can occur in arteries in other areas of your body as well. As the coronary arteries become narrowed or blocked, blood flow to your heart muscle is reduced or stopped.

When your heart muscle doesn't receive enough blood, you may feel chest pain or pressure (angina). If the blood flow is blocked long enough in a coronary artery (about 30 minutes to 2 hours), the portion of the heart muscle that is supplied by that artery will die. Heart muscle death is known as a myocardial infarction (MI) or heart attack.

A heart attack usually is caused by sudden blockage of a heart artery by a blood clot. The clot usually forms in an artery that has been narrowed by fatty deposits.

Heart Attack: Reacting Promptly May Save a Life

A heart attack generally causes chest pain for more than 15 minutes. But a heart attack also can be "silent" and have no symptoms. About half of heart attack victims have warning symptoms hours, days or weeks in advance.

The American Heart Association lists the following warning signs of a heart attack. Be aware that you may not have them at all and that symptoms may come and go.
- Uncomfortable pressure, fullness or squeezing pain in the center of your chest, lasting more than a few minutes.
- Pain spreading to your shoulders, neck or arms.

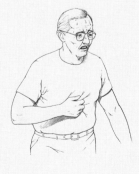

The pain of heart attack varies from person to person, but typically there is a profound squeezing sensation in the chest, accompanied by profuse perspiration. Pain may radiate to the left shoulder and arm, to the back and even to the jaw.

- Light-headedness, fainting, sweating, nausea or shortness of breath.

The more of these symptoms you have, the more likely it is that you are having a heart attack. Whether you suspect a heart attack or think it's just indigestion, act immediately:
- Call 911 first.
- Sit quietly or lie down if you are feeling faint. Breathe slowly and deeply.
- Chew an aspirin, unless you are allergic to it. Aspirin thins the blood and can decrease death rates significantly.

If you observe someone with chest pain, follow the above steps. If the person faints or loses consciousness, begin CPR (see page 2).

Once the heart attack victim arrives at a medical center, he or she may be given clot-dissolving drugs or undergo a procedure called angioplasty, which involves widening blocked arteries to let blood flow more freely to the heart. If the use of clot-dissolving drugs or angioplasty is delayed beyond 2 hours, benefits are substantially reduced.

Specific Conditions

What Is Your Risk of Heart Disease?

Cigarette smoking, high blood pressure and high blood cholesterol are some of the major risk factors for coronary artery disease. Your chances of having a heart attack or dying of heart disease within the next 8 years increase with each risk factor you have. Estimate your risk by adding up the points shown in the yellow-shaded areas.

If you're a man:

1. Do you smoke? No = 0 Yes = 3
2. Find your systolic blood pressure (top number in your reading) and circle the points directly below.

Blood pressure

100	110	120	130	140	150	160	170	180	190	200
1	2	4	5	6	7	8	9	10	12	13

3. Circle the number where your approximate age and blood cholesterol level meet.

Age

Total cholesterol	40	50	60	70
165	4	12	18	21
180	5	13	19	21
195	7	14	19	21
210	8	15	20	21
225	9	16	20	22
240	11	17	21	22
255	12	18	22	22
270	13	19	22	23
285	15	20	23	23
300	16	21	24	23
315	17	22	24	23

If you're a woman:

1. Do you smoke? No = 0 Yes = 1
2. Find your systolic blood pressure (top number in your reading) and circle the points directly below.

Blood pressure

100	110	120	130	140	150	160	170	180	190	200
1	2	3	4	5	6	7	8	9	10	11

3. Circle the number where your approximate age and blood cholesterol level meet.

Age

Total cholesterol	40	50	60	70
165	4	12	18	23
180	5	13	19	23
195	5	13	19	23
210	6	14	20	24
225	7	15	20	24
240	8	15	21	24
255	8	16	21	25
270	9	16	22	25
285	10	17	22	25
300	11	18	23	25
315	11	18	23	26

4. Record Your Points

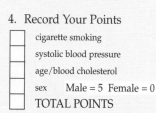

	cigarette smoking
	systolic blood pressure
	age/blood cholesterol
	sex Male = 5 Female = 0
	TOTAL POINTS

5. Estimate Your Risk
   Find your total points to determine your chances (out of 100) of having heart disease within the next 8 years.

Total points	Chances (out of 100)	Total points	Chances (out of 100)
1-10	<1	35	17
11-13	1	36	19
14-17	2	37	21
18-21	3	38	24
22-23	4	39	26
24	5	40	28
25-26	6	41	31
27	7	42	34
28	8	43	36
29	9	44	39
30	10	45	42
31	11	46	46
32	13	47	49
33	14	48	52
34	16	49	55

Note: In this table, the effect on risk from blood cholesterol is limited to total cholesterol. If the assessment also reflected a low level of high-density lipoprotein (HDL) cholesterol, the estimated risk would be higher. This assessment also omits the effects of diabetes mellitus and an abnormal electrocardiogram indicating left ventricular hypertrophy. Women who have diabetes should add 6 points to the total score, and add 4 points if an electrocardiogram shows left ventricular hypertrophy. Men who have diabetes should add 3 points to the total score, and add 2 points for an electrocardiogram that shows left ventricular hypertrophy. (Tables are based on data from the Framingham Heart Study. The table gives the risk for people who have not had a heart attack or cardiovascular bypass surgery.)

■ Lowering Your Risk of Heart Disease

Several risk factors for coronary artery disease can be modified through lifestyle changes or medications. Here's what you can do to reduce your risk:

- Stop smoking. If you smoke, your risk of heart disease is at least two times higher than that of a person who doesn't smoke. For more information on smoking and ways to stop, see page 190.
- Reduce high blood pressure. See page 181.
- Reduce your cholesterol level. See page 212.
- Control diabetes. See pages 173 and 174.
- Maintain proper weight. See page 206.
- Exercise. See page 215.
- Reduce stress. See page 225.

The risk factors listed above may interact with each other to affect your total risk of developing coronary artery disease. The more risk factors you have, the greater your risk of a heart attack.

Controlling these risk factors often involves using medications. But you can usually lower your risk significantly through a careful diet and regular exercise; these efforts sometimes prevent the need for medications.

In addition to a good diet and regular exercise, studies have shown that the following also may lower your risk of heart attack. Discuss with your doctor how each of these factors fits in to lowering your risk.

Aspirin is often recommended to prevent heart attacks. Aspirin reduces the tendency of blood to clot by weakening the activity of platelets (small cell fragments in the blood that stick to each other to form a clot). It may help reduce a clot or even prevent a clot from causing a heart attack. It is inexpensive, generally safe and easy to take. One baby aspirin (which equals one-fourth of a regular-strength adult aspirin) is enough to reduce the risk of a heart attack substantially. In one study, aspirin cut the risk of heart attacks in half. Aspirin does increase the risk of bleeding if an artery to your brain ruptures. Ask your doctor about the risks and benefits of taking aspirin regularly.

Vitamins: Some experts also recommend taking 1 or 2 tablets (400 International Units each) of vitamin E each day to help prevent heart attacks, but recent research has questioned the value of this. Vitamin E is an antioxidant that may help block the buildup of LDL cholesterol (see page 212) in your vessel walls. The value of taking vitamin C to reduce your risk of heart attack has not been clearly shown. However, if you are at increased risk of heart disease, your health care provider may recommend that you take at least 400 micrograms of folic acid (another vitamin) every day.

Estrogen: If you are a woman past menopause, your risk of heart attack increases. Talk to your doctor about your overall risk. Evidence suggests that taking estrogen replacement after menopause will lower your risk of having a heart attack as well as prevent osteoporosis.

Risk-lowering prescription medications: If you've had a heart attack or you have been told by your doctor that you have coronary artery disease, other medicines may lower your risk of heart disease or heart attack. Talk with your doctor about cholesterol-lowering medicines, beta blockers and ACE inhibitors. These medicines, like aspirin, have been shown to lower your risk of heart attack and may be appropriate for you.

Specific Conditions

Hepatitis C

Experts call it the "silent" disease. That's because nearly 4 million Americans have the virus but many of them don't know it. The symptoms can be very subtle.

Could you have the virus and not know it? Or should you be worried that you can "catch" the disease?

If you're in an at-risk group, you should be tested. Treatments are limited, but there are things you can do to manage your lifestyle and live with the virus. If you don't have hepatitis C, there's little concern about acquiring it through casual contact. The main risk is through contact with contaminated blood.

What Is Hepatitis C?

Hepatitis C is a virus that, like hepatitis A and B, causes inflammation of your liver. Hepatitis C ranks second only to alcoholism as a cause of liver disease and is the leading reason for liver transplantation in the United States.

Your liver is one of your body's largest organs. It's a virtual chemical factory, manufacturing vital nutrients and neutralizing toxins.

Generally, hepatitis C is spread through contact with blood contaminated with the virus. In rare cases, it's transmitted sexually. Most people with the virus became infected through a blood transfusion received before 1992 (before improved blood screening tests were available) or through the sharing of contaminated needles during illicit drug use. There's no vaccine to prevent hepatitis C (unlike hepatitis A and B).

If you have hepatitis C, it's likely you've never noticed any symptoms. Most people don't for years, even decades. And if you did have early symptoms, you may have passed them off as a harmless case of the flu. Many people discover that the virus is present purely by accident during a routine blood test.

Attacking Your Liver

About 15 percent to 20 percent of people infected with hepatitis C fight off the virus on their own without liver damage. For the rest, the disease settles in and slowly attacks the liver. Anywhere from 20 percent to 50 percent of people with chronic hepatitis develop cirrhosis (scarring) of the liver, usually within the first 2 decades after infection. Ultimately, liver cancer or liver failure occurs in about half of those who develop cirrhosis.

Should You Be Tested?

Because you can be infected with hepatitis C for years before symptoms appear, you should be tested if you:

- Received a blood transfusion before 1992.
- Used illicit intravenous or intranasal drugs (even once).
- Received an organ transplant before 1992.
- Were exposed to others' blood.
- Had dialysis for kidney failure.

- Received clotting factor concentrates before 1987.
- Had body or ear piercing, tattoos or acupuncture using unsterile equipment.

You should be tested if any of these apply to you.

If you think you may be at risk for hepatitis C, talk to your doctor.

Mayo Clinic Guide to Self-Care

Self-Care

If you're diagnosed with hepatitis C, you may be referred to a liver specialist. Recommended lifestyle changes may include:

- **Eliminating alcohol consumption:** Alcohol use appears to speed progression of liver disease.
- **Avoiding medications that may carry a risk of liver damage:** Your doctor can advise you on what that list might include.
- **Maintaining a healthful lifestyle:** This includes a healthful diet, exercise and appropriate rest.

You'll also want to prevent others from coming in contact with your blood. Cover wounds, don't share your toothbrush or razors and advise health care workers that you have the virus. In addition, don't donate blood, body organs, tissues or semen. Some doctors also advise following safe sex practices.

Medical Help

Early treatment with a combination of medications seems to be the best approach. Physicians often pair interferon alpha, a medication that inhibits duplication of the virus, with another antiviral drug, such as ribavirin.

Researchers are exploring other forms of interferon and other antiviral drugs to enhance the effectiveness of these drugs in treating hepatitis C.

Specific Conditions

High Blood Pressure

High blood pressure (hypertension) is called the "silent killer." Most people with high blood pressure have no symptoms. One-third of the 50 million Americans with the condition are unaware of their risk. The risk lies in the long-term damage the ailment can cause to your heart, brain, kidneys and eyes.

High blood pressure is more common with age. In addition, high blood pressure is more common in blacks than in whites. More men than women have high blood pressure in young adulthood and early middle age, but rates are about equal for ages 55 to 64. Rates for women surpass those for men at age 65 or older.

What Is Blood Pressure?

Have you ever had your blood pressure taken, then wondered what the numbers mean? Knowing and understanding your numbers, then taking steps to control your blood pressure, are critical. Being informed and taking the proper steps can mean the difference between good health and hypertensive heart disease, stroke and kidney disease.

Blood pressure is determined by the amount of blood your heart pumps and the resistance to blood flow in the arteries. Small arteries limit blood flow. In general, the more blood the heart pumps and the smaller the arteries, the higher the blood pressure (that is, your heart must work harder to pump the same amount of blood).

A typical "normal" blood pressure reading, regardless of your age, is 120/80 mm Hg (millimeters of mercury). The top number (120), systolic pressure, is the amount of pressure your heart generates when pumping blood out through your arteries. The bottom number (80), diastolic pressure, is the amount of pressure in the arteries when the heart is at rest between beats.

Your blood pressure normally varies during the day. It rises during activity. It decreases with rest.

In general, the diagnosis of high blood pressure is made if your resting blood pressure is consistently 140/90 mm Hg or higher. Why it reaches or exceeds this level is not always known. In fact, a specific disease or cause is identified in fewer than 1 case in 20. When a cause cannot be determined, high blood pressure is called **essential** or **primary hypertension**.

When a cause is determined, the term **secondary hypertension** is used because the increased pressure is the result of another condition. These specific causes may include medications such as oral contraceptives and kidney disorders such as renal failure, glomerulonephritis and certain adrenal gland problems.

Hypotension (Low Blood Pressure)

Hypotension is low blood pressure. If blood pressure falls to dangerously low levels (shock), the situation can be life-threatening. Shock may result from significant loss of fluid or blood and rarely from serious infections.

Postural hypotension is one potentially dangerous manifestation of low blood pressure. Dizziness or faintness that occurs on standing up quickly from a seated position is the key symptom. (See Dizziness and Fainting, page 34.) It can be caused by medications, pregnancy or illnesses.

Classifying Blood Pressure

Condition	Systolic (Top Number)	Diastolic (Bottom Number)	What to Do
Optimal	Less than 120	Less than 80	
Normal	Less than 130	Less than 85	Recheck in 2 years
High-normal	130-139	85-89	Recheck in 1 year
Hypertension			
Stage 1	140-159	90-99	Confirm within 2 months
Stage 2	160-179	100-109	See doctor within month
Stage 3	180 or more	110 or more	See doctor immediately or within 1 week

Note: "Optimal" blood pressures above apply to all people 18 and older. Blood pressure conditions are diagnosed based on the average of two or more readings taken at two different visits to your doctor, in addition to the original screening visit. (From National Institutes of Health.)

Self-Care

The best strategy is to begin with lifestyle changes such as weight control, diet changes and exercise. If, after 3 to 6 months, your blood pressure has not decreased, your physician may prescribe a medication. Here's what you can do to help yourself:

- **Diet:** Eat a nutritionally balanced diet emphasizing fruits and vegetables and low-fat dairy foods.
- **Salt restriction:** Salt causes the body to retain fluids and so, in many people, can cause high blood pressure. Don't add salt to food. Avoid salty foods such as cured meat, snack foods and canned or prepared foods.
- **Weight reduction:** If your body mass index (BMI) is 25 or more, lose weight. A loss of as few as 10 pounds (4.5 kilograms) may reduce your blood pressure significantly. In some people, weight loss alone is sufficient to avoid the need to take blood pressure drugs. (See Body Mass Index, page 206.)
- **Exercise:** Regular aerobic exercise alone seems to lower blood pressure in some people, even without weight loss.
- **Stop smoking:** The use of tobacco can accelerate the process of atherosclerosis (narrowing of vessels) in people with high blood pressure. Smoking in combination with high blood pressure greatly increases your risk of artery damage.
- **Limit alcohol consumption:** Drinking more than 1.5 ounces of 80-proof liquor, 8 ounces of wine or 24 ounces of beer a day can increase your blood pressure.

The Use of Medications

Your physician will determine which drug or combination of drugs may be best for you. Some drugs work better than others at different ages or in certain races. Your doctor may consider the cost, side effects, the interaction between multiple drugs and how the drugs affect other illnesses. There may be several steps in the process to select medication because the first drug may not lower your blood pressure. A second, third or even fourth drug may be tried either as a substitute or as an additional drug.

Specific Conditions

Sexually Transmitted Diseases

Sexually transmitted disease (STD) is increasing in the United States. Most STDs are treatable, but human immunodeficiency virus (HIV), the cause of acquired immuno-deficiency syndrome (AIDS), has no "current" cure, and death eventually occurs in most cases.

Although HIV can be spread through use of contaminated needles or, rarely, through blood transfusion, it usually is transmitted by sexual contact. The virus is present in semen and vaginal secretions and enters a person's body through small tears that can develop in the vaginal or rectal tissues during sexual activity. Transmission of the virus occurs only after intimate contact with infected blood, semen or vaginal secretions. There have been cases of HIV being passed to health care workers through needlesticks.

STDs such as chlamydia infections, gonorrhea, herpes, venereal warts and syphilis are highly contagious. Many of them can be spread through only one sexual contact. The microorganisms that cause STDs, including HIV, all die within hours once they are outside the body. However, none of these infections are spread through casual contact such as handshaking or sitting on a toilet seat.

The only sure way of preventing STDs and AIDS is through sexual abstinence or a relationship exclusively between two uninfected people. If you have several sexual partners or an infected partner, you place yourself at high risk of contracting an STD.

The Use of Condoms

Correct and consistent use of a latex condom and avoidance of certain sexual practices can decrease the risk of contracting AIDS and other STDs, although condoms do not completely eliminate the risk. Condoms sometimes are made of animal membrane, and the pores in such natural "skin" condoms may allow the AIDS virus to pass through. The use of latex condoms is recommended.

To be effective, a condom must be undamaged, applied before genital contact and remain intact until removed on completion of sexual activity. Extra lubrication (even with lubricated condoms) can help prevent the condom from breaking. Use only water-based lubricants. Oil-based lubricants can cause a condom to break down.

A new condom for females can help reduce the risk of contracting an STD. Most forms of female-directed contraception (for example, the pill) do not provide protection against STDs, although studies indicate that use of the spermicide nonoxynol-9 decreases the frequency of gonorrhea and chlamydial infection. Spermicides in conjunction with a diaphragm also may help kill bacteria.

Risky Behaviors

Different sexual practices carry different degrees of risk of contracting HIV infection. Receptive (passive) anal intercourse is the riskiest because damage to the anal and rectal membranes allows HIV to enter the bloodstream. The passive partner is at much higher risk of contracting HIV than is the active partner, although gonorrhea and syphilis can be acquired from the passive partner's rectum.

Heterosexual vaginal intercourse, particularly with multiple partners, carries a risk of contracting HIV. The virus is believed to be transmitted more easily from the man to the woman than vice versa.

Oral-genital sex is also a possible means of transmission of HIV, gonorrhea, herpes, syphilis and other STDs.

Sexually Transmitted Diseases

If you think you have a sexually transmitted disease (STD), see a physician immediately. If an STD is diagnosed, it is important that you share the information of a confirmed STD with your sexual partner(s). In all cases of STD, abstain from sexual contact until the infection is eliminated completely.

Signs and Symptoms	About the Disease	How Serious Is It?	Medical Treatment
AIDS			
<ul><li>Persistent, unexplained fatigue</li><li>Soaking night sweats</li><li>Shaking chills or fever higher than 100 F for several weeks</li><li>Swelling of lymph nodes for more than 3 months</li><li>Chronic diarrhea</li><li>Persistent headaches</li><li>Dry cough and shortness of breath</li></ul>	AIDS, caused by HIV. Unfortunately, an HIV test is not accurate immediately after exposure, because it takes time for your body to develop or make antibodies. It can take up to 6 months to detect this antibody response	HIV weakens the immune system to the point that opportunistic diseases (ones that your body would normally fight off) begin to affect you. AIDS is a fatal illness, although there have been significant recent advances in the treatment of AIDS	There is no vaccine for AIDS. Treatment includes use of antiviral drugs, immune system boosters and medications to help prevent or treat opportunistic infections. A new class of drugs, called protease inhibitors, has shown promise
Chlamydia infection			
<ul><li>Painful urination</li><li>Vaginal discharge in women</li><li>Urethral discharge in men</li><li>Infection may have no symptoms</li></ul>	Can cause scarring of fallopian tubes in women and prostatitis or epididymitis in men	Touching your eye with infectious secretions can cause eye infection. A mother can pass the infection to her child during delivery, causing pneumonia or eye infection	Antibiotics are prescribed. The infection should disappear within 1 to 2 weeks. All sexual partners must be treated, even though they may not have symptoms. Otherwise, they will pass the disease back and forth between them
Genital herpes			
<ul><li>Pain or itching in the genital area</li><li>Water blisters or open sores</li><li>Genital sores may be present but invisible inside the vagina (women) or urethra (men)</li><li>Recurrent outbreaks</li></ul>	Caused by the herpes simplex virus, usually type 2. Symptoms begin 2 to 7 days after exposure. Itching or burning is followed by blisters and sores. They erupt in the vagina or on the labia, buttocks and anus. In men, on the penis, scrotum, buttocks, anus and thighs. Virus remains dormant in the infected areas and periodically reactivates, causing symptoms	There is no cure or vaccine. The disease is very contagious whenever sores are present. Newborn infants can become infected as they pass through the birth canal of mothers with open sores	Self-care consists of keeping sores clean and dry. The prescription antiviral drug acyclovir helps speed healing. If recurrences are frequent, an oral antiviral antibiotic can be taken daily to suppress the virus.

Specific Conditions

Signs and Symptoms	About the Disease	How Serious Is It?	Medical Treatment

Genital warts

• Warty growths on the genitals, anus, groin, urethra	Venereal warts or genital warts are caused by the human papilloma virus (HPV). They affect both men and women. Persons with impaired immune systems and pregnant women are more susceptible	Generally not serious, but contagious. Women with a history of genital warts have a higher risk of cervical cancer and should get yearly Pap smear	Warts are removed with medication, cryosurgery (freezing), lasers or electrical current. These procedures may require local or general anesthesia

Gonorrhea

• Thick, pus-like discharge from urethra
• Burning, frequent urination
• Slight increase in vaginal discharge and inflammation in women
• Anal discharge or irritation
• Occasionally fever and abdominal pain
	Gonorrhea is caused by bacteria.
	  In men, first symptoms appear between 2 days to 2 weeks after exposure.
	  In women, symptoms may not appear for 1 to 3 weeks. Infection usually affects the cervix and sometimes the fallopian tubes
		Highly contagious, acute infection that may become chronic. In men, it may lead to epididymitis. In women, it can spread to fallopian tubes and cause pelvic inflammatory disease. May result in scarring of the tubes and infertility. Rarely causes joint or throat infection	Many antibiotics are safe and effective for treating gonorrhea. Although treatable, gonorrhea is becoming resistant to some antibiotics. It may be cured with a single injection of ceftriaxone. Oral antibiotics (cefixime, ciprofloxacin) also are effective

Hepatitis B

• Skin and eyes are yellowish • Urine is tea-colored • Flu-like illness • Fatigue and achiness • Fever	Hepatitis B is caused by a virus. Some carriers never have symptoms but are capable of passing the virus to others	A pregnant woman may pass the virus to her developing fetus. Rarely causes liver failure and death	No antiviral treatment. Bed rest is not essential, although it may help you feel better. Maintain good nutrition. Abstain from alcohol use because of damage to the liver. Preventable by vaccination

Syphilis

• Painless sores on the genitals, rectum, tongue or lips • Enlarged lymph nodes in the groin • Rash over any area of the body, especially on palms and soles • Fever • Headache • Soreness and aching in bones or joints	Syphilis is a complex disease caused by a bacterium. Primary stage: painless sores appear in the genital area, rectum or mouth 10 days to 6 weeks after exposure. Second stage, 1 week to 6 months later: red rash may appear anywhere on skin. Third stage, often after years-long latent period: heart disease, mental deterioration	It can be completely cured if the diagnosis is made early and the infection is treated. Left untreated, the disease can lead to death. In pregnant women, it can be transmitted to the fetus, causing deformities and death	Usually treated with penicillin. Other antibiotics can be used for patients allergic to penicillin. A person usually can no longer transmit syphilis 24 hours after beginning therapy. Some people do not respond to the usual doses of penicillin. They must get periodic blood tests to make sure the infectious agent has been destroyed

Mental Health

- Addictive Behavior
- Anxiety and Panic Disorders
- Depression and the "Blues"
- Domestic Abuse
- Memory Loss

In this section, we discuss a range of topics that affect the mental health of millions of Americans and their families. We offer helpful information on how to deal with addictive behavior, anxiety and panic disorders, depression, domestic abuse and memory loss.

Addictive Behavior

You can be addicted to many substances and practices. The main trait of addictive behavior is a compelling need to engage in the activity or to use the addictive substance. In this section, we discuss alcohol, tobacco, drug dependency and compulsive gambling.

■ Alcohol Abuse and Alcoholism

Alcoholism and alcohol abuse cause major social, economic and public health problems. Each year, more than 100,000 people die of alcohol-related causes. The annual cost of lost productivity and health expenses related to alcoholism is more than $100 billion. According to the National Council on Alcoholism and Drug Dependence, more than 13 million Americans abuse alcohol.

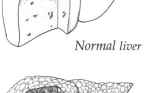

Normal liver

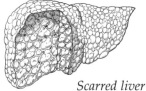

Scarred liver

Excessive alcohol intake can damage body tissues, particularly the liver. Excess use can cause scarring, called cirrhosis.

How Alcohol Works in Your Body

The form of alcohol in the beverages we drink is ethyl alcohol (ethanol), a colorless liquid that in its pure form has a burning taste. Ethanol is produced by the fermentation of sugars, which occur naturally in grains and fruits such as barley and grapes.

When you drink alcohol, it depresses your central nervous system by acting as a sedative. In some people, the initial reaction may be stimulation, but as drinking continues, sedating or calming effects occur. By depressing the control centers of your brain, it relaxes you and reduces your inhibitions. The more you drink, the more you are sedated. Initially, alcohol affects areas of thought, emotion and judgment. In sufficient amounts, alcohol impairs speech and muscle coordination and produces sleep. Taken in large enough quantities, alcohol is a lethal poison—it can cause life-threatening coma by severely depressing the vital centers of your brain.

Excessive use of alcohol can produce several harmful effects on your brain and nervous system. It also can severely damage your liver, pancreas and cardiovascular system. Alcohol use in pregnant women can damage the fetus.

Alcohol Intoxication

The intoxicating effects of alcohol relate to the concentration of alcohol in the blood. For example, if you are not a regular drinker and your blood alcohol concentration is more than 100 mg/dL (milligrams of alcohol per deciliter of blood), you may be quite intoxicated and have difficulty speaking, thinking and moving around. As your blood alcohol concentration increases, mild confusion may give way to stupor and, ultimately, coma. Alcoholics and regular drinkers develop a tolerance for alcohol.

How much food you have eaten and how recently you ate before drinking affect how you respond to alcohol. Size, body fat and tolerance to the effects of alcohol also play significant roles. Drinking equal amounts of alcohol may have a greater effect on a woman than on a man. Women generally have a higher blood alcohol concentration per drink because of their smaller size and less dilution of the alcohol. They also may metabolize alcohol more slowly than men.

Most states define legal intoxication as a blood alcohol concentration of at least 70 to 100 mg/dL, or 0.1 percent. Even at concentrations much lower than the legal limit, some people lose coordination and reaction time.

Mayo Clinic Guide to Self-Care

What Is Alcohol Abuse?

Drinking problems in people who do not have all the characteristics of alcoholism are often referred to as "alcohol abuse" or "problem drinking." These individuals engage in excessive drinking that results in health or social problems but are not dependent on alcohol and have not fully lost control over the use of alcohol.

What Is Alcoholism?

Alcoholism is a chronic disease. It is often progressive and fatal. It is characterized by periods of preoccupation with alcohol and impaired control over alcohol intake. There is continued use despite adverse consequences and distortion in thinking. Most alcoholics deny there is a problem. Other signs include:

- Drinking alone or in secret
- Not remembering conversations or commitments
- Making a ritual of having drinks before, with or after dinner and becoming annoyed when this ritual is disturbed or questioned
- Losing interest in activities and hobbies that used to bring pleasure
- Irritability as usual drinking time nears, especially if alcohol isn't available
- Keeping alcohol in unlikely places at home, at work or in the car
- Gulping drinks, ordering doubles, becoming intoxicated intentionally to feel good or drinking to feel "normal"
- Having problems with relationships, employment or finances or legal problems

■ Treating Alcoholism and Alcohol Abuse

Most alcoholics, and alcohol abusers, enter treatment reluctantly because they deny the problem. They often must be pressured. Health or legal problems may prompt treatment. Intervention helps an alcoholic recognize and accept the need for treatment. If you're concerned about a friend or family member, discuss intervention with a professional.

Self-Administered Alcoholism Screening Test

To screen for alcoholism, Mayo Clinic developed the Self-Administered Alcoholism Screening Test (SAAST) in 1982. The SAAST consists of 37 questions. The test can identify 95 percent of alcoholics who are ill enough to be hospitalized.

The SAAST tries to identify behaviors, medical symptoms and consequences of drinking in the alcoholic. Here is a sample of questions from the test:

1. Do you have a drink now and then?
2. Do you feel you are a normal drinker (that is, drink no more than average)?
3. Have you ever awakened the morning after drinking the previous evening and found that you could not remember a part of the evening?
4. Do close relatives ever worry or complain about your drinking?
5. Can you stop drinking without a struggle after one or two drinks?
6. Do you ever feel guilty about your drinking?
7. Do friends or relatives think you are a normal drinker?
8. Are you always able to stop drinking when you want to?
9. Have you ever attended a meeting of Alcoholics Anonymous (AA) because of your drinking?
10. Have you gotten into physical fights when drinking?

These responses suggest you are at risk for alcoholism: 1. Yes; 2. No; 3. Yes; 4. Yes; 5. No; 6. Yes; 7. No; 8. No; 9. Yes; 10. Yes.

If you answered three or four of the questions with the responses listed, you likely have a drinking problem and need professional evaluation.

■ Individualized Treatment

A wide range of treatments are available to help people with alcohol problems. Treatment should be tailored to the individual. Treatment may involve an evaluation, a brief intervention, an outpatient program or counseling or a residential inpatient stay.

It is important to first determine whether you are alcohol-dependent. If you have not lost control over your use of alcohol, your treatment may involve reducing your drinking. If you are an alcohol abuser, you may be able to modify your drinking. If you have alcoholism, cutting back is ineffective and inappropriate. Abstinence must be a part of the alcoholic's treatment goal.

For people who are not dependent on alcohol but are experiencing the adverse effects of drinking, the goal of treatment is reduction of alcohol-related problems, often by counseling or a brief intervention. A brief intervention usually involves alcohol-abuse specialists who can establish a specific treatment plan. Interventions may include goal setting, behavioral modification techniques, use of self-help manuals, counseling and follow-up care at a treatment center.

The most common residential alcoholism treatment programs in the United States are based on the "Minnesota Model." This includes abstinence, individual and group therapy, participation in Alcoholics Anonymous, educational lectures, family involvement, work assignments, activity therapy and use of counselors (many of whom are recovering alcoholics) and multiprofessional staff. (Contact your insurance provider to determine whether residential treatment is included in your coverage.)

In addition to residential treatment, there are many other approaches including acupuncture, biofeedback, motivational enhancement therapy, cognitive-behavioral therapy and aversion therapy. Aversion therapy involves pairing the drinking of alcohol with a strong aversive response such as nausea or vomiting induced by a medication. After repeated pairing, the alcohol itself causes the aversive response and that decreases the likelihood of relapse. For obvious reasons, aversion therapy tends to be unappealing, although it is often effective.

Coping With Teenage Drinking

Although it may take years for many adults to develop alcohol dependence, teenagers can become addicted in months. Use among teens increases dramatically during the 10th and 11th grades. Each year in the United States, more than 2,000 young people between the ages of 15 and 20 die in alcohol-related automobile accidents, and many more are left disabled. Alcohol also is often implicated in other teenage deaths, including drownings, suicides and fires.

For young people, the likelihood of addiction depends on the influence of parents, peers and other role models, susceptibility to advertising, how early in life they begin to use alcohol, their psychological need for alcohol and genetic factors (family or parental alcoholism) that may predispose them to addiction.

Look for these signs:
- Loses interest in activities and hobbies
- Appears anxious, irritable
- Has difficulties or changes in relationships with friends; joins a new crowd
- Grades drop

To prevent teenage alcohol use:
- Set a good example regarding alcohol use.
- Communicate with your children.
- Discuss the legal and medical consequences of drinking.

The Minnesota Model

Here is what you might expect from a typical residential treatment program based in part on the "Minnesota Model."

- **Detoxification and withdrawal:** Treatment may begin with a program of detoxification. This usually takes about 4 to 7 days. Medications may be necessary to prevent delirium tremens (DTs) or other withdrawal seizures.
- **Medical assessment and treatment:** Common medical problems related to alcoholism are high blood pressure, increased blood sugar and liver and heart disease.
- **Psychological support and psychiatric treatment:** Group and individual counseling and therapy support recovery from the psychological aspects of alcoholism. Sometimes, emotional symptoms of the disease may mimic psychiatric disorders.
- **Recovery programs:** Detoxification and medical treatment are only the first steps for most people in a residential treatment program.
- **Acceptance and abstinence are emphasized:** Effective treatment is impossible unless you can accept that you are addicted and unable to control your drinking.
- **Drug treatments:** An alcohol-sensitizing drug called disulfiram (Antabuse) may be useful. If you drink alcohol, the drug produces a severe physical reaction that includes flushing, nausea, vomiting and headaches. Disulfiram will not cure alcoholism nor can it remove the compulsion to drink. But it can be a strong deterrent. Naltrexone, a drug long known to block the narcotic "high," recently has been found to reduce the urge to drink in recovering alcoholics. Unlike disulfiram, however, naltrexone does not cause a reaction within a few minutes of taking a drink. Naltrexone can produce side effects, particularly liver damage.
- **Continuing support:** Aftercare programs and Alcoholics Anonymous help recovering alcoholics maintain abstinence from alcohol, help to manage any relapses and help with needed lifestyle changes.

FOR MORE INFORMATION

- Alcoholics Anonymous, General Service Office, 475 Riverside Drive, New York, NY 10115. (Refer to your telephone book for local phone number.)
- Al-Anon Family Group Headquarters, Inc., 1600 Corporate Landing Parkway, Virginia Beach, VA 23454-5617; (888) 425-2666.
- National Council on Alcoholism and Drug Dependence, 12 West 21st Street, New York, NY 10010; 24-hour referral (800) NCA-CALL.

Treatment for Hangover: Avoid Alcohol Altogether

Even small amounts of alcohol can cause unpleasant side effects. Some people develop a flushed feeling, whereas others are sensitive to the chemical tyramine found in red wines, brandy and cognac.

The classic hangover, although well-studied, isn't fully understood. It's probably due to dehydration, by-products from the breakdown of alcohol, liver injury, overeating and disturbed sleep.

The best treatment for hangovers is to avoid alcohol altogether. The next best thing is to drink in moderation.

But if you have a hangover, it's too late to do much to improve your health and function. A lot of hangover remedies have been tried, but there isn't much evidence that they help—and they may hurt.

If you have a hangover, follow this advice:
- Rest and rehydrate. Drink bland liquids (water, soda, some fruit juices or broth). Avoid acidic, caffeinated or alcohol-containing beverages.
- Use over-the-counter pain medication with care. See page 265.

Smoking and Tobacco Use

When you inhale the smoke of a cigarette, you're letting loose a chemical parade that will march through some of your body's vital organs—brain, lungs, heart and blood vessels. Your body is exposed to chemicals that cause cancer and addiction.

Although the link between smoking and lung cancer is well known, smoking harms other organs and tissues. Approximately one-fifth of all deaths in the United States are due to smoking.

Nicotine, one of the key ingredients in tobacco, stimulates brain chemicals that can lead to addiction. It triggers your adrenal glands to produce hormones that stress your heart by increasing blood pressure and heart rate.

The carbon monoxide you inhale from tobacco smoke replaces oxygen in your blood cells, robbing your heart, brain and the rest of your body of this life-giving element. Smoking also deadens your senses of taste and smell so food isn't as appetizing as it once was.

Cigarette smoke delivers more than 40 known cancer-causing chemicals, tiny amounts of poisons such as arsenic and cyanide and more than 4,000 other substances to your body. One of the most powerful chemicals is nicotine. It's the nicotine that keeps you smoking. Nicotine is addictive; it can be as addictive as cocaine. It increases the amount of a brain chemical called dopamine, which makes you feel good. Getting that "dopamine boost" is part of the addiction process.

How to Stop Smoking

Many smokers yearn to stop, but find it hard because of nicotine's powerful addictive hold. In fact, most people will need more than one attempt before they successfully stop. Here are some suggestions to help you stop smoking:

Do your homework. Examine the wide range of self-help materials available from the American Cancer Society, the American Lung Association, your physician and your library. Look into smoking-cessation programs. Talk to ex-smokers. Find out how they stopped and what they found helpful.

Make small changes. Limit places where you smoke by smoking in only one room in your home or even outside. Practice not smoking by not smoking in the car. Begin an exercise program if you are capable (see page 215).

Pay attention to your smoking. As you prepare to stop smoking, pay attention to your behavior. When do you smoke? Where? With whom do you smoke? List your key triggers to smoking. Plan to cope with them when you stop. Practice coping with these situations without smoking.

Seek help. Participate in a formal program. The more help you get, the better your chance of success. Studies show that people who try to stop through formal programs are up to 8 times more likely to succeed than those who try on their own.

Be motivated. The key to stopping is commitment. When Mayo Clinic studied the results of its own programs, it found that smokers who were more motivated to stop were twice as likely to be successful in stopping as those who were less motivated. List your reasons for stopping. To increase your motivation, add to the list regularly.

Set a stop date. Make it a day with low stress. Tell your friends, spouse and coworkers your intention. They can provide support through trying times.

Mayo Clinic Guide to Self-Care

■ Nicotine Replacement Therapy

The best tested treatments currently available to help people stop smoking are based on delivering nicotine to the brain—by means other than smoking or medications that alter brain chemistry. A growing number of over-the-counter and prescription medications are available to help in your attempt to stop smoking.

Over-the-Counter Medications

Nicotine patch: The patch delivers nicotine through your skin and into your bloodstream. Studies have shown that people who properly use the patch are twice as likely to stop smoking. To use the patch, place it on the least hairy areas of your body (your chest, upper arms, back or abdomen) in the morning. Rotate locations when you apply the next day's patch. Remove the old patch before putting on a new one. Length of use varies with individual needs. Usually 6 to 8 weeks is necessary to firmly establish the required behavior changes. Strengths vary by brand; read label instructions carefully. Heavier smokers may need to use more than one patch at a time—under the direction of a health care provider. **Caution:** About 10 percent to 20 percent of people get an itchy rash at the site of the patch. If it is a minor redness, use a small amount of hydrocortisone cream on the area after the patch is removed. If it is irritated, you will need to stop using the patch or switch to another brand. Do not smoke while wearing a patch.

Nicotine gum: This is not chewing gum. It is a gum like resin that delivers nicotine to the blood through the lining of your mouth. Studies show that people who properly use the gum are more successful than those who try to stop smoking without it. Two strengths are available: 2 and 4 milligrams. Heavier smokers may need the higher dose. To use the gum, put a piece in your mouth and bite it gently a few times until its unusual taste is released. Then park the gum between your cheek and gum. Repeat the process every few minutes. A piece should last about 30 minutes. Use the gum when you feel the urge to smoke or in situations when you know the urge will be present. Initially, you may use up to 10 to 12 pieces a day. Gradually decrease the number over a period of weeks as you develop ways to deal with smoking triggers. **Caution:** Rapid chewing and swallowing the saliva inactivates the nicotine and may cause nausea. Read labels carefully.

Prescription Medications

Nicotine nasal spray: The nicotine in the nasal spray is sprayed directly into each nostril where the nicotine is absorbed through nasal membranes into veins, transported to the heart and then sent to the brain. It is a somewhat quicker delivery system than the gum or patch, although it is not nearly as quick as a cigarette. The usual dose—one spray into each nostril—is 1 milligram. People typically are directed to start with 1 to 2 doses per hour; the minimum is 8 doses per day and the maximum is 40 doses per day. For most people, use of the spray should be reduced 6 to 8 weeks into the treatment. During the early days of treatment, the spray can be irritating to the nose, causing a hot, peppery feeling along with coughing and sneezing. These symptoms subside in 5 to 7 days.

The nicotine inhaler: It's shaped something like a cigarette. You puff on it, and it gives off nicotine vapors in your mouth. The nicotine is absorbed through the lining of the mouth and into your bloodstream and goes to the brain, relieving withdrawal symptoms.

Bupropion is an antidepressant drug. Bupropion tablets increase the level of dopamine, the brain chemical that is also boosted by smoking. As with many medications, it has side effects, including insomnia and dry mouth. If you have a history of seizures, do not use this drug. Two other prescription medications can be effective alternatives but are considered "secondline" medications. One is clonidine, an older blood pressure medication, and the other is nortriptyline, an older antidepressant. Your doctor may recommend one of them if other medications don't work, or if you experience side effects.

Smokers who combine medication treatment with visits to a health care provider for support and counseling are much more successful than those who try to quit on their own. Only about 5 percent of smokers stop without professional help. The newest U. S. Public Health Service guideline recommends use of combination treatments (for example, a combination of two nicotine medications or a nicotine medication and bupropion along with professional help).

■ Coping With Nicotine Withdrawal

Below is a list of common withdrawal symptoms and some suggestions for coping with them. Withdrawal can last from a few days to a few weeks. It's important to try new behaviors.

Problem	Solutions
Craving	• Distract yourself • Do deep-breathing exercises (see page 225) • Realize that the craving will pass
Irritability	• Take a few slow, deep breaths • Image an enjoyable outdoor scene and take a mini-vacation • Soak in a hot bath
Insomnia	• Take a walk several hours before going to bed • Unwind by reading • Take a warm bath • Eat a banana or drink warm milk • Avoid beverages with caffeine after noon • See chapter on sleep disorders, page 44
Increased appetite	• Make a personal survival kit. Include straws, cinnamon sticks, coffee stirrers, licorice, toothpicks, gum or fresh vegetables • Drink lots of water or low-calorie liquids
Inability to concentrate	• Drink lots of water • Take a brisk walk—outside if possible • Simplify your schedule for a few days • Take a break
Fatigue	• Get more exercise • Get an adequate amount of sleep • Take a nap • Try not to push yourself for 2 to 4 weeks
Constipation, gas, stomach pain	• Drink plenty of fluids • Add fiber to your diet: fruit, raw vegetables, whole-grain cereals • Gradually change your diet • See constipation, page 58; gas, page 60

Source: Mayo Nicotine Dependence Center.

Mayo Clinic Guide to Self-Care

■ Teenage Smoking: What Can Be Done?

What's the harm in children "experimenting" with cigarettes?

Cigarette smoking is rapidly addictive. Most teenagers underestimate the health risks of smoking and overestimate their ability to stop once they start. Many teenagers believe that they can stop smoking anytime they choose. The reality is that among high school seniors who smoke from one to five cigarettes a day, 70 percent will still be smoking 5 years later. More than half of those who smoke in high school have unsuccessfully tried to stop.

Teenagers start smoking earlier than many parents realize. Ten percent of current adult smokers began when they were between 9 and 10 years old and half of teenagers who start to smoke begin by 14 years of age. Almost 20 percent of eighth graders have smoked in the past 30 days. Among high school seniors, the rate is 30 percent. The younger a child begins smoking, the greater the chance that he or she will become a heavy smoker as an adult. Also, teenagers who smoke are more likely to experiment with marijuana and other illegal drugs.

Here are some strategies parents might try:

- **Talk with your teenagers. Ask whether their friends smoke.** The risk of your child smoking is 13 times higher if his or her best friends smoke. Most teenagers smoke their first cigarette with a friend who already smokes.
- **Learn what your children think about smoking.** Ask them to read this information so you can discuss it together.
- **Help your child explore personal feelings about peer pressures and smoking.** Use nonjudgmental questions and rehearse with them how they could handle tough situations.
- **Encourage your teenager to enjoy maximal energy and health.** The active, vivacious lifestyles portrayed in many cigarette advertisements are actually more representative of nonsmokers. People who smoke have colds and other respiratory infections more frequently.
- **Note the social repercussions.** Smoking gives you bad breath and makes your hair and clothes smell.
- **Set a personal example of not smoking.** If you currently smoke, one of the best reasons to stop is for the sake of your children. Never smoke in the presence of your children.
- **Work with your schools.**

The Dangers of Secondhand Smoke

The health threat to the nonsmoker from exposure to tobacco smoke is well documented. Secondhand smoke exposure is associated with lung cancer and heart disease in nonsmokers. Most states have enacted laws limiting smoking in public places.

People with respiratory or heart conditions and the very young and very old in general are at special health risk when exposed to secondhand smoke. Infants are three times more likely to die of sudden infant death syndrome if their mothers smoke during and after pregnancy.

Children younger than 1 year who are exposed to smoke have a higher frequency of admissions to hospitals for respiratory illness than children of parents who do not smoke. Secondhand smoke increases a child's risk of getting ear infections, pneumonia, bronchitis or tonsillitis.

◼ Drug Dependency

Dependency on drugs, whether prescription or illegal, is dangerous because of its long-term physical effects, its disruptive effect on family and work and the risks associated with sudden withdrawal. Illegal drugs are hazardous not only by their nature but also because of the risk of contamination with toxic or infectious substances. In most cases, help is essential to quitting.

Common Drugs of Abuse

Glue: Young children may sniff glue, which is a central nervous system depressant. At first, a few sniffs may give a "high," but the child develops a tolerance in a matter of weeks. The initial symptoms mimic alcoholic inebriation, including slurred speech, dizziness, breakdown of inhibitions, drowsiness and amnesia. The child may have hallucinations, lose weight and lose consciousness.

Central nervous system stimulants (amphetamines and cocaine): Known as "uppers," amphetamines produce an extraordinarily strong psychological addiction that amounts to a compulsion. Abusers develop a high degree of tolerance to the euphoric effects, which last for several hours. Cocaine triggers the release of chemicals in your body which stimulate your heart to pump faster and harder. These reactions result in the rush of euphoria, the illusion of control and heightened sexual drive. Even a modest dose of cocaine can kill you. Injecting or smoking cocaine (called "crack") can be more dangerous because a greater amount of it goes into your bloodstream.

Opioids: Opium is produced from the milky discharge from seeds of the poppy plant. Opioids include opiates (substances naturally produced from opium, such as heroin and morphine) and synthetic substances that have morphine-like action. Physicians may prescribe them as pain relievers, anesthetics or cough suppressants (such as codeine and methadone). Signs of abuse include depression, anxiety, impulsiveness, low frustration tolerance and the need for immediate gratification.

Marijuana and hashish: Marijuana is made from the leaves and flowers of the hemp plant, *Cannabis sativa.* Hashish comes from the concentrated resin of the same plant. Your body absorbs the psychoactive substances in these drugs. If you are acutely intoxicated with marijuana or hashish, you feel relaxed and euphoric. These compounds affect your concentration and perceptual and motor functions. Chronic users have an increased heart rate, redness of the eyes and a decrease in lung function. Withdrawal symptoms include aggression, irritability, stomach discomfort and anxiety.

Hallucinogens: LSD (lysergic acid diethylamide) produces profound changes in mood and thought processes, resulting in hallucinations and a state resembling acute psychosis. Acute panic reactions may occur, as may rapid heart rate, hypertension and tremors. The most common street preparation of PCP (phencyclidine) is called "angel dust," a white granular powder. In low doses (5 mg), PCP produces excitement, incoordination and absence of sensation (analgesic). In high doses, it can cause drooling, vomiting, stupor or coma. When there is acute psychosis associated with PCP, the person is at high risk for suicide or violence toward others.

Designer drugs have become increasingly popular in the '90s. They are formulated to achieve specific effects and to chemically modify existing drugs to avoid criminal prosecution under existing laws. Common names include "ecstasy," "Adam," "Eve" and "China white." Use of these drugs produces intoxication and has caused serious medical conditions, including movement disorders and death.

Medical Help

Drug users may require an intervention on the part of family and friends. The drug user may require hospitalization for detoxification. Follow-up outpatient programs (support groups, day care or residential) lasting weeks or months may be necessary to prevent a relapse.

FOR MORE INFORMATION
- National Institute on Drug Abuse, (800) 662-4357.
- Narcotics Anonymous (NA), World Office, P.O. Box 9999, Van Nuys, CA 91409-9999; (818) 773-9999.

How to Identify Drug Use Among Teenagers

These clues are only possible indications that your teenager is using drugs:
- **School:** The child suddenly shows an active dislike of school and looks for excuses to stay home. Contact school officials to see if your child's attendance record matches what you know about his or her absent days. An A or B student who suddenly begins to fail courses or receives only minimally passing grades may be using drugs.
- **Physical health:** Listlessness and apathy are possible indications of drug use.
- **Appearance** is extremely important to adolescents. A significant warning sign can be a sudden lack of interest in clothing or looks.
- **Personal behavior:** Teenagers enjoy their privacy. However, be wary of exaggerated efforts to bar you from going into their bedrooms or knowing where they go with their friends.
- **Money:** Sudden requests for more money without a reasonable explanation for its use may be an indication of drug use.

What can you do?

Adolescents need to feel that there is an open line of communication with their parents. Even in the face of your child's reluctance to share feelings, continue to express an interest in listening to your child talk about his or her experiences.

▇ Compulsive Gambling

Gambling odds, as the saying goes, are stacked in favor of the house. But that doesn't stop people from trying. The amount gambled yearly in the United States—estimated at more than $500 billion—easily outpaces government expenses on Medicare and Medicaid combined.

Most people who wager don't have a problem. But a minority—an estimated 1 percent to 2 percent of the general population—become compulsive gamblers. People in this group lose control of their betting, often with serious and sometimes fatal consequences.

What Is Compulsive Gambling?

The American Psychiatric Association (APA) classifies compulsive gambling as an impulse-control disorder. To meet the APA's diagnostic criteria for compulsive gambling, a person must show persistent gambling behavior as indicated by at least five of the following criteria:

1. Being preoccupied with gambling (for example, being preoccupied with reliving past gambling experiences, handicapping or planning the next venture, thinking of ways to get money with which to gamble).
2. Needing to gamble with increasing amounts of money to achieve desired excitement.
3. Having repeated unsuccessful efforts to cut back or stop gambling.
4. Being restless or irritable when attempting to cut down or stop gambling.
5. Gambling as a way of escaping problems or of relieving a dysphoric mood (feelings of helplessness, guilt, anxiety, depression).
6. After losing money gambling, often returning another day to get even ("chasing" one's losses).
7. Lying to family members, therapist or others to conceal extent of involvement with gambling.
8. Having committed illegal acts such as forgery, fraud, theft or embezzlement to finance gambling.
9. Having jeopardized or lost a significant relationship, job or educational or career opportunity because of gambling.
10. Relying on others to provide money to relieve a desperate financial situation caused by gambling.

Medical Help

The best therapy probably resembles the best therapy for other forms of addiction. That involves education and development of a therapeutic relationship with another person or group of people with the intent to stop gambling.

- **Group therapy** provides support and encouragement and helps reduce the use of defense mechanisms. People who have "been there" can see through a person's denial and help confront the problem.
- **Medications** to ease the process of recovery are being investigated. Some of the drugs being considered are those that have been helpful in treating diseases such as alcoholism, obsessive-compulsive disorders and depression.
- **Gamblers Anonymous** provides a 12-step program patterned after that of Alcoholics Anonymous. For people who wonder whether they may have a gambling problem, Gamblers Anonymous publishes a list of 20 questions as a screening tool and provides a list of local chapters. You also may find state-sponsored help groups in your local telephone directory. Gamblers Anonymous has more than 1,200 U.S. locations and 20 international chapters.

Signs of an Uncontrollable Urge to Gamble

You may have a gambling addiction if:
- You take time from work and family life to gamble.
- You gamble in secret.
- You feel remorse after gambling and repeatedly vow to quit. You may even quit for a while and then start again.
- You don't plan to gamble. You just "end up" gambling. And you gamble until your last dollar is gone.

- You gamble with money you need to pay bills or solve financial problems. You lie, steal, borrow or sell things to get gambling money.
- When you lose, you gamble to win back your losses. When you win, you gamble to win more. You dream of the "big win" and what it will buy.
- You gamble when you feel "down" or when you feel like celebrating.

Anxiety and Panic Disorders

It can happen at any time. Suddenly, your heart begins to race, your face flushes and you have trouble breathing. You feel dizzy, nauseated, out of control—some people even feel like they are dying. Each year, thousands of Americans have an experience like this. Many, thinking they're having a heart attack, go to an emergency room. Others try to ignore it, not realizing that they've experienced a panic attack.

Panic attacks are sudden episodes of intense fear that prompt physical reactions in your body. Ten to 20 percent of Americans will have an attack like this at some time in their lives. Once dismissed as "nerves" or stress, a panic attack is now recognized as a potentially disabling but treatable condition.

Tripping an Alarm System

Panic attacks typically begin in young adulthood and can happen throughout your life. An episode usually begins abruptly, peaks within 10 minutes and lasts about half an hour. Symptoms can include a rapid heart rate, sweating, trembling and shortness of breath. You may have chills, hot flashes, nausea, abdominal cramping, chest pain and dizziness. Tightness in your throat or trouble swallowing is common.

If panic attacks are frequent, or if fear of having them affects your activities, you may have a condition called panic disorder. Women are more likely than men to have panic attacks. Researchers aren't sure why or what causes panic attacks. Heredity may play a role—your chance of having panic attacks increases if you have a close family member who has had them.

Many researchers believe your body's natural fight-or-flight response to danger is involved. For example, if a grizzly bear came after you, your body would react instinctively. Your heart and breathing would speed up as your body readied itself for a life-threatening situation. Many of the same reactions occur in a panic attack. No obvious stressor is present, but something trips your body's alarm system.

Other health problems—such as an impending heart attack, hyperthyroidism or drug withdrawal—can cause symptoms similar to panic attacks. If you have symptoms of a panic attack, seek medical care.

Treatment Options

Fortunately, treatment for panic attacks and panic disorder is very effective. Most people are able to resume everyday activities. Treatment may involve:

- **Education:** Knowing what you experienced is the first step in learning to manage it. Your doctor may give you information and teach you coping techniques.
- **Medication:** Your doctor may prescribe an antidepressant, which usually is effective for preventing future attacks. In some cases, a tranquilizer may be given alone or with other medications. Effectiveness varies. The duration of treatment depends on the severity of your disorder and your response to treatment.
- **Therapy:** During sessions with a psychiatrist or psychologist, coping skills and management of anxiety triggers are taught. Most people need only 8 to 10 sessions. Long-term psychotherapy usually isn't necessary.
- **Relaxation techniques:** See page 225.

FOR MORE INFORMATION

- National Mental Health Association, 1021 Prince Street, Alexandria, VA 22314-2971; (800) 969-6642; Internet address: http://www.nmha.org.

Depression and the "Blues"

Almost everyone has the blues from time to time—a period of several days or a week in which you seem to be in a "funk." This condition usually goes away and you resume your normal patterns. Nevertheless, having the blues is troublesome, and there are steps you can take to avoid them.

Having the blues is not the same as having clinical depression. The blues are temporary and usually go away after a short time.

Depression is a persistent medical problem, but one that can be treated. It may improve eventually, but leaving it untreated typically means it will persist for many months or longer. If you are depressed, you may find little, if any, joy in life. You may have no energy, feel unworthy or guilty for no reason, find it difficult to concentrate or be irritable. You might wake up after only a few hours of sleep or experience changes in appetite—eating less than usual or eating too much. You may experience a sense of hopelessness or even consider suicide (see page 200). A person with depression may have some, most or all of these symptoms.

The following list shows the different signs for depression and the blues.

Signs of depression

- Persistent lack of energy
- Lasting sadness
- Irritability and mood swings
- Recurring sense of hopelessness
- Continual negative view of the world and others
- Overeating or loss of appetite
- Feelings of unworthiness or guilt
- Inability to concentrate, poor memory
- Recurrent early morning awakening or other changes in sleep patterns
- Inability to enjoy pleasurable activities

Signs of the blues

- Feeling down for a few days but still able to function normally in daily activities
- Occasional lack of energy, or a mild change in sleeping patterns
- Ability to enjoy some recreational activities
- Stable weight
- A quickly passing feeling of hopelessness

Self-Care for the Blues

If your mood falls into the "blues" column, try these things:

- Share your feelings. Talk to a trusted friend, spouse, family member or your spiritual counselor. They can offer you support, guidance and perspective.
- Spend time with other people.
- Engage in activities that have interested you in the past, particularly activities that you have enjoyed.
- Regular moderate exercise may lift your mood.
- Get adequate rest and eat balanced meals.
- Don't undertake too much at one time. If you have large tasks to do, break them into smaller ones. Set goals you can accomplish.
- Look for small opportunities to be helpful to someone less fortunate.

Causes of Depression

Every year in the United States, more than 17 million adults have a depressive illness. Occasionally, it is a side effect of a prescription drug, illness or poor diet. Imbalances of certain brain chemicals may be a factor. But often the cause is unclear.

You are at a higher risk for depression if a blood relative has had it. Depression also may recur. If you've had it once, you're at a higher risk to develop it again. Don't let these factors control your life. But be aware of them in assessing your mood. And don't delay seeking medical attention if you notice recurrent depressive symptoms. Also, if you're being treated for depression by one clinician, let your other health care providers know so confusion and medication interactions can be avoided.

Depression also may be preceded by a severe shock or stress in life, such as the death of a loved one (see below) or the loss of a job, or it can arise when things are going very well. Certainly it's normal to feel sad after losses or setbacks. But if that sadness doesn't stop fairly quickly, a serious depression likely has developed.

Depression may not go away by itself. Don't expect to snap out of it all of a sudden or expect to be able to beat your depression through sheer determination. If depressive symptoms last more than a few weeks, or if you're feeling hopeless or suicidal, it's time to seek help. Don't blame yourself for feeling depressed. It's not your fault, and it's not a sign of weakness.

Contact your family doctor or ask for a referral to a psychiatrist. A psychiatrist, just as your family physician, is trained as a medical doctor and can help you exclude significant medical illnesses that might be contributing to your symptoms.

If your symptoms have been mild—but persistent—a psychologist (who is trained in various types of "talking therapy" but does not have a medical degree) may be very helpful. Discussing feelings with a family member or close friend is helpful, but it's no substitute for seeking professional help.

If you know someone who is depressed, invite him or her to take part in normal social activities. Gently but firmly encourage participation. But don't overdo it. The role of friends and family in helping people with depression is to encourage and support professional care. The problem shouldn't be trivialized, but rather it should be viewed as an opportunity to help, because depression can be treated successfully in most cases. Offer reassurance that things will get better, but don't expect a depressed person to improve suddenly. Don't minimize a depressed person's feelings. Instead, listen carefully to what he or she says.

Seasonal affective disorder, another form of depression, seems to be related to light exposure. It occurs more in northern climates in winter, when days are shorter. It affects women more than men and sometimes is treated with increased light exposure during the day, obtained with a light box (a source of bright broad-spectrum light).

Coping With Loss: Practical Suggestions

- **Express your feelings.** Write a book of memories, or even a letter to the person who died.
- **Ask for help.** When we experience sudden loss, our friends may not know how to respond. We can relieve others and help ourselves by asking for specific kinds of help.

- **Stay involved.** People who grieve may need to remind themselves about exercise, diet and rest.
- **When indicated, evaluate for depression.** If the grief is extremely severe in the short run or persistent over the long run (6 months or more), then consider depression as a possible cause.

■ Treatment Options

Most people who have depression improve a great deal when treated with antidepressant medicines. There are more than a dozen such medicines, some of which work in different ways. A physician, frequently a psychiatrist or family doctor, will select a medicine likely to be helpful. Discuss potential side effects with your physician. If you experience symptoms that concern you, call the physician who prescribed the medication. Common side effects may include dry mouth, rash, dizziness, constipation or jitteriness.

Other treatment methods include psychotherapy—talking about your feelings—and programs with a psychiatrist, psychologist or other qualified professional. There are various kinds of psychotherapy, some involving just the patient and the therapist, others involving a group of people with the same general problem who meet to discuss their situation under the guidance of a therapist.

Treatment takes time. Although some signs of change may be evident in as little as 2 weeks, full benefit may require 6 weeks or more. That lengthy process can be discouraging, so it's important for friends and family to provide support and encouragement during this time when medications may need ongoing adjustment.

Someone who is being treated should not expect a sudden dramatic change in mood and activity. Look for gradual improvement in sleep and a slow improvement in appetite and level of energy. The person's mood and overall sense of well-being will also show gradual positive shifts.

Aside from making sure that the person providing the treatment is qualified, it's important to feel comfortable with your clinician. He or she should listen to you describe your problem, ask questions, discuss findings and recommendations and explain possible risks and alternatives to the treatments being recommended.

Warning Signs of Potential Suicide

It is important to keep in mind that these warning signs are only guidelines. There is no one type of suicidal person. If you are concerned, seek help immediately.

- **Withdrawal:** Unwilling to communicate and appears to have an overwhelming urge to be alone.
- **Moodiness:** An emotional high one day followed by being down in the dumps. Sudden, inexplicable calm.
- **Life crisis or trauma:** Divorce, death, an accident or the loss of self-esteem that may occur after loss of a job or a financial setback may produce suicidal thinking.

- **Personality change:** A change in attitude, personal appearance or activities. An introvert suddenly becomes an extrovert.
- **Threats:** The popular assumption that people who threaten suicide don't do it is not true.
- **Gift giving:** The person "bequeaths" cherished belongings to friends and loved ones.
- **Depression:** The person appears to be physically depressed and may be unable to function socially or in the workplace.
- **Risk taking:** The suicidal urge may be manifested in sudden participation in high-speed driving or unsafe sex.

FOR MORE INFORMATION

- National Mental Health Association, 1021 Prince Street, Alexandria, VA 22314-2971; (800) 969-6642; Internet address: http://www.nmha.org.

Domestic Abuse

Beatings, forced sex, being afraid of violence from a spouse or partner or living in fear that your spouse or partner will harm or abuse your children: All of these situations are examples of domestic abuse.

Women predominantly, but not exclusively, suffer domestic abuse. Between 2 million and 4 million women are battered and 1,500 women are murdered annually by a husband, ex-husband or partner. Domestic violence can happen among all races, ages, income and religious groups.

Battering is the use of physical force to control and maintain power over another person. Domestic abuse also may involve intimidation, psychological abuse, harassment, humiliation and threats.

Symptoms of Abusive Behavior

You may be in an abusive relationship if you:

- Have ever been hit, kicked, shoved or threatened with violence
- Feel that you have no choice about how you spend your time, where you go or what you wear
- Have been accused by your partner of things you've never done
- Must ask your partner for permission to make everyday decisions
- Go along with your partner's decisions because you're afraid of his anger

Self-Care

How to Respond

- If you are concerned about the potential for physical abuse, talk to someone as soon as possible. Local crisis hotlines are one option. Social service agencies are another. Confide in a friend, physician or member of the clergy.
- If you are in an abusive relationship, have a flight plan. Be prepared to take your children, house keys and important papers. It's important to be alert. Be ready to leave at a moment's notice.
- Keep cash on hand in case of an emergency.
- Keep a list of phone numbers of friends who may be able to help you.
- Know the number of a women's shelter.

Professional Help

Some people are reluctant to discuss these issues because it's embarrassing to talk openly about such matters with strangers. But by calling a social service agency or confiding in a counselor, feelings of embarrassment or shame can be discussed.

If police are called, request a timely and serious response. Some jurisdictions have a mandatory arrest law, which means that an abuser will be removed from the home while the case is adjudicated.

If you go to a shelter, expect to be safe and to receive counseling. You should also inquire about legal assistance (for instance, the possibility of obtaining a restraining order that would legally bar the abuser from having contact with you).

Counseling also should be available as a means to provide support and discussion of your feelings. Counselors should discuss with you the decision as to whether to pursue legal action.

FOR MORE INFORMATION

- National Domestic Violence Hotline, (800) 799-7233.
- National Organization for Victim Assistance, (202) 232-6682.

Memory Loss

All of us experience short-term memory loss. We can't remember where we put the car keys, or we forget the name of a person we just met. This is normal. But if memory loss is persistent, you need to see a health care professional.

We were born with billions of brain cells. As we age, some of these brain cells die and are not replaced. As we grow older, our bodies also produce less of the chemicals that our brain cells need to work. Although short-term and long-term memory aren't usually affected, recent memory can deteriorate with age.

The three types of memory are described below:

- **Short-term memory:** This is your temporary memory. You may look up a number in the phone book, but after you dial the number you forget it. Once you've finished using the information, it vanishes.
- **Recent memory:** This is memory that preserves the recent past, such as what you ate for breakfast today or what you wore yesterday.
- **Long-term memory:** This is memory that preserves the distant past, such as recollections from childhood.

Memory loss (dementia) can be caused by many things: a side effect of medications, a head injury, alcoholism or a stroke. Hearing and vision problems can affect memory. Pregnant women sometimes have short-term memory problems.

Alzheimer's disease is the most common form of dementia. Symptoms include gradual loss of memory for recent events and inability to learn new information; a growing tendency to repeat oneself, misplace objects, become confused and get lost; a slow disintegration of personality, judgment and social graces; and increasing irritability, anxiety, depression, confusion and restlessness.

Self-Care to Improve Your Memory

- **Establish a routine.** Managing your daily activities is easier when you follow a routine. (Choose a set time to do household chores: clean the bathroom on Saturday; water the plants on Sunday.)
- **Exercise your "mental muscles."** Play word games, crossword puzzles or other activities that challenge your mental abilities.
- **Practice.** When you walk into a room, make a mental inventory of people you recognize. When you meet someone, repeat his or her name in conversation.
- **Nudge the numbers.** For example, if your wife's birthday is October 3, do something to remind you, such as hum the song "Three Coins in a Fountain."
- **Make associations.** When driving, look for landmarks to associate with your route and name them out loud to imprint them on your memory ("turn at the high school to get to Bob's house").
- **Try not to worry.** Fretting about memory loss can make it worse.
- **Write lists.** Keep track of important tasks and appointments. For example, pay the water bill on a certain day each month.

Medical Help

Consult a health care provider if you are concerned about memory loss.

FOR MORE INFORMATION

- The Alzheimer's Association, 919 N. Michigan Ave., Suite 1100, Chicago IL 60611-1676; (800) 272-3900; Internet address: http://www.alz.org.

Staying Healthy

This section is filled with practical information designed to help you maintain and improve your health by establishing and sustaining a healthful lifestyle.

Handwashing

With today's high-tech approach to health care, it's easy to forget the simplest way to avoid infection—handwashing. With a little soap and water, you often can prevent what may take lots of time and money to cure.

Why Is It Important?

Germs accumulate on your hands as you perform daily activities. By not washing your hands, you can acquire or pass on a host of ailments, from the common cold to more serious diseases such as an intestinal infection (dysentery) or inflammation of the liver (hepatitis).

Most cases of diarrhea and vomiting are caused by inadequate handwashing.

Overall, infections claim more lives than any other disease except heart disease and cancer.

Pneumonia and flu are the sixth leading cause of death in the United States.

Americans annually spend more than $20 billion to fight infections. More important than the dollar figure are the pain and suffering that often could be prevented by a few pennies' worth of soap.

What's Proper Handwashing?

Thorough handwashing isn't simple. You must apply soap or detergent to your hands and rub vigorously for at least 10 seconds to suspend the germs (microorganisms). Then rinse them away.

Water temperature isn't essential. Water warm enough (about 110 F) to cut through grease is best. Water hot enough to kill germs can harm your hands.

Germs tend to accumulate around your cuticles, beneath your fingernails and in the creases of your hands, so concentrate on these areas. Rinse all soap from your hands to remove as many microorganisms as possible.

When Should You Wash?

It's impossible to keep your hands germ-free, but there are times when it's critical to wash your hands.

Always wash:

- Before you handle or eat food
- After you visit the bathroom
- After changing a diaper
- After playing with a pet
- After handling garbage
- After handling money
- After blowing your nose, sneezing or coughing into your hand
- After handling uncooked food (especially meat)

Handwashing and Hospitals

We all can improve when it comes to regular, vigorous handwashing. Certainly it's a matter for concern among health care professionals.

Infections acquired in the hospital (nosocomial infections) are just too common. The Centers for Disease Control and Prevention reports that annual direct costs of these infections average $4 billion.

What to do?

Remember that caregivers are often busy. Sometimes they forget to wash their hands. If you're the patient, a friendly reminder should be welcome.

Weight: What's Healthy for You?

Many overweight people are stymied by trying to lose weight. We're all bombarded by diets and schemes. Weight loss sells! Being significantly overweight has risks. Success at weight loss requires the key ingredients of knowledge, commitment, reasonable eating and regular exercise.

For most overweight Americans, weight loss is a healthy goal. Losing weight often means a reduced risk of heart disease, diabetes and high blood pressure. However, many people, often women, who aren't fat are trying to lose pounds. For them, losing weight offers no healthful benefits and may even be detrimental.

The Risks of Being Overweight

Your desirable weight is the weight at which you're as healthy as possible. And your weight is only one part of the lifestyle picture that contributes to your long-term health.

Being overweight may place you at risk for:

- Increased blood pressure
- Heart disease
- Type 2 diabetes
- Deteriorating joints
- Chronic low back pain
- Gallstones
- Respiratory problems
- Abnormal blood fats

Anyone who wants to be thinner meets a challenge. Of people who lose weight, as many as 95 percent regain the weight within 5 years. So, what should you do? First, determine whether you are really overweight. If so, develop a safe and healthful weight loss program.

Staying Healthy

Your body has a nearly unlimited capacity to store fat. Losing weight reduces crowding of your organs and the strain on your lower back, hips and knees.

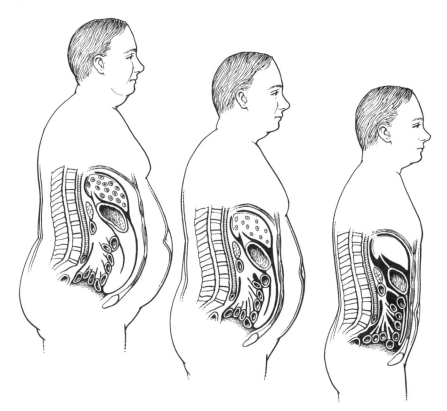

■ Determining Your Body Mass Index

What is a healthy weight? If you have high blood pressure, or if you're at risk, it's not critical that you become "thin." But you should try to achieve or maintain a weight that improves control of your blood pressure and also lessens your risks for other health problems.

Three do-it-yourself evaluations can tell you whether your weight is healthy or whether you could benefit from losing a few pounds.

Body Mass Index

The first step in determining your healthy weight is to figure out your body mass index (BMI). You can do that by using the chart shown below.

A BMI of 19 to 24 is desirable. If your BMI is 25 to 29, you're overweight. You're considered obese if you have a BMI of 30 or more. Extreme obesity is a BMI of more than 40.

You're at increased risk for development of a weight-related disease, such as high blood pressure, if your BMI is 25 or greater.

What's your BMI?

Body mass index (BMI)

BMI	Healthy		Overweight					Obesity				
	19	**24**	25	26	27	28	29	30	35	40	45	50
Height							Weight in pounds					
4'10"	91	115	119	124	129	134	138	143	167	191	215	239
4'11"	94	119	124	128	133	138	143	148	173	198	222	247
5'0"	97	123	128	133	138	143	148	153	179	204	230	255
5'1"	100	127	132	137	143	148	153	158	185	211	238	264
5'2"	104	131	136	142	147	153	158	164	191	218	246	273
5'3"	107	135	141	146	152	158	163	169	197	225	254	282
5'4"	110	140	145	151	157	163	169	174	204	232	262	291
5'5"	114	144	150	156	162	168	174	180	210	240	270	300
5'6"	118	148	155	161	167	173	179	186	216	247	278	309
5'7"	121	153	159	166	172	178	185	191	223	255	287	319
5'8"	125	158	164	171	177	184	190	197	230	262	295	328
5'9"	128	162	169	176	182	189	196	203	236	270	304	338
5'10"	132	167	174	181	188	195	202	209	243	278	313	348
5'11"	136	172	179	186	193	200	208	215	250	286	322	358
6'0"	140	177	184	191	199	206	213	221	258	294	331	368
6'1"	144	182	189	197	204	212	219	227	265	302	340	378
6'2"	148	186	194	202	210	218	225	233	272	311	350	389
6'3"	152	192	200	208	216	224	232	240	279	319	359	399
6'4"	156	197	205	213	221	230	238	246	287	328	369	410

Modified from National Institutes of Health Clinical Guidelines on the Identification, Evaluation, and Treatment of Overweight and Obesity in Adults, 1998.

Waist Circumference

This measurement is second to your BMI in importance. It indicates where most of your fat is located. People who carry most of their weight around their waists are often referred to as "apples." Those who carry most of their weight below their waist, around their hips and thighs, are known as "pears."

Generally, it's better to have a pear shape than an apple shape. Fat accumulation around your waist is associated with an increased risk for high blood pressure, in addition to other diseases such as diabetes, coronary artery disease, stroke and certain types of cancer. That's because fat in your abdomen is more likely to break down and accumulate in your arteries, although the exact mechanism for how this occurs hasn't been proved.

To determine whether you're carrying too much weight around your abdomen, measure your waist circumference. Find the highest point on each of your hip bones and measure across your abdomen just above those highest points. A measurement of more than 40 inches (102 centimeters) in men and 35 inches (88 centimeters) in women signifies increased health risks, especially if you have a BMI of 25 or more.

■ Tips on Losing Weight

To lose weight, you need to modify your lifestyle. You will need to make changes in your diet and physical activity level. Commit to losing weight, lose weight slowly and work to gradually change your eating and exercise habits. It's long-term changes that spell success.

Self-Care

- **Don't start a weight-control program when you're depressed** or going through major life changes. Such ventures are often doomed to failure from the outset.
- **Set reasonable weight loss goals** (long- and short-term). If you want to lose 40 pounds, start with a goal of losing 5 pounds.
- **Check your food intake carefully.** Most adults underestimate how many calories they are eating. It's usually reasonable to cut 500 to 1,000 calories per day from what you're currently eating to produce a weight loss of 1 to 2 pounds per week. Diets that restrict you to fewer than 1,200 calories a day may not meet your daily nutritional needs. Refer to Eating Well, page 209.
- **Learn to enjoy more healthful foods.** See the food pyramid for healthful diet recommendations, page 210. Keep healthful foods on hand, both for meals and snacking. Plan snacks.
- **Limit fat to less than 30 percent of your diet**—20 percent if possible. But don't overdo it. Your body needs some fats. You can lower your fat intake dramatically by eating less meat and avoiding fried foods, fat-laden desserts and fatty add-ons such as margarine, mayonnaise and salad dressing.
- **Don't skip meals.** Eating at established times keeps your appetite and food selections under better control. Eating breakfast helps increase your metabolism early in the day, and thus you burn more calories.
- **Eat more fresh or frozen vegetables and fruits.** They can help you feel full and don't contain a lot of calories.

- **Keep diet records.** People who write down everything they eat are more successful at long-term weight maintenance. Also, keep an exercise log.
- **Record the factors that influence your weight control efforts.** Note when you have the urge to eat. Is it tied to your mood, time of day, varieties of food available, a certain activity? Do you eat without thinking much about what you're doing, such as while watching television or reading a newspaper?
- **Consider what you drink.** Limit regular soft drinks. Alcohol, also high in calories, can increase your appetite and decrease your willpower. Low-fat milk and juices should be within limits—they have calories too. Drink water. Occasional soft drinks are OK.
- **Limit sugar and sweets.** Both are high in calories and low in other nutrients. Sweets such as candy and desserts also can be high in fat.
- **Eat slowly.** You'll eat less, because you'll feel fuller.
- **Focus on eating.** Don't do anything else while you eat (such as reading or watching television).
- **Serve yourself and other family members from the stove,** rather than placing the entire dish of food on the table.
- **Use a smaller plate,** serve yourself smaller portions and put down your fork or spoon between bites.
- **Try to ride out food cravings** when they hit. They usually pass in minutes.
- **Don't weigh yourself too often**—weekly is fine.
- **Use a daily multivitamin** if you're dieting, especially if you limit your calories to 1,400 per day. Avoid expensive, high-dose or "weight-loss formulas."

The health of some people is greatly affected as a result of being overweight (morbidly obese). For them, radical steps, such as medications to suppress appetite, fasting or surgery, may be necessary to prevent premature death. Any of these approaches must always be done under the careful supervision of a physician. But, without a change in eating habits, even these radical steps may fail.

■ Physical Activity: The Key to Burning Calories

Exercise is an important part of any weight loss program. But make any changes gradually, especially if you are out-of-shape. If you're older than 40 or a smoker or have had a heart attack or have diabetes, consult your physician before you start a new exercise program. An exercise stress test may be necessary to assess your risks and limitations.

- **Try to find one or more activities that you enjoy** and can do regularly. Begin slowly, and increase gradually to your goal. Your goal is to maintain moderate activity for 30 minutes or more every day.
- **Your activity does not need to be overly strenuous** to produce positive results. You can achieve your goal through moderate, regular exercise like walking.
- **Vary your exercises** to improve overall fitness and to keep it interesting.
- **Find an exercise buddy.** It may help you stick to your schedule.
- **Little things can add up.** Park at the far end of the parking lot. Take the stairs rather than the elevator. Get off the bus a stop or two early and walk.
- **Keep a log of your activity.**
- **Stick with your exercise schedule.** Don't eliminate time for exercise.
- Refer to the chapter Exercise and Fitness, page 215, for more information.

Eating Well

The food you eat is the source of energy and nutrition for your body. And, of course, eating is a pleasurable experience for most people. Getting enough food is rarely a problem, but getting good nutrition can be a challenge. To feel well, ward off disease and perform at a peak level, you need balanced nutrition.

Many chronic diseases (heart disease, cancer and stroke) are, in part, caused by eating too much of the wrong kinds of food. For most people, the best approach to good nutrition is to follow the principles of food selection advised by the government. The latest revision of the Dietary Guidelines for Americans advises you to do the following:

- Aim for a healthy weight (see pages 205 – 208, 211).
- Be physically active every day.
- Let the Food Guide Pyramid guide your food choices.
- Choose a variety of grains daily, especially whole grains.
- Choose a variety of fruits and vegetables daily.
- Keep food safe to eat.
- Choose a diet that is low in saturated fat and cholesterol and moderate in total fat.
- Choose beverages and foods that limit your intake of sugars.
- Choose and prepare foods with less salt.

If you do drink alcoholic beverages, do so in moderation.

Select Fruits and Vegetables for a Healthy Diet

Most of the foods in a healthy diet will come from fruits, vegetables and the carbohydrate food groups — all of which contain only plant-based items.

Practically all fruits are desirable, but some fruits are better than others. Whole fresh and frozen fruits are best because they are higher in fiber and lower in calories than canned fruits, fruit juices and dried fruits. Dried fruits are relatively high in calories because their water content has been removed in the drying process. With the water gone, the volume the fruit occupies is much smaller. A quarter-cup of raisins contains the same calories — about 100, as almost 2 cups of grapes. The grapes are more filling because they occupy a greater volume. Choosing the grapes allows you to consume almost eight times more food than choosing the raisins would allow. In addition to grapes, other excellent choices include apples, bananas, blueberries, cantaloupes, cherries, grapefruits, honeydew melon, kiwi and mangos.

Vegetables are also highly desirable options, including salad greens, asparagus, green beans, broccoli, cauliflower, zucchini, summer squash, carrots, eggplant, mushrooms, onions, tomatoes and many more. Some vegetables can be considered carbohydrates because they are starchy, containing more calories than typical vegetables, and they function more like a carbohydrate in your body. Starchy vegetables include corn, potatoes, sweet potatoes and winter squash.

The Food Guide Pyramid

The Food Guide Pyramid was developed by the U.S. Department of Agriculture. The pyramid incorporates many principles that add up to a plan for eating low-fat foods that are high in fiber and rich in important vitamins, minerals and other nutrients. All of these factors contribute to optimal health and energy, help you control your weight and reduce your risk of heart disease and some types of cancer. The arrangement of the food groups in a pyramid emphasizes the kinds of foods to eat more of and those to limit.

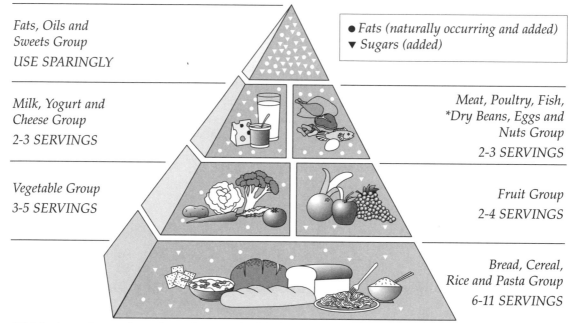

Fats, Oils and Sweets Group
USE SPARINGLY

● *Fats (naturally occurring and added)*
▼ *Sugars (added)*

Milk, Yogurt and Cheese Group
2-3 SERVINGS

*Meat, Poultry, Fish, *Dry Beans, Eggs and Nuts Group*
2-3 SERVINGS

Vegetable Group
3-5 SERVINGS

Fruit Group
2-4 SERVINGS

Bread, Cereal, Rice and Pasta Group
6-11 SERVINGS

Eat dry beans frequently as alternatives to animal foods.

How Many Servings Do You Need Each Day?

	Women and Some Older Adults	Children, Teenage Girls, Active Women, Most Men	Teenage Boys, Active Men	Pregnant and Breast-Feeding Women
Calorie level*	About 1,600	About 2,200	About 2,800	About 1,800-2,800
Bread group	6	9	11	9
Vegetable group	3	4	5	4
Fruit group	2	3	4	3
Milk group	2-3†	2-3†	2-3†	3
Meat group	2 for a total of 5 oz	2 for a total of 6 oz	3 for a total of 7 oz	3 for a total of 7 oz

*These are the calorie levels if you choose low-fat, lean foods from the five major food groups and use foods from the fats, oils and sweets group sparingly.

†Teenagers and young adults to age 24 need 3 servings.

From Mayo Clinic Diet Manual, seventh edition, 1994. Also from the U.S. Department of Agriculture Food Guide Pyramid.

■ The Mayo Clinic Healthy Weight Pyramid™

If weight is an issue for you, the Mayo Clinic Healthy Weight Pyramid can show you where to focus when selecting foods that promote healthy weight. You'll also reduce your risk of weight-related diseases (see page 205). What's more, you'll never be hungry if you follow this approach to daily dining.

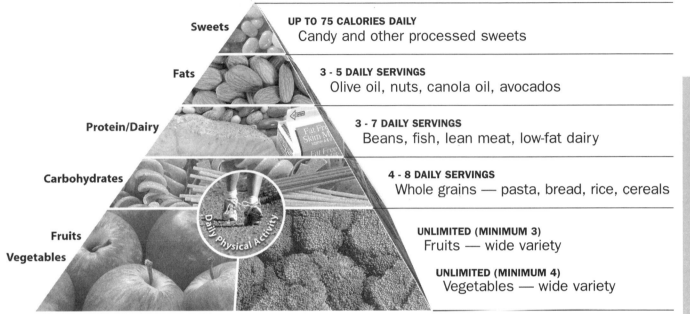

Sweets
UP TO 75 CALORIES DAILY
Candy and other processed sweets

Fats
3 - 5 DAILY SERVINGS
Olive oil, nuts, canola oil, avocados

Protein/Dairy
3 - 7 DAILY SERVINGS
Beans, fish, lean meat, low-fat dairy

Carbohydrates
4 - 8 DAILY SERVINGS
Whole grains — pasta, bread, rice, cereals

Fruits
UNLIMITED (MINIMUM 3)
Fruits — wide variety

Vegetables
UNLIMITED (MINIMUM 4)
Vegetables — wide variety

Daily Physical Activity

© *Mayo Foundation for Medical Education and Research. See your doctor before you begin any healthy weight plan.*

■ Caffeine

Caffeine occurs naturally in coffee, tea and chocolate. Caffeine frequently is added to soft drinks and over-the-counter drugs, including headache and cold tablets, stay awake medications and allergy remedies.

Although relying on caffeine is not recognized medically as a drug addiction, you may come to depend on caffeine as a "pick-me-up." You may feel somewhat drowsy or have a mild headache until you have your caffeinated beverage. Signs that you may be using too much caffeine include difficulty sleeping, headaches, tiredness, irritability, nervousness, vague depression or frequent yawning.

Self-Care

If caffeine is bothering you, try the following:

- If you drink more than 4 servings per day of caffeine-containing beverages, decrease your intake gradually (1 serving per day).
- When you are thirsty, drink decaffeinated beverages or water.
- Mix decaffeinated coffee in with your regular coffee before brewing.
- Substitute regular instant coffee, which contains less caffeine than brewed coffee.
- Switch to tea or other beverages. Be careful when switching to herb teas, however. Some types, particularly homemade varieties, can have the same effects as coffee, or worse.
- Symptoms should begin clearing in 4 to 10 days.

Lowering Your Cholesterol

Cardiovascular disease remains the leading cause of death in this country. Many of the 1 million deaths occur because of narrowed or blocked arteries (atherosclerosis). Cholesterol plays a significant role in this largely preventable condition.

Atherosclerosis is a silent, painless process in which cholesterol-containing fatty deposits accumulate in the walls of your arteries. These accumulations occur as bumps called plaques. As plaque builds up, the interior of your artery narrows and the flow of blood is reduced.

What Is Cholesterol?

Cholesterol is in every cell of your body, and every cell needs it. But your risk for cardiovascular disease goes up considerably if you have too much of this waxy, fatty substance in your blood.

Weight loss, a low-fat diet and other lifestyle changes can help bring your cholesterol down. But sometimes, they aren't enough. Your cholesterol level may still put you at risk of heart attack or stroke.

Fortunately, there's now an array of powerful drugs available that can rapidly reduce your cholesterol and, ultimately, the health risks it poses.

Why You Need Cholesterol

Cholesterol is just one kind of fat (lipid) in your blood. It's often talked about as if it were a poison, but you can't live without it. It's essential to your body's cell membranes, to the insulation of your nerves and to the production of certain hormones. It also helps you digest food.

Your liver makes about 80 percent of the cholesterol in your body. You take in the rest when you eat animal products.

Like nutrients from digested food, cholesterol is transported throughout your body by your bloodstream. For this to happen, your body coats cholesterol with a protein. The cholesterol-protein package is called a "lipoprotein" (lip-oh-PRO-teen). Low-density lipoprotein (LDL) cholesterol is often referred to as "bad" cholesterol. Over time, it can build up in your blood vessels with other substances to form plaque. That can cause a blockage, resulting in heart attack or stroke. In contrast, high-density lipoprotein (HDL) cholesterol is often called "good" cholesterol because it helps "clean" cholesterol from your blood vessels.

Drug Therapy

If, despite dietary changes and exercise, you still have too much bad cholesterol or not enough good (see Understanding Your Cholesterol Test, page 214), your physician may consider drug therapy. Medications can change your blood levels of cholesterol or triglycerides, another type of lipid in your blood.

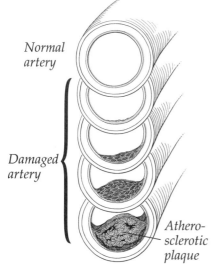

Normal artery

Damaged artery

Athero-sclerotic plaque

An excess of LDL cholesterol particles in your blood increases your risk for a buildup of cholesterol within the wall of your arteries. Eventually, bumps called plaques may form, narrowing or even blocking your artery.

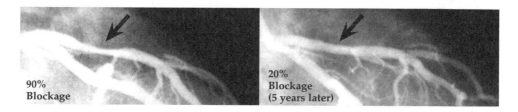

Coronary artery angiograms taken 5 years apart show the kind of results that can be achieved with cholesterol-lowering drugs.

90% Blockage

20% Blockage (5 years later)

By reducing LDL cholesterol or other lipids, the drugs can help prevent plaque buildup or even reduce it. And within a few months of taking them, they can help stabilize plaque already in your blood vessels. This may prevent plaque from cracking or breaking off, which can cause an obstruction or blood clot.

Types of drugs available include:

- **Resins:** Cholestyramine (Questran) and colestipol (Colestid), both known as "resins," have been in use for about 20 years. They lower cholesterol indirectly by binding with bile acids in your intestinal tract. Bile acids are made in your liver from cholesterol and are needed for food digestion. By tying up bile acids, the drugs prompt your liver to make more bile acids. Because your liver uses cholesterol to make the acids, less cholesterol is available to reach your bloodstream.
- **Triglyceride-lowering drugs:** Gemfibrozil (Lopid) or large doses of niacin, a vitamin, can reduce triglyceride production and remove triglycerides from circulation.
- **Statins:** These drugs, introduced in the late 1980s, are fast becoming the most widely prescribed drugs to lower cholesterol. You may have seen them advertised and already know their names: fluvastatin (Lescol), lovastatin (Mevacor), simvastatin (Zocor), pravastatin (Pravachol) and atorvastatin (Lipitor).

Taken in tablet or capsule form, statins work directly in your liver to block a substance your liver needs to manufacture cholesterol. That depletes cholesterol in your liver cells and causes the cells to remove cholesterol from circulating blood.

Depending on the dose, statins can reduce your LDL cholesterol by up to 40 percent. That's usually enough to bring your LDL levels within recommended guidelines. Statins also may help your body reabsorb cholesterol from plaques, slowly unplugging blood vessels.

Statins are the only type of lipid-lowering drug proved to reduce your risk of death from cardiovascular disease. Along with niacin, statins also have been shown to reduce your risk of having a second heart attack.

Do You Need Medication?

If your doctor knows you have cardiovascular disease (you've had a heart attack, for example), he or she likely will prescribe medication and lifestyle changes right away if your LDL cholesterol is more than 100 milligrams per deciliter (mg/dL). The decision isn't as clear if you have high cholesterol without known cardiovascular disease.

At first, your doctor may simply recommend exercise, a low-fat diet and other changes. But if these aren't effective, drug therapy is an option, particularly if you have other risk factors for cardiovascular disease.

Why Do You Have High Cholesterol?

Your genes and your lifestyle choices influence how much and what kind of cholesterol you have. Your liver may make too much LDL cholesterol or may not "clean" enough of it from your blood. Or, your liver may not make enough HDL cholesterol.

Smoking, a high-fat diet and inactivity also can increase LDL levels and reduce HDL levels. They also affect levels of other blood lipids.

The best way to find out how much and what kind of cholesterol you have is to go to your doctor and have a blood lipids test. Home tests give you only your total cholesterol. They can't tell you how much "good" or "bad" cholesterol you have.

Drug therapy, along with lifestyle changes, is often recommended for people without established cardiovascular disease if:

- Your LDL cholesterol is more than 190 mg/dL after lifestyle changes, or
- Your LDL cholesterol is more than 160 mg/dL after lifestyle changes and you have two or more risk factors.

Weighing Your Options

Which lipid-lowering drug your doctor recommends for you depends on many factors. These include how much "good" or "bad" cholesterol you have and whether other lipids in your blood are high. Your age also may be a factor. Sometimes your doctor may recommend a combination of drugs.

The effectiveness of lipid-lowering drugs varies from person to person. There isn't one drug that's best for everyone. Nor is it necessary to take the newest drug if your current medication is effective.

A Long-Term Program

The decision to take any kind of lipid-lowering drug is a serious matter. Once you start, you must typically take the drug the rest of your life. That can be expensive. Lipid-lowering drugs can cost $200 or more a month. You also need to have your liver checked regularly. Rarely, the drugs can cause liver damage, which is why they're not recommended if you have liver disease.

Other side effects for most lipid-lowering drugs usually aren't serious, but may be bothersome enough to keep you from taking the medication. The statins, for example, can cause muscle pain when taken in combination with other drugs, such as gemfibrozil, antifungal medications or the popular antibiotic erythromycin. However, this side effect is rare.

The resins can cause constipation and bloating, or decrease the effectiveness of other medications taken at the same time. Niacin sometimes causes irritating skin flushing and can increase your blood sugar level, aggravate a stomach ulcer or trigger an attack of gout. And gemfibrozil can cause gallstones.

In addition, because lipid-lowering drugs have been available for only about 20 years, physicians haven't been able to study their safety when used over a lifetime.

As with any medication, carefully weigh the advantages of taking a drug against not taking it. If you have cardiovascular disease or are at high risk for it, lipid-lowering drugs are one of the most important treatment options you have.

Understanding Your Cholesterol Test

Test	Desirable	Borderline	Undesirable
Total cholesterol	Below 200	200-239	240 and above
LDL cholesterol	Below 130	130-159	160 and above
HDL cholesterol	Above 45	40-45	Below 40
Triglycerides	Below 150	150-199	Above 200

Levels are given in milligrams per deciliter. Levels are for people **without** known cardiovascular disease. If you have established cardiovascular disease, your physician may have different guidelines for you.

Exercise and Fitness

Regular exercise three or four times a week reduces risk of death from all causes, including heart disease and cancer, by about 70 percent. With routine exercise, you may reach a level of fitness comparable to an inactive person 10 to 20 years younger.

The benefits of exercise include the following:

- **Heart:** Exercise increases your heart's ability to pump blood and decreases your resting heart rate. Your heart can pump more blood with less effort.
- **Cholesterol:** Exercise improves cholesterol levels.
- **Triglycerides:** Exercise can lower your triglyceride level.
- **Blood pressure:** Exercise can lower blood pressure and is especially helpful if you have mild hypertension. Regular exercise also can help prevent as well as reduce high blood pressure.
- **Diabetes:** If you have diabetes, exercise can lower your blood sugar. Exercise can help prevent adult-onset diabetes.
- **Bones:** Women who exercise have a better chance of avoiding osteoporosis, provided that they do not become so active that menstruation stops.
- **General:** Regular exercise also relieves stress, improves your overall sense of well-being, helps you sleep better and improves concentration.

■ Aerobic vs. Anaerobic Exercise

Aerobic exercise (which literally means "to exercise with oxygen") occurs when you continuously move large muscle groups such as your leg muscles. This exercise places increased demands on the heart, lungs and muscle cells. It is not so intense, however, that it causes pain (from lactic acid buildup). If you're exercising in a good aerobic range, you should be breaking a sweat and breathing faster but still be able to exercise comfortably for 20 to 40 minutes. Aerobic exercise improves your overall endurance. Walking, biking, jogging and swimming are familiar aerobic exercises.

Anaerobic exercise ("to exercise without oxygen") occurs when the demands made on a muscle are great enough that it uses up all of the available oxygen and starts to burn stored energy without oxygen. This alternate path for burning energy produces lactic acid. As lactic acid builds up in muscles it causes pain. That's one reason why you can't carry on anaerobic exercises very long. Weight lifting is a classic example. Anaerobic exercise can be healthful but it builds strength more than endurance. If you are just starting an exercise program, supplement your aerobic exercise with light anaerobic exercises. Work with light weights or set machines at light resistance to avoid injuries.

What It Means to Be Fit

You're fit if you can:
- Carry out daily tasks without fatigue and have ample energy to enjoy leisure pursuits
- Walk a mile or climb a few flights of stairs without becoming "winded" or feeling heaviness or fatigue in your legs
- Carry on a conversation during light to moderate exercise such as brisk walking

If you sit most of the day, you're probably not fit. Signs of deconditioning include feeling tired most of the time, being unable to keep up with others your age, avoiding physical activity because you know you'll quickly tire and becoming short of breath or fatigued when walking a short distance.

■ Starting a Fitness Program

Consult your health care provider before you begin an exercise program if you smoke, are overweight, are older than 40 years and have never exercised or have a chronic condition such as heart disease, diabetes, high blood pressure, lung disease or kidney disease. The risks of exercise stem from doing too much, too vigorously, with too little previous activity.

If you are medically able to begin a program, here are some helpful hints:

- **Begin gradually**. Don't overdo it. If you have trouble talking to a companion during your workout, you probably are pushing too hard.
- **Select the exercise that is right for you.** It should be something you enjoy—or at least find tolerable. Otherwise, in time you will avoid it.
- **Do it regularly but moderately** and never exercise to the point of nausea, dizziness or extreme shortness of breath. Your goals should be:
  - *Frequency:* Exercise at least three or four times a week.
  - *Intensity:* Aim for about 60 percent of your maximal aerobic capacity. For most people, 60 percent capacity means moderate exertion with deep breathing, but short of panting or becoming overheated.
  - *Time:* Set a goal of at least 20 to 30 minutes a session. If time is a factor, three 10-minute sessions can be as beneficial as one 30-minute workout. If you're not used to exercise, start at a comfortable length of time and gradually work up to your goal.
- **Always warm up and cool down.** Stretch in warm-up to help loosen muscles; stretch in cool-down to increase flexibility.

How Many Calories Does It Use Up?

Exercise that's equivalent to burning about 1,000 calories a week significantly lowers your overall risk of a heart attack. The chart shows the range of energy used while performing various activities for 1 hour. The more you weigh, the more calories you use.

Activity (1-Hour Duration)	Calories Used* 120- to 130- lb Person	Calories Used* 170- to 180- lb Person	Activity (1-Hour Duration)	Calories Used* 120- to 130- lb Person	Calories Used* 170- to 180- lb Person
Aerobic dancing	290-575	400-800	Racquetball	345-690	480-690
Backpacking	29-630	400-880	Rope skipping	345-690	480-960
Badminton	230-515	320-720	Running, 8 mph	745	1,040
Bicycling (outdoor)	170-800	240-1,120	Skating, ice or roller	230-460	320-640
Bicycling (stationary)	85-800	120-1,120	Skiing (cross-country)	290-800	400-1,120
Bowling	115-170	160-240	Skiing (downhill)	170-460	240-640
Canoeing	170-460	240-640	Stair climbing	230-460	320-640
Dancing	115-400	160-560	Swimming	230-690	320-900
Gardening	115-400	160-560	Tennis	230-515	320-720
Golfing (carrying bag)	115-400	160-560	Volleyball	170-400	240-560
Hiking	170-690	240-960	Walking, 2 mph	150	210
Jogging, 5 mph	460	640			

For other body weights, you can calculate approximate calories used by selecting the numbers of calories used from the second column. Multiply it by your weight and divide by 175. For example, if you weigh 220 lb, jogging uses $\frac{640 \times 220}{175}$ = 804 calories/hour.

Walk Your Way to Fitness

Less than half of American adults exercise regularly. Yet a brisk walk, 30 to 60 minutes each day, can help you attain the fitness level associated with a longer, more healthful life.

Exercise doesn't have to be intense. Even walking slowly can lower your risk of heart disease. Faster, farther or more frequent walking offers greater health benefits.

First Things First

The best walking program takes advantage of your fitness goals while being safe, convenient and fun. Here are tips to get the most out of walking:

- **Set realistic goals.** What do you want to gain from regular exercise? Be specific. Are you 45 and concerned about warding off a heart attack? Are you 75 and wanting to enjoy more recreational activities and prolong your independence? Do you want to lose weight? Lower your blood pressure? Relieve stress? Maybe you just want to feel better.

  Walking can help you achieve these goals. Decide what's most important to you. Then be specific about how you can reach that goal. Don't say, "I'm going to walk more." Say, "I'm going to walk from 7 to 7:30 on Tuesday, Thursday and Saturday mornings."

- **Buy good shoes.** You don't need to spend a lot of money on shoes designed specifically for walking. You do need to wear shoes that provide protection and stability.

- **Dress right.** Dress in loose-fitting, comfortable clothes. Choose materials appropriate for the weather—a windbreaker for cool and windy days, layers of clothing in cold weather. Wear bright colors trimmed with reflective fabric or tape. Avoid rubberized material; it doesn't allow perspiration to escape. Protect yourself from the sun with sunscreen, sunglasses or a hat.

- **Drink water.** When you exercise, you need extra water to maintain your normal body temperature and cool working muscles. To help replenish the fluids you lose during exercise, drink water before and after activity. If you walk for more than 20 minutes, drink one-half to a cup of water every 20 minutes, especially in hot weather.

- **See your doctor.** If you're age 40 or older or have a chronic health problem, review your exercise goals with your doctor before starting.

Planning Your Program

If you put out a little more physical effort than usual, your body responds by improving its capacity for exercise. By gradually increasing the amount of exercise you do, and allowing the adaptive processes to occur, you can improve your fitness level in 8 to 12 weeks. To condition your heart and lungs safely, plan these aspects of your program:

- **Intensity**: Remember, exercise doesn't have to be strenuous to be healthful. But what is a desirable range of exercise intensity for you? Here are two simple tools to help you find out:
  1. Talk test. While you walk, you should be able to carry on a conversation with a companion. If you can't, you're probably pushing too hard. Slow your pace.
  2. Perceived exertion. This refers to the total amount of physical effort you experience. The perceived exertion scale accounts for all sensations of exertion, physical stress and fatigue.

Perceived Exertion Scale

On this scale, a rating of 6 indicates minimal exertion, such as sitting comfortably in a chair. A rating of 20 corresponds to maximum effort, such as jogging up a steep hill.	6
	7 Very, very light
	8
	9 Very light
	10
Aim for a rating of 13. In general, it corresponds to 70 percent of the maximal exercise capacity. We consider this to be nearly ideal for most people. When you use the scale, don't become preoccupied with any one factor such as leg discomfort or labored breathing. Instead, try to concentrate on your overall feeling of exertion.	11 Fairly light
	12
	13 Somewhat hard
	14
	15 Hard
	16
	17 Very hard
	18
	19 Very, very hard
	20

- **Frequency:** Walk at least three times a week. For conditioning and health benefits, your goal is eventually to walk 3 to 4 hours a week.
- **Duration:** Walk for at least 20 to 30 minutes. If you've never exercised regularly or you haven't exercised for a long time, start at a level that's comfortable for you. It may be no more than 5 minutes.

A 12-Week Schedule

Use this schedule to enhance what walking you're already doing or to start a regular program.

Week	Time (min)	Days/week	Total hours/week
1	20	3	1
2	20	3	1
3-4	25	3	1.25
5-6*	30	3-4	1.5-2
7-8	35	4-5	2-3
9-10	40	4-5	3-3.5
11-12	40	5-6	3.5-4

*Here's another way to build up your goal of walking 3 to 4 hours a week. Continue walking 3 to 4 days a week. But gradually extend each walk until you're walking between 45 and 60 minutes.

■ Stretching Exercises for Walkers

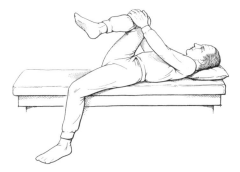

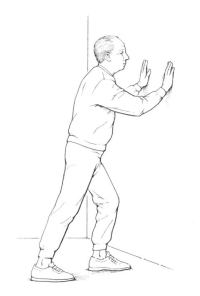

Upper thigh stretch: *Lie on a table or bed with one leg and hip as near the edge as possible and your lower leg hanging relaxed over the edge. Pull your other thigh and knee firmly toward your chest until your lower back flattens against the table. Hold for 30 seconds. Relax. Repeat with other leg.*

Calf stretch: *Stand an arm's length from wall. Lean into wall. Place one leg forward with knee bent. Keep other leg back with knee straight and heel down. Keeping back straight, move hips toward wall until you feel a stretch. Hold 30 seconds. Relax. Repeat with other leg.*

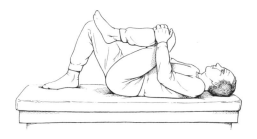

Lower back stretch: *Lie on a firm surface, such as the floor or a table, with your hips and knees bent and feet flat on the surface. Pull your left knee toward your shoulder with both hands (if you have knee problems, pull from the back of your thigh). Hold for 30 seconds. Relax. Repeat with other leg.*

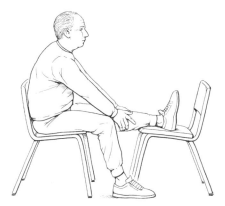

Hamstring stretch: *Sit in chair with one leg on another chair. Keep back straight. Slowly bend pelvis forward at the hip until you feel a stretch in the back of your thigh. Hold 30 seconds. Relax. Repeat with other leg.*

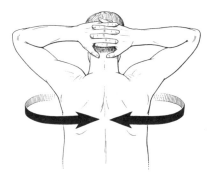

Chest stretch: *Clasp your hands behind your head. Pull elbows firmly back while inhaling deeply. Hold for 30 seconds (keep breathing). Relax.*

Staying Healthy

In addition to the time you spend walking, be sure to warm up and cool down. Use the stretching and flexibility exercises that are illustrated on the previous page.

A good exercise program includes three phases:

- **Warm-up:** Before each walk, spend about 5 minutes preparing your body for walking. These five gentle exercises gradually increase your heart rate, body temperature and blood flow to your muscles. Stretching also develops and maintains adequate muscle and joint flexibility.
- **Conditioning:** Walking develops your aerobic capacity by increasing your heart rate, depth of breathing and muscle endurance. You'll also burn calories. Calories burned depend on how fast and how long you walk and how much you weigh (see How Many Calories Does It Use Up?, page 216).
- **Cool-down:** After each walk, spend about 5 minutes cooling down with the same exercises you use to warm up. This phase allows your heart rate and muscles to return to normal. It also develops flexibility.

Stepping Out Safely

Congratulations. You've committed to a regular walking program. You're confident of the benefits you'll gain. But as you prepare, beware of the terrible too's—doing:

- too much
- too hard, with
- too little preparation

Foot or heel pain is a common result. Problems such as these can derail your walking program and sap your motivation. Here's how to walk without wearing yourself out:

- **Progress gradually.** If you haven't been physically active in the past 2 months, start conservatively. In the first 2 to 3 weeks, choose an intensity at the lower end of the perceived exertion scale. Gradually increase intensity only after you're walking comfortably for your desired length of time.
- **Listen to your body.** Expect to feel some muscle soreness after adding time to your schedule. However, gasping for breath and feeling sore joints are signals to slow down. Muscle stiffness lasting several days means you went too far.

See your doctor immediately if you notice any symptoms suggesting heart or lung disease, such as chest pain, chest pressure, unusual fatigue lasting several hours, heart irregularity or unusual shortness of breath during or immediately after exercise.

- **Replace worn-out shoes.** After 500 miles or a year of regular wear, your shoes may start to break down. Invest in a new pair when soles start to separate from uppers. Check for loss of stability by lining up your shoes side by side. Then look to see if either shoe tilts to the right or left.
- **Choose your course carefully.** Check out the route you plan to walk. Avoid paths with cracked sidewalks, potholes, low-hanging limbs or uneven turf. Don't walk at night along a road. When possible, walk with a companion, and always carry personal identification.
- **Don't overdo it.** If exercise begins to feel like an obligation, try taking a day off from your schedule each week. Use the time to do some other recreational activity that you enjoy.

Choosing a Walking Shoe

When buying walking shoes, look for quality in these features:

- **Toe box:** Helps prevent calluses on the tops and sides of your toes. Look for a rounded, roomy toe compartment.
- **Exterior:** Provides comfort and durability. Look for full-grain leather or other breathable materials.
- **Interior:** Offers comfort and protection. Look for a padded heel collar to reduce chafing, a padded tongue and ankle to protect the front of your foot and a smooth, absorbent lining. Check for removable insoles that you can air out or replace.
- **Heel counter:** Stabilizes your foot through its roll forward. Keeps it from rolling from side to side. For more support, look for a heel counter that extends all around the side of the shoe toward the arch.
- **Rocker shape:** Provides flexibility and proper heel strike. Look for a natural heel-to-toe curve. Heel should be slightly beveled.
- **Insole:** Also called a sock liner. It adds a measure of cushioning and support.

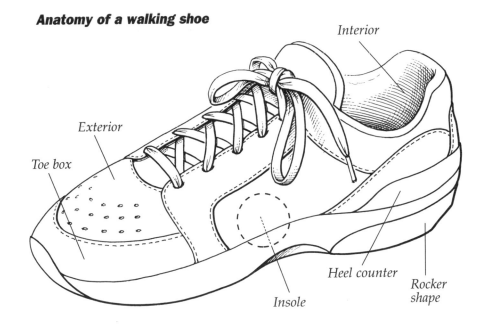

Anatomy of a walking shoe

Interior

Exterior

Toe box

Insole

Heel counter

Rocker shape

Walking shoes range in price from $40 to $120. Least expensive, basic models offer proper design and quality materials. Lightweight models run 2 to 3 ounces lighter than other styles. Less weight means a lighter walk but also less support and durability. Performance models are the most expensive. They're geared toward more style-conscious walkers or more aggressive walkers who may need ultimate durability.

Screening and Immunizations

Adult Screening Tests and Procedures

Test or Procedure	Purpose	Recommendation
Blood cholesterol test	Detect people at high risk of coronary artery disease	• Baseline test in your 20s. If values are within desirable ranges, every 5 years. See page 214
Blood pressure measurement	Early detection of high blood pressure	• Every 2 years or as your health care provider recommends
Colon cancer screening (several tests are available)	Detect cancers and growths (polyps) on the inside wall of the colon which may become cancerous	• Flexible sigmoidoscopy, every 3 to 5 years after age 50 • Colon X-ray, every 3 to 5 years after age 50, in combination with proctoscopy or sigmoidoscopy • Colonoscopy, every 5 years after age 50. Replaces the need for other tests and is the most definitive method, but it also has more risk and is the most expensive
Complete physical examination*	Detect conditions before symptoms develop Preventive care reduces your risk of developing certain diseases	• Twice in your 20s • Three times in your 30s • Four times in your 40s • Five times in your 50s • Annually after 60 • More frequently if you have a chronic medical condition or take medications
Dental checkup	Detect cavities of teeth and problems of the gums, tongue and mouth	• At least once a year or as your dentist recommends
Electrocardiogram (ECG)	Identify injury to heart or irregular rhythms	• Baseline by age 40. As needed or recommended thereafter
Eye examination	Detect vision problems	• Every 4 to 5 years, or as recommended by your doctor
Mammogram (breast X-ray)	Early detection of breast cancer	• Yearly in women older than 50. Yearly in women in their 40s may be appropriate. See page 145
Pap smear	Detect abnormal cells that could develop into cancer	• Every 1 to 3 years based on your risk and as recommended by your health care provider. See page 151
Prostate-specific antigen (PSA)	Measure amount of a protein secreted by the prostate gland. High levels can indicate prostate cancer	• Consider the test if you have a strong family history of prostate cancer or as recommended by your health-care provider. The PSA level also can be increased if the prostate is enlarged or inflamed but not cancerous

*Components of a "complete physical" depend on your age, sex, past illnesses, your risks based on your behavior and your family history of diseases.

Adult Immunization Schedule

Vaccine	Recommendation
Diphtheria/tetanus booster	• Every 10 years. After a deep or dirty wound if the most recent booster was more than 5 years ago. Boosters should be given as soon as possible after the injury
Hepatitis A (2-shot series)	• Travelers and people in high-risk groups (chronic liver disease, men with male sex partners, intravenous drug users, people who have had contact with someone who has hepatitis A)
Hepatitis B (3-shot series)	• Health care workers, high-risk groups (persons with multiple sexual partners, sexual partner who is a carrier) and others who might be exposed to infected blood or body fluids
Influenza	• Every year for persons 50 or older and others at high risk, such as health care workers and people with chronic illnesses
Measles/mumps/rubella (2 shots recommended)	• Adults born after 1956 without proof of previous immunization or immunity
Pneumococcal vaccination	• Age 65 or older or any adult with a medical condition that increases the risk of infection. Persons who are generally healthy may need only one shot. Those less healthy and people who received their first shot before age 65 may need shots more often
Varicella (chickenpox) (2-shot series)	• Susceptible adults (health care workers without immunity or adults without known disease who are exposed to chickenpox)

Pediatric and Adolescent Schedule

The following chart includes the recommended schedule of vaccines used at the Mayo Clinic; it is a modification of recommendations endorsed by the American Academy of Pediatrics and the federal Centers for Disease Control and Prevention. You should check with your personal physician or health care provider regarding the timing of immunizations for your child.

Age	Vaccine	Age	Vaccine
2 months	PCV, HBV-Hib, DTaP, IPV	15 months	PCV, DTaP-Hib
4 months	PCV, HBV-Hib, DTaP, IPV	3 years	MMR (Hearing/Vision optional)
6 months	PCV, DTaP	5 years	DTaP, IPV (Hearing/Vision optional)
9 months	HBV, IPV	11 years	Td (HBV, MMR, Varivax if not previously given)
12 months	MMR, Varivax	17 years	Meningococcal vaccine

Abbreviations

PCV — Pneumococcal conjugate vaccine
HBV-Hib — Hepatitis B-*Haemophilus influenzae* type b vaccine
DTaP — Diphtheria-tetanus-acellular pertussis vaccine
IPV — Poliovirus vaccine inactivated (Salk)

HBV — Hepatitis B vaccine
MMR — Measles/mumps/rubella vaccine
Varivax — Chickenpox vaccine

Keeping Stress Under Control

Many factors can cause stress, often because they are related to changes in our lives. These changes can be events that we consider happy, such as a vacation or a job promotion, as well as negative changes, such as the death of a loved one or the loss of a job.

When we respond to stress with anxiety, tension or worry, that response is not just "mental." When we feel threatened in some way, chemical "messengers" are released, producing physical changes such as rapid pulse, quick breathing and dry mouth. These changes prepare the body for "fight or flight." If we react to stress for long periods, it may contribute to physical or emotional illness.

■ Signs and Symptoms of Stress

Physical	Psychological	Behavioral
Headaches	Anxiety	Overeating/loss of appetite
Grinding teeth	Irritability	Impatience
Tight, dry throat	Feeling of impending danger or doom	Argumentative
Clenched jaws	Depression	Procrastination
Chest pain	Slowed thinking	Increased use of alcohol or drugs
Shortness of breath	Racing thoughts	Increased smoking
Pounding heart	Feeling of helplessness	Withdrawal or isolation
High blood pressure	Feeling of hopelessness	Avoiding or neglecting
Muscle aches	Feeling of worthlessness	responsibility
Indigestion	Feeling of lack of direction	Poor job performance
Constipation/diarrhea	Feeling of insecurity	Burnout
Increased perspiration	Sadness	Poor personal hygiene
Cold, sweaty hands	Defensiveness	Change in religious practices
Fatigue	Anger	Change in family or close relationships
Insomnia	Hypersensitivity	
Frequent illness	Apathy	

Self-Care

- **Learn to relax.** Techniques such as guided imagery, meditation, muscle relaxation and relaxed breathing can help you relax (see page 225). Your goal is to lower your heart rate and blood pressure while reducing muscle tension.
- **Discuss your concerns** with a trusted friend. Talking helps to relieve strains and put things in perspective, and it may lead to a healthy plan of action.
- **Plan your work** in a step-by-step manner. Accomplish small tasks.
- **Deal with your anger.** Anger needs to be expressed, but carefully. "Count to 10," compose yourself and respond to the anger in a more effective manner.
- **Get away.** A change of pace can help develop a new outlook.
- **Be realistic.** Set realistic goals. Prioritize. Concentrate on what's important. Setting our goals unrealistically high invites failure. Decide on your priorities and concentrate on the things of most importance to you.

Self-Care

- **Avoid self-medication.** At times we may seek to use medication or alcohol for a feeling of relief. Such substances only mask the problem.
- **Get plenty of sleep, exercise and nutritious food.** A healthy body promotes good mental health. Sleep helps us tackle problems in a refreshed state. Exercise helps burn off the excess energy that stress can produce.
- **Seek help.** Contact your physician or a mental health professional if stress is building or you're not functioning well.

Relaxation Techniques to Reduce Stress

Progressive Muscle Relaxation

- Sit or lie in a comfortable position and close your eyes. Allow your jaw to drop and your eyelids to be relaxed but not tightly closed.
- Mentally scan your body, starting with your toes and working slowly to your head. Focus on each part individually; imagine tension melting away.
- Tighten the muscles in one area of your body and hold them for a count of 5, relax and move on to the next area.

Visual Imagery

- Allow thoughts to flow through your mind but do not focus on any of them. Suggest to yourself that you are relaxed and calm, that your hands are warm (or cool if you are hot) and heavy, that your heart is beating calmly.
- Breathe slowly, regularly and deeply.
- Once you are relaxed, imagine you are in a favorite place or in a spot of great beauty.
- After 5 or 10 minutes, rouse yourself from the state gradually.

Relaxed Breathing

With practice, you can breathe in a deep and relaxing way. At first, practice lying on your back while wearing clothing that is loose around your waist and abdomen. Once you have learned this position, practice while sitting and then while standing.

- Lie on your back on a bed.
- Place your feet slightly apart. Rest one hand comfortably on your abdomen near your navel. Place the other hand on your chest.

- Inhale through your nose. Exhale through your mouth.
- Concentrate on your breathing for a few minutes and become aware of which hand is rising and falling with each breath.
- Gently exhale most of the air in your lungs.
- Inhale while slowly counting to 4, about 1 second per count. As you inhale gently, slightly extend your abdomen, causing it to rise about 1 inch. (You should be able to feel the movement with your hand.) Do not pull your shoulders up or move your chest.
- As you breathe in, imagine the warmed air flowing into all parts of your body.
- Pause 1 second after inhaling.
- Slowly exhale to a count of 4. While you are exhaling, your abdomen will slowly fall.
- As air flows out, imagine that tension also is flowing out.
- Pause 1 second after exhaling.
- If it is difficult to inhale and exhale to a count of 4, shorten the count slightly and later work up to 4. If you feel light-headed, slow your breathing or breathe less deeply.
- Repeat the slow inhaling, pausing, slow exhaling and pausing 5 to 10 times. Exhale. Inhale slowly: 1, 2, 3, 4. Pause. Exhale slowly: 1, 2, 3, 4. Pause. Inhale: 1, 2, 3, 4. Pause. Exhale: 1, 2, 3, 4. Pause. Continue on your own.

If it's difficult to make your breathing regular, take a slightly deeper breath, hold it for a second or two and then let it out slowly through pursed lips for about 10 seconds. Repeat this once or twice and return to the other procedure.

Protecting Yourself

Nearly 1 in every 20 deaths in the United States results from accidents. Accidents are the most common cause of death in people younger than 35. Half of all childhood deaths are due to accidents. Many of these accidents could be avoided. In the following pages, we offer various safety tips. This information is not comprehensive, but it may alert you to other potentially dangerous circumstances in your everyday life. For a discussion of workplace safety, see page 231.

■ Reduce Your Risk on the Road

Approximately 50,000 people die on our roads and highways every year. Many more are severely injured. To reduce your risk, follow these suggestions:

- **Always wear a seat belt,** even if you are traveling only a short distance. Most accidents occur within a few miles of home.
- **Place children in car seats.** (See the article below.)
- **Drive defensively.** Be aware of other cars at all times.
  - Don't tailgate. Allow 1 car length of space for every 10 miles per hour of speed.
  - Keep windows and mirrors clean. Keep all lines of vision clear. Don't rely on mirrors—turn your head and check blind spots. Avoid "road rage."
- **Consider the weather.** Carry food, blankets and protective clothing. Keep your gas tank as full as possible. Do not leave your car in an emergency. If your engine is running, roll windows down an inch or two to avoid a buildup of carbon monoxide.
- **Don't drive while impaired.** Don't drive after consuming alcohol or when you have taken medications that make you drowsy or impair your reaction time.
- **Avoid distractions.** Keep children in their seatbelts. Do not let the radio, a conversation on a cellular phone or a roadside attraction distract you.
- **Keep your car properly serviced** at the recommended intervals (at least every 6 months or 7,500 miles, whichever comes first) and before extended traveling.
- **Carry an emergency kit** (flashlight, first-aid supplies, jumper cable, a quarter for a phone call, flares, candle and matches).

Air Bags and Infant Car Safety Seats Don't Mix

The force of an air bag's deployment can kill or severely injure infants or small children. Seat them all in back. Here's some advice for safely transporting your children:

- For infants who weigh less than 20 pounds or are younger than 1 year of age, use infant car safety seats—or convertible infant-toddler safety seats. In a collision, the rigid seat supports your baby's back, neck and head. Secure your infant's child safety seat properly in the back seat of your car.
- For children who weigh 20 to 40 pounds or are younger than 4 years, use a child safety seat, anchored correctly, in the back seat. The safety seat's straps should hold the upper third of your child's chest securely.

For children who weigh more than 40 pounds but who are too small to wear a lap and shoulder belt properly, use a car booster seat to obtain correct positioning of the lap and shoulder belt.

■ Preventing Falls

Trips and falls pose a danger to young children and the elderly. In fact, falls are the leading cause of accidental death among people older than 65. Falls may be caused by faulty balance, poor vision, illness, medications and other factors. The best self-care is to develop a plan that reduces risk and prevents injury in the first place.

Self-Care

Here are some tips to prevent falls:
- **Have your vision and hearing checked regularly.** If vision and hearing are impaired, you lose important cues that help you maintain balance.
- **Exercise regularly.** Exercise improves your strength, muscle tone and coordination. This not only helps prevent falls but also reduces the severity of injury if you do fall.
- **Be wary of drugs.** Ask your doctor about the drugs you take. Some drugs may affect balance and coordination.
- **Avoid alcohol.** Even a little alcohol can cause falls, especially if your balance and reflexes are already impaired.
- **Get up slowly.** A momentary decrease in blood pressure, due to drugs or aging, can cause dizziness if you stand up too quickly.
- **Maintain balance and footing.** If you feel dizzy, use a cane or walker. Wear sturdy, low-heeled shoes with wide, nonslip soles.
- **Eliminate loose rugs or mats.**
- **Install adequate lighting,** especially night lighting.
- Block steps for infants and toddlers; install handrails for elderly.

■ Lead Exposure

One of every 11 children in the United States has dangerous levels of lead in his or her bloodstream, according to the U.S. Environmental Protection Agency (EPA). Children are more sensitive to lead poisoning than adults. The federal Centers for Disease Control and Prevention recommends having your child tested for lead poisoning at age 1, or at 6 months if you think your home has high levels of lead. Children older than 1 year should be tested every couple of years, or every year if the residence contains lead paint or you use lead in your job or hobby.

Here are some potential sources of lead poisoning:
- **Soil:** Lead particles that settle on the soil from paint or gasoline used years ago can stay there for many years. High concentrations of lead in soil can be found around old homes and in some urban settings.
- **Household dust:** This can contain lead from paint chips or soil brought in from outside.
- **Water:** Lead pipes, brass plumbing fixtures and copper pipes soldered with lead can release lead particles into tap water. If you have such plumbing, let cold water run 30 to 60 seconds before drinking it. Hot water absorbs more lead than cold water. The EPA warns against making baby formula from hot tap water in old plumbing systems.
- **Lead paint:** Although now outlawed, lead paint is still on walls and woodwork in many older homes. When sanding or stripping in an older home, wear a mask and keep children away from dust and chips.

Carbon Monoxide Poisoning

Carbon monoxide is a poisonous gas produced by incomplete burning of fuel. It has no color, taste or odor. Carbon monoxide builds up in red blood cells, preventing oxygen from being carried and starving your body of oxygen.

An estimated 10,000 people are affected by carbon monoxide poisoning each year in the United States. However, a few simple measures can help prevent poisoning.

- **Know the signs and symptoms.** They include headache, fever, red-appearing skin, dizziness, weakness, fatigue, nausea, vomiting, shortness of breath, chest pain and trouble thinking. Symptoms of carbon monoxide poisoning often come on slowly and may be mistaken for a cold or the flu. Clues include similar symptoms being experienced by everyone in the same building or improvement of symptoms when you leave the building for a day or more and then a return of the symptoms when you come back to the building.
- **Be aware of possible sources.** The most common sources are gas and oil furnaces, wood stoves, gas appliances, pool heaters and engine exhaust fumes. Cracked heat exchangers on furnaces, blocked chimneys, flues or appliance vents can allow carbon monoxide to reach living areas. An inadequate supply of fresh air to a furnace also can allow carbon monoxide to build up in living spaces. Tight home construction also may increase your risk because less fresh air gets in.
- **Get a detector.** The detectors sound a warning when carbon monoxide builds up. Look for UL 2034 on the package.
- **Know when to take action.** If the alarm sounds, ventilate the area by opening doors and windows. If anyone is experiencing poisoning symptoms, evacuate immediately and call 911 from a nearby phone. If no one is experiencing symptoms, continue to ventilate, turn off all fuel-burning appliances and have a qualified technician inspect your home.

Indoor Air Pollution

The U.S. Environmental Protection Agency (EPA) rates indoor air pollution among the top four environmental health risks. (Others are outdoor air pollution, toxic chemicals in the workplace and contaminated drinking water.)

Indoor air's most dangerous pollutants include the following:

- **Tobacco smoke:** Smoking causes lung cancer. Even if you don't smoke but live with someone who does, you have a 30 percent higher risk of lung cancer than someone who lives in a smoke-free home. Air-filtering devices help, but remove mainly smoke's solid particles, not the gases.
- **Radon:** This naturally occurring gas is made by the radioactive decay of uranium in rocks and soil. You can easily overlook radon because you can't see, taste or smell it. Yet, radon can seep into your home and other buildings through basement cracks, sewer openings and joints between walls and floors. After chronic exposure at high levels, radon may lead to lung cancer. To check your home's radon level, buy a radon detector. If your radon level is high, call the EPA radon hot line: (800) SOS-RADON.

Mayo Clinic Guide to Self-Care

Your Health and the Workplace

- **Health, Safety and Injury Prevention**
- **Balancing Work and Home**
- **Stress Relievers**
- **Coping With Technology**
- **Pregnancy and Work**
- **Retirement Planning**

This section focuses on ways to improve your success and well-being in the work environment. You'll find practical information on a variety of fundamental health and safety issues. There's advice on balancing your work with home, family and a possible pregnancy. We include tips to reduce or deal with stress and strategies to dodge or deal with computer-related pains and strains. The section ends with need-to-know facts on retirement planning.

Health, Safety and Injury Prevention

■ Back Care Basics

Your back moves in many directions and is used in weight-bearing activities. Therefore, your lower back is a common site for pain.

Self-Care

Take care of your lower back:
- **Exercise regularly.** Activity can improve your overall fitness and extremity strength and help you shed excess pounds, all of which may protect your back. Include abdominal strengthening in your routine. Abdominal muscles help support and protect the back.
- **Listen to your body.** If your back hurts, stop and rest, or change your activity. During a period of pain, continue gentle stretches but stop abdominal and back strengthening exercises.
- **Perfect your posture.** Good posture actually reduces wear and tear on your back's muscles and joints.
- **Avoid high-risk moves.** Too much twisting, bending and reaching fatigue your back and leave it vulnerable to injury.
- **Lift with your legs.** Always bend your knees when you lift.
- **When you're in pain:** Pay attention to the first twinge; don't ignore it! Most back problems respond well to simple measures such as rest, gentle stretches, cold compresses and over-the-counter pain relievers. Avoid bending and stooping, but stay active, walking as much as possible.

Medical Help

You should notice steady improvement within the first 2 weeks. Check with your doctor if your back pain continues longer or if it is accompanied by weakness, numbness or shooting pains in your legs. **If new bladder or bowel control problems appear, see a physician immediately.**

For more information, see page 50.

■ Carpal Tunnel: No Strain, No Pain

You may have more in common than you think with the butcher, the baker and the candlestick maker. If your hobby or work involves working with your hands, you need to guard against carpal tunnel syndrome.

Warning Signs
This preventable and treatable condition has distinct warning signs:
- Numbness, or a tingling sensation in your hands or thumb, index and middle fingers (but not your little finger).
- Discomfort in the forearm or hand after forceful or repetitive use.
- Awakening with these same symptoms during the night.

Mayo Clinic Guide to Self-Care

What Causes Carpal Tunnel Syndrome?

The carpal tunnel is a passageway between your wrist and hand that contains and protects nerves and tendons. When the tissues in the carpal tunnel become swollen or inflamed, they put pressure on a nerve that provides sensation to your thumb and index, middle and ring fingers. Excess pressure on this nerve may cause you to experience any of the above-mentioned symptoms. If the condition is left untreated, nerve and muscle damage can occur.

Who's at Risk?

You are—if your work or hobbies involve heavy or repetitive wrist or finger motion, forceful pinching or gripping or working with vibrating tools. However, most people do these activities without injury.

Women are at higher risk than men. Some health conditions can increase your risk, including obesity, diabetes, hypothyroidism, rheumatoid arthritis and pregnancy. Fortunately, carpal tunnel syndrome related to pregnancy almost always improves after childbirth.

Avoiding the Problem

Quick breaks, massage, ibuprofen, aspirin or other over-the-counter anti-inflammatory medications can relieve your symptoms temporarily. But your best bet is to take these precautions:

- Take a five-minute break every hour. Stop your activity; gently stretch your hands and fingers back. Alternate tasks when possible.
- Watch your form. Avoid bending your wrist all the way up or down. A relaxed middle position is best.
- Relax your grip. Avoid using a hard grip when driving your car, painting or writing. Oversized grips on pens, pencils and tools may allow a softer grasp.

Medical Help

Try the measures listed above, but if pain, numbness or weakness persists for more than a couple of weeks, see your doctor. Splints, therapy, injection or prescription medications may be recommended. Occasionally, surgery is necessary.

For more information, see page 96.

■ Coping With Arthritis at Work

One in seven Americans has some form of arthritis. The most common type, affecting 20 million Americans, is osteoarthritis, in which cartilage breaks down from overuse or injury. It's typically a problem in workers older than 55 and will likely be troubling on the job when it involves the base of the thumb, shoulder, back, hip or knee. It may become hard to walk, bear weight, perform overhead activities or use fine motor skills.

The second most common form is rheumatoid arthritis. It affects 2 million Americans. Inflammation, rather than mechanical cartilage failure, causes most joint damage. The body's immune system attacks organs of the body, especially the lining of the joints, causing them to become inflamed.

Here are tips on dealing with arthritis at work:

- Know and accept your limitations; sometimes long-term changes are necessary.
- Communicate special needs to your employer. Minor adaptations of your work environment or more frequent short breaks from work may take care of your problem.
- Check on a flexible work schedule; allow time to warm up and loosen joints before starting work.
- Try to organize your work activities to minimize significant repetitive motion; alternate heavy lifting with standing or sitting.
- Consider special equipment, such as pencil grippers, arm supports and floor mats for prolonged standing.
- Exercise, balanced with work and relaxation, is appropriate. But avoid any activity that hurts the joint for 2 or more hours after you've stopped.

Exercises for Office Workers

Sitting at work for 8 hours a day can cause office workers syndrome—fatigue, stress, back pain, even blood clots. These stretches will help (and may even improve your job performance).

Three 5-minute stretch breaks a day will perk you up, relax your muscles and enhance your flexibility. Here are six exercises you can do without leaving your desk. (Note: Hold each stretch for 10 to 20 seconds. Repeat each exercise once or twice on both sides.)

1. Stretch your fingers out as far as you can. Hold for 10 seconds. Relax. Now bend your fingers at the knuckles and squeeze.
2. Slowly tilt your head to the left until you feel a stretch on the side of your neck. Repeat to the right and forward.
3. Hold your left arm just above the elbow with your right hand. Gently pull your elbow across your chest toward the right shoulder while turning your head to look over the left shoulder.
4. Raise your left elbow above your head and put your left palm on the back of your neck. Now grasp your left elbow with your right hand. Gently pull your elbow behind your head and toward your right shoulder until you feel a nice stretch in your shoulder or upper arms.
5. Hold your left leg just below the knee. Gently pull your bent leg toward your chest. Step two: Hold it with your right arm and pull it toward your right shoulder.
6. Cross your left leg over your right leg. Cross your right elbow over your left thigh. Gently press your leg with your elbow to twist your hip and lower and middle parts of your back. Look over your left shoulder to complete the stretch.

Lifting Techniques

Your back has three natural curves—inward at your neck, outward at your shoulder blades and inward again at the small of your back.

Whether you're toting your toddler or lugging lumber for a home improvement project, maintaining the proper alignment of these curves while lifting and working can prevent back injury.

- Think through your task. Clear space for proper lifting. Make sure the pathway and your destination are clear of obstacles, too. Would the task be easier if you used a cart or dolly? When possible, push a heavy load rather than pull.
- Lift with your legs. Position your feet shoulder-width apart. Bend at your knees, not your waist. Straddle your load and allow your powerful leg muscles to do the work.
- Hug that load. Carrying a load close to your body puts less force on your lower back (see page 54).
- If you twist, you'll shout. Instead, turn by pivoting your feet.

Even at rest, you can help keep your back healthy:
- Sitting: Choose a chair that supports your lower back and keeps your knees and hips level.
- Sleeping: A firm mattress lets you move freely, avoiding morning stiffness or backache.
- Standing: For time-consuming tasks, alternate resting one foot on a low stool or shelf.

Shape Up for Lifting

Strengthen the muscles of your lower back and abdomen—they support and protect your spine. Keep trim, too. You're more likely to get back injuries if you carry excess weight around your middle.

Oh, My Aching Back

Acute back pain usually resolves within 2 weeks. Stay active, but avoid a lot of lifting and bending. Apply ice the first day or two you feel pain. After 48 to 72 hours, use heat. Use of over-the-counter pain relievers may be helpful.

Warning: Seek medical help if you have:
- Shooting pain down one or both legs (especially below the knees)
- Weakness
- New bowel or bladder control problems (incontinence, constipation)

Note: X-rays are usually not helpful or necessary to diagnose a back pain problem.

For more information, see page 50.

■ Safety in the Workplace

Protect yourself and others by following these safety rules and commonsense guidelines:

- **Protective eye wear:** If your job carries a risk of eye injury, your employer is required by law to provide you with protective glasses, and you are required to wear them. If they interfere with your efficiency, try another design.

- **Protection from noise:** In conditions of excessively loud noise, your employer should regularly measure noise levels or provide protective devices. Specially designed earmuffs are available. Some types close out the outside world; others are fitted with earphones and a microphone that enable you to communicate with other workers. Commercially available earplugs made of foam, plastic or rubber or custom-molded plugs also effectively decrease your exposure to excessive noise. Don't use cotton balls. They can get stuck deep in your ear canal.
- **Fumes, smoke, dust and gas hazards:** Many respiratory symptoms can result from exposure to toxic fumes, gases, particles and smoke in the workplace. The exposure may be long-term with low levels of chemicals; accidental exposure also may occur in which high levels of industrial toxic chemicals are inhaled for a short time. Wear proper clothing, air-filtration masks, eye gear and other appropriate protection. Be sure ventilation is adequate.

If you are pregnant or are trying to become pregnant, avoid any exposure to hazardous chemicals.

If you suspect that there may be dangerous smoke, fumes, dust or chemical exposure in your workplace, discuss the matter with your physician. Many permanent respiratory ailments develop slowly as a result of industrial exposure over a period of years. Small exposures that may seem harmless can result in chronic disease. If you think that you or your coworkers are at unnecessary risk, consult with your company safety office, or contact OSHA or your union.

Medication and alcohol use: Do not consume alcohol before or during working hours. Do not operate machinery when you are taking medications that might make you drowsy. If taking medications, ask your physician or pharmacist how they might affect your job.

■ Sleeping Tips for Shift Workers

Changing your normal rhythm of waking and sleeping, as a result of switching shifts, requires a period of adjustment. If you have ever flown across multiple time zones, you know what can happen when your body's internal clock is disrupted. Insomnia, mental and physical fatigue, indigestion and an overall feeling of ill health are common.

If your job requires constant changing of shifts, your body will have more difficulty adjusting and readjusting as you get older. Some studies suggest that too frequent shift changes over a lengthy period can put you at an increased risk of coronary artery disease or peptic ulcer.

Here are some strategies to try:
- Work a shift for 3 weeks rather than rotating to a different schedule every week.
- Change the sequence. A more normal sleep pattern results when the shift sequence is day-evening-night rather than the day-night-evening.
- Tolerance to shift rotation varies among people. If you have difficulty making the adjustment, consider changing your job. If you experience severe insomnia, ask your physician about a short-acting sleeping pill.

For more information, see page 44.

■ Drugs, Alcohol and Work

Illegal street drugs and alcohol can affect your health and safety in the workplace, as well as the safety of your coworkers. The problem is extensive. Consider the following statistics:

- Seventy-five percent of illegal drug users are employed.
- Alcoholism causes 500 million lost workdays a year.
- Drug- and alcohol-related problems are one of the four top reasons for workplace violence.
- The risk of an accident is 5 times greater in people coming to work under the influence of drugs or alcohol.
- People using drugs or alcohol miss nearly 10 times as much work as coworkers who do not use drugs or alcohol.
- Drug users, as a group, use medical benefits at a rate 8 times higher than non-users.
- A Gallup poll of employees found that 97 percent agreed that workplace drug testing is appropriate under certain circumstances, and 85 percent believed that urine testing may deter illicit drug use.

Self-Assessment

To determine if you have a problem with alcohol or drugs, ask yourself the following questions:

- Have I used an illegal drug in the past 6 months?
- Have I misused a prescription drug because of its effect (to sleep or calm myself, or for pleasure)?
- Have I done something unsafe or taken risks while under the influence of alcohol or drugs, such as driving a car, operating heavy equipment or making decisions that affect the safety of others?
- Have I used alcohol within 12 hours of going to work?
- Has my drug or alcohol use negatively affected my relationships, my health or my ability to work?

   If you answered "yes" to any of these questions, you are showing signs of substance abuse and should take action.

Self-Care

- If you or a family member is dependent on alcohol, refer to Alcohol Abuse and Alcoholism on page 186.
- If you or a family member has problems with drug addiction, refer to Drug Dependency on page 194.
- Many large corporations offer confidential employee assistance programs to help workers deal with drug and alcohol abuse. Inquire about their availability through your personnel or human resources department.
- If your company does not offer an alcohol or drug rehabilitation program, contact your health care provider or a mental health professional for a confidential referral.

Workplace Health

Balancing Work and Home

Five Tips to Save Your Sanity

Is life a circus these days? Try these five tips to save your sanity:

- Identify the activities on your schedule that are absolutely necessary and satisfy you most. Is your schedule weighted toward these things? Or does it neglect them in favor of things that are unnecessary and unfulfilling? Create a schedule emphasizing the things that matter.
- Organize household tasks efficiently. Doing daily laundry and running errands in "batches" are good places to start. A weekly family calendar of important dates helps avoid "deadline panic."
- Eliminate time-consuming misunderstandings by communicating clearly and listening carefully. In your complicated life, you have to talk with everyone from your partner to your child care provider. Be good at it.
- Fight the guilt. Remember: Having a family and a job is normal—for both women and men. If nothing helps, tell your kids how you're feeling. Chances are they'll understand.
- Save "alone time" each day for an activity you enjoy. Really. Recast the frantic hour right after work as quiet family snack time. It'll keep hungry kids at bay and help everyone decompress for the evening.

Balance doesn't mean doing everything. Develop your own idea of balance and take steps to live it.

For more information, see pages 224 and 239.

A Sick Child and a Demanding Job

"My daughter had a lot of colds and ear infections when she was a toddler, so I went through periods where I missed 2 or 3 days of work each month," recalls Joanne of Minneapolis. "I'm a teacher, so having to find a substitute for all those days was a real hassle. And I can still remember what my principal said to me so many times: 'Your daughter's sick, again?'"

This statement sums up the challenge that working parents face when their children become sick. For some, a child's illness also means lost pay. Count on it: Your child is going to get sick. By preparing for it now, you can promote your child's health— and keep your boss happy.

- **Before your child gets sick,** try to find people who can help with caregiving.
  Options may include:
  Grandparents or other relatives
  Friends
  Neighbors
  Retired people
  Members of places of worship
  College students
  Other parents who stay at home or run home-based businesses

As you search for alternative caregivers, ask everyone you know. Perhaps your school secretary or child's teachers will have suggestions. When talking with alternative caregivers, you can offer value in exchange. Some people want money, but others might be willing to work on an exchange system. In return for child care, you could offer to do household chores, run errands or babysit on evenings or weekends. If possible, line up several people you can call. Have a plan A—and plans B and C.

- **Work it out with your partner.** The burden of caring for sick children can fall especially hard on women. "In a lot of families, it's either covertly or overtly suggested that it's the mom who stays home with the sick child," says Jill A. Swanson, M.D., head of the community pediatric and adolescent medicine section at Mayo Clinic, Rochester, Minnesota. "Sometimes moms need to say to dads, 'Hey, it's your turn.' Moms need to know that it's OK to ask others to share this responsibility."

It pays to discuss this issue ahead of time with a spouse or partner. While children are young, one of you might be able to work a part-time job or a job with flexible hours. You also can trade "shifts." For example, perhaps your partner can stay home in the morning while you work and then trade roles with you in the afternoon to lessen the impact on either job.

- **Consider child care centers for sick children.** Some child care centers are designed specifically for sick children. Children's hospitals may offer this service. In other cases, regular child care centers provide a separate area for sick children.

Some parents prefer not to use such services, reasoning that a sick child belongs at home with mom or dad. But others say there are circumstances in which sick-child centers can do the job. For example, a child with a contagious condition may have only mild symptoms and basically feel fine, even though he or she is forced to stay away from school. Perhaps all the child needs is a nap and some quiet play, and a parent's presence is not required.

Before you decide to use sick-child centers, visit one or two with your child. Ask about costs and policies, and determine whether you feel comfortable with the personnel and setting.

Remember that sick-child centers are only for children with mild symptoms. When children are quite ill, they may need the kind of attention only a parent can provide—at home.

- **Aim for a flexible work life.** Try to structure your work so that you have more flexibility for child care. Technology—such as E-mail, cellular phones, fax machines—offers more opportunities for this than ever before. Ask about such options when you look for your next job. And ask about allowances for emergency child care.

- **Work it out with your employer.** Another option is to negotiate. If you present solutions instead of ultimatums, your employer might respond positively. Be willing to bring work home or work extra hours during evenings and weekends. Ask colleagues if you can delegate tasks to them. Offer to trade shifts with another employee. Show that you intend to complete your work even when your children get sick.

Some companies recognize that it's in their interest to help parents care for sick children. This insight has led to a number of creative solutions:

Some companies give employees a number of paid, non-vacation days off to use for any purpose, including sick-child care. Some employers help locate sick-child centers for employees and even subsidize the costs.

Other companies allow employees to use sick leave or vacation days when caring for children. In some cases, employees can "donate" their unused sick leave to a coworker.

Perhaps your company lacks a policy on sick-child care simply because no one has asked for it. Once you bring this issue to light, you and your employer may be able to work together—especially if other parents voice similar concerns. Everyone loses when conflicts between work and family drain a productive employee. Searching for mutual solutions can turn up a win-win scenario.

- **Know your benefits and rights.** Your union contract or employee benefits package might include policies on caring for sick children. In the United States, the Family and Medical Leave Act requires employers to grant leave so that employees can care for sick family members. Remember, however, that the time off mandated under the law is unpaid and that there are conditions you must meet to be covered by this act.
- **Take the long-range view.** There's a saying: "On our deathbed, few of us will wish we'd spent more time at the office." A broader perspective can help you make choices about child care that align with your long-term goals.

■ Morning Madness

For most families—especially those in which both parents work outside the home—morning is one of the most stressful times of the day. Reduce morning stress as follows:

- Make sure everyone gets adequate rest. Set realistic bedtimes for your children and enforce them. Begin heading to bed 30 to 60 minutes before you want lights out.
- Keep everyone moving. To get children in and out of the bathroom, set a timer and create a rotation schedule.
- Avoid distractions. Don't allow the kids to watch television until everyone is ready to go.
- Take an extra 10 minutes for yourself (such as for coffee or meditation) before the kids get up. If you still feel rushed, try setting the alarm for 15 minutes earlier.

Don't take total responsibility for getting everyone out the door. Let your children help by having them lay out their clothes, prepare their lunches and pack their backpacks the night before. Children tend to be more cooperative if they feel like they are a part of the process.

Stress Relievers

■ Burned Out? Get a Tune-Up

If you dread going to work or feel burned out or stressed over a period of weeks, you are facing a situation that could affect your professional and personal relationships and even your livelihood. Overwhelming frustration or indifference toward your job, persistent irritability, anger, sarcasm and a quickness to argue are indicators of a condition that needs to be dealt with. Here are strategies you can use:

- Take care of yourself. Eat regular, balanced meals, including breakfast. Get adequate sleep and exercise.
- Develop friendships at work and outside the office. Sharing unsettling feelings with people you trust is the first step toward resolving them. Limit activities with "negative" friends who reinforce bad feelings.
- Take time off. Take a vacation or a long weekend. Plan private time each week when you do not answer calls or pages. During the workday, take short breaks.
- Set limits. When necessary, learn to say "no" in a friendly but firm manner.
- Choose battles wisely. Don't rush to argue every time someone disagrees with you. Keep a cool head, and save your argument for things that really matter. (Better yet, try not to argue at all.)
- Have an outlet. Read, do a hobby, exercise or get involved in some other activity that gets your mind off work and is relaxing.
- Seek help. If none of these steps relieve your feelings of stress or burnout, ask a health care professional for advice.

Burnout buster: Throw away all but the important papers on your desk, transferring any tasks to a master list. Throughout the day, scan that list and work on tasks in priority order.

■ Coworker Conflict: Five Steps to Make the Peace

The best way to deal with differences is directly, that is, talking with the person with whom you have a conflict. However, the mood of that discussion is crucial. Here are some helpful tips:

- **Discuss the matter privately.** Choose neutral territory, at a specific time that each can agree on. Approach the other person in a nonthreatening manner, such as "I would like to talk something over with you. I'm feeling . . . ." Another opening line is, "I would like to check something out with you when you have a chance to talk."
- **Don't blame the other person.** Use "I" statements. It will make the other person feel less defensive or angry.
- **Listen closely to the other person.** Understanding the other person's point of view may help you feel less stressed or angry.
- **Focus on ways to resolve the problem.** Don't get sidetracked in an argument.
- **Seek help.** Talk with an employee assistance counselor who can help develop ground rules for such discussions and promote respectful communication.

Workplace Health

Five Fast Tips for Managing Time

- Create a reading file of articles ripped from or marked in newspapers and journals.
- Throw away all but the important papers on your desk. Prepare a master list of tasks. Pitch files older than 6 months.
- Throughout the day, scan your master list and work on tasks in priority order.
- Use a planner. Store addresses and telephone numbers there. Copy master list items onto the page for the day on which you expect to do them. Evaluate and prioritize daily.
- For especially important or difficult projects, reserve an interruption-free block of time behind closed doors.

Get to Know Your Boss and You'll Get Along Better

If you and your boss mix like oil and water, don't despair. To revive your relationship, work on getting to know him or her better. Here's how:

- Ask yourself, "What does my boss really need?" Is it more important to him or her that you stay on schedule while producing fair-to-good results, or is sacrificing a deadline OK if it means making a project perfect? Does your boss like to know your every move, or does he or she feel taxed with information overload when you provide updates? Learn your boss's preferences and use the information to make your boss's life and yours easier.
- Know what your boss expects. If the person you report to isn't forthcoming about expectations, be direct in asking what they are.
- Determine your boss's personal style. Formal or informal? Big picture or details? Without becoming a clone, try to adapt your behavior.

Talk to your boss. A frank yet diplomatic talk may be all it takes to move a relationship from strained to satisfactory.

Halt Hostility: Talk It Out

"It's OK to feel anger—even when you're on the job," says Dr. Richard E. Finlayson of Mayo's Department of Psychiatry and Psychology. "The question is," he adds, "are you handling anger properly?"

To head off hostility, the most important thing to do is to talk to someone to release tension and possibly gain a new perspective.

When a conflict is already brewing:

- Talk about *solutions* as well as problems. Work with others to rectify the situation.
- Try to put off your anger until you've heard all the facts.
- If you feel an outburst coming on, take a break. Count to 10, breathe deeply, go for a walk—whatever it takes to cool off and avoid doing something you might regret later.
- Use "active listening" skills and calmly repeat back what you've heard. ("Let me make sure I understand you. . . .")
- When an angry confrontation seems inevitable, seek a neutral third party to help talk it through.

Handling Office Gossip

A changing company in which job futures might seem uncertain is sure to fuel speculation among the staff. And when there is a lack of real information, the tongues of wondering employees will wag.

In these types of situations, says Connie L. Tooley, Mayo Clinic employee assistance coordinator, trust levels drop and employees fill in the blanks.

Rumors thrive in this setting. They may offer a diversion for the participants but are often painful or destructive to the person at the center of the chatter. Tooley and her counterparts in Mayo's Employee Assistance Program say you can control gossip.

Take responsibility. For example, identify yourself in the role of a listener instead of a backbiter. If the conversation turns to rumors, say you're not comfortable with the discussion. If you overhear something, walk away. You can even resolve to say only positive things instead of sustaining the negative.

Healthy Ways to Handle Demanding Workloads

If you're like most people in the workplace, you're busy figuring out how to handle more work with fewer resources.

Long before job demands create undue pressure, recognize the signs of workplace stress. Mayo Clinic behavioral medicine specialist Dr. Barbara K. Bruce notes signs of stress to watch for: headaches, abdominal upset, disrupted sleep, fatigue, lack of patience and loss of sense of humor.

Once you know the tension's mounting, take healthful steps to fend it off. How? Don't be a workaholic. Do take care of relationships. "So-called workaholics," Bruce says, "are 'productive' to the exclusion of other parts of their lives. Often as work demands climb, we spend less and less time with friends and family. This contributes to the increased stress and exhaustion—and ultimately decreases productivity."

Research shows that social support acts as a buffer for stress. So relationships (with spouses, coworkers and others) are very important.

Listen Up: Train Yourself to Be a Good Listener

Use the EARS formula to train yourself to listen better.

E = Encourage your partner. Nod, ask questions, indicate with your body language that you're following what's being said. Focus all your attention on your partner. Don't fiddle with items on your desk or lose eye contact.

A = Acknowledge your partner. Restate or repeat his or her point of view to check out whether you're getting the message. Say, "So, you think we should . . . ." Don't assume you understand your partner until he or she agrees with your restatement.

R = **Respond to your partner.** Ask questions to get more information. Say, "Tell me more." Often, your partner will open up and get to the real issue at this point. Don't be too quick to give your opinion or a hasty answer.

S = **Slow down.** Involve your partner in coming up with a solution or considering options. Two brains are generally better than one. End the conversation on a positive note—one that encourages, not discourages, further communication.

■ When You Become the Boss

You used to be "one of the guys." Then, you're promoted. It's a difficult situation. You have new and expanded responsibilities. You may be supervising a person who wanted the promotion you received. Develop a plan to gain the support of your former coworkers. Help your former peers through the change, set clear limits, change your relationships with them—and get the work done. Not so easy!

To get started on creating the new order, meet with each person. Use this six-step agenda to guide your conversation.

1. **Acknowledge the awkwardness.** Say, "We've worked together for a long time. This change may take some getting used to. I want it to work well."

2. **Ask for support.** Say, "I want your help in making this transition an easy one. Can I count on you?"

3. **Ask for input.** Say, "What do you think my highest priority should be? What else should I keep in mind?" Then listen.

4. **Ask for a situation report.** Say, "Bring me up to speed on all of your projects (or areas of responsibility)."

5. **Set goals with the person.** Get the spotlight off your relationship and on the work to be done. Focus on productivity and output. If possible, limit the time frame to this quarter, or even this month. Make the goals measurable, and be specific about what you expect.

6. **Appreciate and acknowledge** the person's contributions, unique abilities and importance to the team or department.

Coping With Technology

■ Hunched by Lunchtime?

If your job makes you feel like the Hunchback of Notre Dame, you may need some ergonomic advice. "Ergonomics" is a long word with a big impact on your health. Ergonomists study ways to fit work to the worker.

If you work at a computer, knowing about ergonomics is a must. Here are some basics:

- Sit comfortably upright. Avoid slouching.
- Keep your keyboard at elbow height or slightly lower.
- Place your monitor as far away as possible, making sure you can still read the text.
- Check your shoulders from time to time. Are they tense? Consciously relax them.
  Stand while you work. You'll be in prominent company. Ernest Hemingway, Virginia Woolf, Winston Churchill and Thomas Jefferson used desks raised for standing.

Remember the phrase "get up and move." For example, stand while you're on the phone. Print out computer files, move to a new location and proofread on paper instead of the monitor.

■ Tuning Out Technology?

Have you felt the urge to kill your computer? You're not alone. Nearly 60 percent of workers are technophobic. "Technophobia" (fear of technology) isn't a disease that requires medical attention. It's a general term describing an attitude or reaction, one that produces symptoms of anxiety.

More specifically, people fear looking stupid, appearing inadequate, being monitored by Big Brother, losing control, being at the mercy of a machine, relying on anything mechanical because it might fail, damaging the machine or the data and losing face-to-face contact.

People fear for their job security. Self-confidence dwindles. When an electronic device fails to operate properly, whom can they blame? The manufacturer, the machine or themselves? Two-thirds blame themselves.

Technophobia may result in outright rejection of new gadgets, reluctance to learn, ineffectiveness on the job and increased absenteeism. The phobia prevents 75 percent of employees from using information technology properly. Most people bumble along, using only 10 to 25 percent of the capabilities of any software program. And a whopping 75 percent secretly wonder, "What is software, anyhow?"

To tackle technophobia:

- Practice!
- Play a game with your computer.
- Get a coach—maybe a coworker.
- Use your "help desk," if provided.
- Read a "dummies" book.
- List the benefits to hang on your wall.
- Tackle one thing at a time.
- Take a weekend course.
- Celebrate achievements along the way.
- Practice!

■ Computers and Neck Pain

Try these suggestions:

- Adjust your screen to eye level so you don't have to slouch or stretch to see. Pushing the monitor back can give you greater depth of focus as well as more work space.
- Make sure your eyeglasses allow you to see the screen without tilting your head.
- Sit in a desk chair that supports your upper spine and your lower back. A chair with arm supports may help relieve neck tension.
- Take 30-second micro-breaks every hour to stretch and exercise your neck.
- Use a speaker phone or headset. Don't type while cradling the phone on your shoulder.

■ Computer Screens and Eyestrain

There you sit, peering at your video display terminal (VDT). If you're one of a growing number of people for whom using a computer is integral to their work, you may be peering for the umpteenth hour today. And like many computer users, you may be experiencing eyestrain as a result.

Symptoms may include:

- Sore, tired, burning, itching or dry eyes
- Blurred or double vision
- Distance vision blurred after prolonged staring at monitor
- Headache, sore neck
- Difficulty shifting focus between monitor and source documents
- Difficulty focusing on the screen image
- Color fringes or afterimages when you look away from the monitor
- Increased sensitivity to light

Eyestrain associated with VDTs isn't thought to have serious or long-term consequences, but it is disruptive and unpleasant. Although you probably can't change every factor that may cause eyestrain, here are some things you can try to ease the strain:

- Change your work habits.
- Take eye breaks. Look away from the screen and into the distance or at an object several feet away for 10 seconds every 10 minutes.
- Change of pace. Try to move around at least once every 2 hours, giving both your eyes and your body a needed rest. Arrange noncomputer work as breaks from the screen. Consider standing while doing such work.
- Wink 'em, blink 'em ... Dry eyes can result from prolonged computer use, especially for contact lens wearers. Some people blink only once a minute when doing computer work (once every 5 seconds is normal). Less blinking means less lubrication from tears, resulting in dry, itchy or burning eyes. So blink more often. If that doesn't help, you may want to consider using an eyedrop form of artificial tears available over-the-counter.
- ... and nod. If possible, lean back and close your eyes for a few moments once in a while. You may not want to do this at your desk and risk being accused of sleeping on the job.

Mayo Clinic Guide to Self-Care

Everything in Its Place

Monitor: Position your monitor 18 to 30 inches from your eyes. Many people find that putting the screen at arm's length is about right. If you have to get too close to read small type, consider using larger font sizes for characters on your screen. This is usually an easy adjustment in preferences offered in word processing and Internet-browser software.

The top of the screen should be at eye level or below so that you look down slightly at your work. Place the monitor too high and you'll have to tilt your head back to look up at it, a recipe for a sore neck—and for dry eyes, because you may not close your eyes completely when you blink. If you have your monitor on top of your central processing unit (CPU), consider placing the CPU to one side or on the floor.

Dust on the screen cuts down contrast and may contribute to glare and reflection problems. Keep it clean.

Keyboard: Put your keyboard directly in front of the monitor. If you place it at an angle or to the side, your eyes will be forced to focus separately, a tiring activity.

Source documents: Put reading and reference material on a copy stand beside the monitor and at the same level, angle and distance away. That way, your eyes aren't constantly readjusting as they go back and forth.

Ambient (surrounding) light and glare: To check glare, sit at your computer with the monitor off. You will be able to see the reflected light and images you don't normally see—including yourself. Note any intense glare. The worst problems likely will be from sources above or behind you, including fluorescent lighting and sunlight.

If possible, place your monitor so that the brightest light sources are off to the side, parallel with your line of sight to the monitor. Consider turning off some or all overhead lights. If you can't do that, tilting the monitor downward a little may reduce glare. Closing blinds or shades also may help. A hood or glare-reducing screen is an option, but be sure you aren't sacrificing the intensity of whites on your screen. Adjustable task lighting that doesn't shine into your eyes as you look at the screen can reduce eyestrain. Overall, the surrounding light should be darker than the whitest white on your screen.

Glasses: The correct correction can help. If you wear glasses or contacts, make sure the correction is right for computer work. Most lenses are fitted for reading print and may not be optimal for computer work. For example, many bifocal wearers are constantly craning their necks to look through the bottom half of the lenses, bringing on backache or neckache. Glasses or contact lenses designed to focus correctly for computer work may be a worthwhile investment.

See an eye care professional if you have:

- Prolonged eye discomfort
- A noticeable change in vision
- Double vision

Pregnancy and Work

Know Your Rights

Many women work throughout their pregnancy and during their children's infancy. In fact, more than half of all women with children younger than 6 have paying jobs. But it's important to remember that Superwoman is fiction. It can be stressful to juggle a demanding job, the physical changes during pregnancy, housework and child care.

Here we offer you some general tips. But remember, each pregnancy, delivery and parenting experience is different. If your pregnancy is uncomplicated, you can probably work right up to delivery. It's generally good for you to work, even if your job is physically strenuous. Several federal and state laws can help you make decisions about working during your pregnancy and after your baby is born. Whenever state laws are more generous, they take priority over federal laws.

The Pregnancy Discrimination Act of 1978 makes it illegal to discriminate against pregnant employees. Women with pregnancy-related disabilities are entitled to the same disability leave, job protection or reassignment offered other disabled employees. Federal offices or businesses employing fewer than 15 employees are exempt.

The Family and Medical Leave Act of 1993 requires employers of 50 or more persons to provide up to 12 weeks of unpaid leave a year for:

- The birth, adoption or foster care of a child
- Care for a sick child, spouse or parent
- Your own serious health condition

You must have worked at least 1,250 hours for that employer in the past year to be eligible. Employers may ask you to use available sick leave, vacation, personal or family leave for part of the time. You are entitled to the same insurance benefits as when you were working. You may return to the same or an equivalent job. The law includes fathers, and it requires a 30-day notice, when possible.

Tips for Making Work Time More Pleasant

- When you're pregnant, you need more sleep than usual, especially for a physically demanding job. Limit outside activities temporarily.
- To combat morning sickness:
  - Get a good night's sleep; rise early enough to dress without rushing.
  - Keep crackers or other bland food at work for frequent nibbling.
  - Avoid nausea-triggering odors—even if it means politely asking a coworker to avoid wearing a certain aftershave or cologne temporarily.
- Use comfortable, adjustable office equipment.

Workplace Cautions If You're Pregnant

Discuss safety concerns with your doctor. These conditions may include:
- Heavy, repetitive lifting, prolonged standing, vibrations from large machines.
- Frequent shift changes.
- An overheated workplace.
- Exposure to lead, mercury, X-rays, drugs for treating cancer, anesthetic gases and organic solvents (benzene, for example). Federal law requires industries to have on file and available to employees Material Safety Data Sheets that report on hazardous substances in the workplace.
- Exposure to infections. You can limit your risk by wearing gloves, washing your hands frequently and eating away from your workplace.

Returning to Work After the Birth

- After your baby is born, you need to be comfortable with your decision about returning to work. Share your feelings with your partner and your doctor.
- If you decide to return to work, enlist your partner's help: getting baby up and ready, preparing meals, cleaning the house and doing laundry.
- It's important to schedule time for yourself. Ask a friend, relative or babysitter to watch your baby while you spend time with your partner, go to lunch, shop, exercise or just relax at home.
- It's common to feel guilty about returning to work. You feel pulled both ways. You worry about missing first steps or first words. You wonder how you'll continue breast-feeding. You want your baby to receive the best possible care.
- Talk with your employer and partner about extending your leave as long as possible. Investigate part-time, flex-time, job-sharing or telecommuting options for easing back into work. Share your creative ideas about managing your work in your absence.
- Separation anxiety is normal for babies between 6 and 13 months old. Although clingy at first, your baby will adapt rapidly to a new routine.

Tips for Continuing Breast-Feeding When You Work

- Ask your employer for a quiet, private place (perhaps an empty office with a door lock) where you can express your breast milk. If your employer has on-site child care or if your caregiver is nearby, you may nurse your baby during an extended break or lunchtime.
- Borrow or rent a breast pump. Electric pumps are generally more effective for milk expression than hand pumping. Double-breasted pumps are fast (10 to 15 minutes) and help maintain your milk supply.
- Introduce your baby to bottles with breast milk early in your maternity leave. Substitute a bottle for one feeding a day. You may need to try several nipples to find one your baby takes easily. Sometimes it's easier to have your partner give the bottle.

- Empty your breasts once or twice during the workday. Use an insulated bag with cold packs to transport the milk. Use it for two or three feedings the next day. If you can't express your milk at work, do so before leaving in the morning and on returning and an additional time or two on the weekend. Breast milk will keep for 5 days in the refrigerator. Give the bottle straight from the refrigerator or warmed under the tap. Don't heat breast milk in a microwave. The immunity that breast milk provides can be destroyed, and the hot milk could burn your baby.
- Limit the amount of formula the caregiver offers in your absence so your baby nurses well on your return, maintaining your milk supply.
- Talk with your hospital's lactation consultant, or call a La Leche League representative listed in the telephone book.

Child Care Choices

Child care varies widely, and no choice is best for everyone. Each has its advantages and challenges. Ask friends, coworkers and health care providers for referrals. Begin at least 3 months before you need care; openings in good programs may be scarce. Many communities list child care resource and referral agencies in the telephone book. Otherwise, Child Care Aware (800-424-2246) can direct you, or contact National Association of Child Care Resources and Referral Agencies (202-393-5501).

- Visit and interview all the caregivers. Ask about training and experience.
- Ask whether drop-in visits are allowed. Most quality programs encourage parents to visit freely.
- Discuss emergency care and whether the provider has training in infant CPR (cardiopulmonary resuscitation).
- Discuss hours, late policies, diaper preferences, no-smoking policy and emergency procedures.

Retirement Planning

Remember when retirement meant a gold watch and time on your hands? Now it often means volunteering at the crisis shelter, scheduling trips to the Grand Canyon and squeezing in visits with the kids.

About 35 million Americans are at or close to retirement age—a new stage of life that can be as rewarding and fulfilling as the preceding ones. Healthful lifestyles and medical advances mean more years of better health to enjoy retirement than ever before.

Is retirement satisfying? A lot depends on you.

From Employee to Retiree

Before Social Security came into effect about 60 years ago, people worked as long as they could or until they died. Retirement in our culture is relatively new.

With its newness can come lack of preparation and experience. Retirement isn't something that happens overnight. It helps to view it as a process that unfolds in stages, says Virginia Richardson, social work professor at Ohio State University. At each stage, you can take steps to increase your satisfaction.

Stage 1: Pre-retirement: This stage covers life from about ages 40 to 60—a time to take stock of yourself and what you can do to prepare for a long life. This applies to you whether or not you'll retire from paid employment. "There's plenty of evidence to show that people who think about and prepare for retirement adjust better," says Richardson.

Three factors usually determine adjustment:

1. Financial security: Save and invest wisely now, even though discipline and risk are required. Attending pre-retirement classes can help you estimate your retirement income and whether it will be enough for the lifestyle you envision. Starting early gives you time to make changes if the figures don't add up.

2. Good health: Controlling your weight with regular exercise and a healthful diet, plus preventive medical care, can pay off later with continued good health and vitality.

3. Positive attitude: Optimism about the future is a tonic for a satisfying retirement.

To develop a positive attitude:

- Envision life after work: How are you going to occupy the time that used to be filled by your job? Busy work and hobbies aren't enough. Think of retirement as an opportunity for continued growth and enrichment.

Planning to Retire? Stay Connected and Keep Moving

Recent research supports common sense: If you want to stay healthy in retirement, then keep up your circulation—and stay in circulation.

In one study, exercise and emotional support were the strongest predictors of health in older adults. Researchers saw a possible link between lack of social contact and lower amounts of certain hormones. Those chemical changes may affect the immune system.

To multiply your benefits, combine social and physical activity. Join an exercise class. Walk with a friend. Bike with your family. Do anything that keeps you active socially and physically.

- Scrutinize yourself: If your identity, self-esteem and social network are tied to your career or your spouse's work, you could have trouble adjusting. Explore new ways to achieve a sense of accomplishment, structure and status.
- Don't ignore your emotions: Acknowledge feelings of grief, anger or sadness about aging and leaving your job. If these emotions persist, consider counseling.

Stage 2: Decision time: Will you retire early? How do you want to live? The more control you have over these decisions, the better you'll adjust to not working. To exercise control:

- Rehearse for retirement: Plan what you'd like to do with your free time and try it out on weekends and vacations. Gradually reduce your work hours or responsibilities. If your spouse has died, investigate activities for singles that are available during the hours you now work.
- Reassess marriage roles: If you're a homemaker, will having your spouse around help or hinder your daily routine? Start now to share household tasks. If you've had a career, how can you become more comfortable at home from 9 to 5? How will your routines change if you retire and your spouse doesn't?

Stage 3: Retirement: Sometimes circumstances take retirement out of your control. If you're forced to retire due to a layoff or illness, or if you can't afford to retire, retirement may be stressful.

Even the best planned retirement can have emotional bumps. Dr. Richardson found that feelings of loss, the blues, restlessness, anxiety, mild depression or preoccupation with the past are normal for many people during the first 6 months. If you have these feelings, expect them to end and that you'll have renewed vitality by the end of the first year. If not, or if the feelings seem overwhelming, talk to your doctor.

More than 90 percent of voluntary retirements, however, are satisfying. Here's what experts recommend for a smooth retirement:

- Stay active: Setting goals and sticking to a schedule maintain continuity and structure. For example, get up each morning at a regular time, take a walk, then read the newspaper and eat breakfast. Join a service club. Become a volunteer.
- Emphasize intellectual pastimes: Work crossword puzzles or play Scrabble to help keep your mind sharp. Mental abilities don't inevitably decline with age. "Use it or lose it" applies to your mind as well as your body.
- Travel: It doesn't have to be far or expensive. Travel organizations that meet the needs of older adults are a growing specialty.
- Go back to school: Finish your degree, start a new one or just take classes for fun. Most universities and colleges have noncredit continuing education programs.

A concept that combines travel with education is Elderhostel. As a participant, you live on a college campus while taking noncredit courses in everything from astronomy to Shakespeare. For example, one of the courses involves studying Southwest Indian pottery for 1 week at the College of Santa Fe. For information, write: Elderhostel, 75 Federal St., Boston, MA 02110 or call (617) 426-8056.

- Volunteer: You'll not only feel a sense of accomplishment but also fill a desperate need in this time of tight budgets. Museums, schools, hospitals, libraries and social agencies are some of the places where your experience and help are welcome.

Plan and work at your retirement. It could be the best job you've ever had.

The Healthy Consumer

In this section, we answer questions related to the healthy consumer, such as, How can you best communicate and work with your physician? What can you learn from your family's medical history? How effective are home medical testing kits? What should you include in the family's home medicine chest and first-aid kit? What are the potential health risks associated with travel? We also discuss proper use of medications and include easy-to-understand descriptions of cold remedies and over-the-counter pain medications that are mentioned throughout this book.

- **You and Your Health Care Provider**
- **Dealing With the Health Care System**
- **Home Medical Testing Kits**
- **Your Family Medical Tree**
- **Medications and You**
- **Vitamin and Mineral Supplements**
- **Alternative Medicine and Your Health**
- **The Healthy Traveler**

You and Your Health Care Provider

If you don't already have a main doctor, often called a primary care doctor, now is the time to find one. This is the physician who helps you make most of your medical decisions and who oversees the care you get from specialists. If you wait until you're sick and in a rush for relief, you may be forced to turn over serious treatment decisions to a doctor you don't know and who doesn't know you. That kind of uncertainty can make matters worse. When you're sick is not the time to scan the Yellow Pages looking for a doctor.

You'll probably want to choose one of three kinds of doctors as your main doctor — a family practitioner, an internist or a geriatrician. A family practitioner provides health care for people of all ages. An internist treats adults, and may have had additional training in a specialty such as heart diseases. A geriatrician is trained in family practice or internal medicine, and has had additional training in caring for older adults.

To receive a medical license, all doctors have to graduate from an accredited medical school and go through at least one year of training afterward. That's the minimum. But for your care, you need a doctor specially trained and experienced in treating adults — one who has completed work beyond the minimum. This extra work is usually called a residency and involves 2 to 6 years of supervised training. This extra training makes a doctor eligible for certification by the board of a given medical specialty. Afterward, the doctor must pass the certifying exam. Family practitioners, internists and geriatricians have all gone through this extra training.

Before you start looking for a doctor, think about what you most want in a doctor. Make a list, identifying the essentials as well as other features that would be nice but aren't absolutely necessary.

At the top of your list, put these three essentials:
- Trust
- Ability to communicate
- Availability

You need to be able to trust your doctor's advice about your health care. You need a doctor who will take time to listen to your concerns and who will talk to you with words you can easily follow. You'll want a doctor who's not too rushed to explain the medical term for your diagnosis or to help you understand why you need certain tests. If you can't trust or understand your doctor, you'll probably not take the medical advice you get as seriously as you need to. And your health could suffer.

Make sure your doctor is easily accessible. Some insurance programs may try to assign you a doctor who practices in another town. Find a good doctor as close to home as possible. You'll be more willing to go see the doctor when you need to if his or her office is nearby.

As you work on your list, think about other doctors you've had. Consider what you liked and didn't like about them. Perhaps you liked the doctors who were friendly and emotionally involved in your care and didn't like the doctors who were strictly business and bossy.

If you're a woman, you may prefer a woman doctor. If you're a man, you may prefer a man doctor. If you have a chronic health problem, such as diabetes, you

---

might want a doctor who has a subspecialty in that area.

Here are a few other questions to consider as you expand your list:

- Do you want a doctor practicing alone or in a group?
- How far away is the doctor's office from your home?
- Does the doctor accept Medicare or other insurance you have?
- Is the doctor allowed to admit patients to the hospital you prefer?
- Is the doctor part of a health maintenance organization (HMO)? If so, what restrictions does this imply?

How to Find a Doctor

Once you have an idea about what kind of doctor you want, identify several candidates. If you're on a managed care insurance plan, you may be limited to the doctors on the insurance company's list. If so, call the insurer to make sure you have the most current list.

Narrow Your Search

The best way to find a doctor is by word of mouth from trusted friends. So ask your friends, family, work colleagues and other trusted health care providers for recommendations. Be sure to ask what they like about the doctor, as well as any problems they've noticed. This can help you zero in on selected doctors.

Call the Doctor's Office

Once you've selected two or three doctors, call their offices. Tell the receptionist you're looking for a doctor and you'd like to speak with someone who could answer a few questions about the doctor and the office procedures. Take note of how the assistants respond to you because if you choose this doctor, you'll be working with these people. Are they courteous and helpful, or do they seem abrupt and inconvenienced by your call?

A good place to start is to find out if the doctor is accepting new patients. Next, ask if the doctor accepts your medical insurance plan.

Here are a few other questions you might consider asking:

- What's the doctor's special field of practice?
- What are your office hours?
- How many days a week does the doctor see patients?
- Are evening or weekend appointments possible?
- If I call the office with a medical question, can I speak with the doctor?
- How does the doctor arrange to answer medical questions after hours?
- How far in advance do people have to make an appointment? (If longer than a month, the doctor is probably overloaded. You might want to look elsewhere.)
- How long do people generally have to wait in the office? (Expect a wait of less than 20 minutes.)
- How willing is the doctor to refer people to a specialist?
- How long will you be able to visit with the doctor? (Some HMOs restrict total time to less than 30 minutes.)

Verify Credentials

Before you invest time and money in visiting a doctor, make a phone call or visit a Web site to confirm the doctor's credentials. If your doctor is board certified in a specialty, such as family practice, internal medicine or geriatrics, you can confirm this by checking with the American Board of Medical Specialties. You can call this organization at 866-275-2267 or log on to the Web site *www.abms.org.* The American Medical Association also has a Web site that identifies specialists. It's called AMA Physician Select, *www.ama-assn.org/ aps/amahg.htm.*

To determine if any disciplinary action has been taken or may be pending against a doctor, call your state medical licensing board. For the number, look under state government listings in your phone book or call directory assistance. Keep in mind, however, that even the best doctors occasionally have legal problems. So don't let this be the only factor in your decision.

Visit the Doctor's Office

After deciding on your first choice of a doctor, make an appointment. You'll probably have to pay for the visit, even if all you want to do is get to know the doctor. With that in mind, you might as well schedule a checkup. Let the assistant doing the scheduling know that this is your first visit and that you'd like a little extra time to talk with the doctor.

As you did in your initial phone call to the doctor's office, when you arrive for your appointment pay attention to how the office staff treats you. Also make note of how long you have to wait. If it's longer than 20 minutes, ask about the reason for the delay. The office staff may have overlooked your name on the list. Or perhaps the doctor is delayed at the hospital, and you may choose to reschedule the appointment.

When you meet the doctor, feel free to ask about:

- His or her medical background
- Why he or she chose to practice in a certain field of medicine
- Whether he or she treats many people in your age group and with your particular medical problem (if you have any)

Trust Your Instincts

If you don't feel compatible with the doctor, try the next one on your list. You're more likely to follow the advice of a doctor with whom you feel comfortable. Doctors know it. So don't worry about offending them. Concentrate on your needs.

■ Specialists You May Need

How do you know when you need a specialist or other health care provider, such as a physical therapist, a physician extender or a nurse practitioner? Generally, your main doctor will refer you to a specialist when you have a problem that warrants it. If you're concerned that you have medical problems not being adequately cared for by your main doctor, you might want to seek a specialist whose training and experience matches the problem.

Knowledge about diseases and treatment is growing so fast that specialties and subspecialties have emerged to help manage this information. A family doctor or internist, for example, can't possibly keep up on all the new findings in each area of health care from head to toe. Specialists are sometimes needed to perform many of the different diagnostic tests and to interpret the data. You and your main doctor will find it reassuring to have so many sources for specialized help with any complex health care problems that may lie ahead.

If you visit a specialist, ask that the records of your diagnosis and treatment be sent to your main doctor, who needs to keep track of your overall health care. Ask for a copy of the records for yourself. Also, next time you visit your main doctor, be sure to give a report of what the specialist did for you.

Specialists

Here's a list of specialists you might need along with the systems, diseases, conditions or therapies that they can help you with:

Allergist, immunologist. Allergies and diseases of the immune system
Anesthesiologist. Administers and monitors anesthetics
Audiologist. Tests hearing and treats hearing disorders
Cardiologist. Disorders of the heart, blood vessels and circulation
Dermatologist. Skin diseases, which can be deadly
Emergency medicine specialist. Evaluates and treats trauma, emergencies
Endocrinologist. Problems with the glands, including diabetes
Family physician. Total involvement with all family members and conditions
Gastroenterologist. Digestive diseases
Geneticist. Specialist in inherited diseases
Gynecologist. Specialist in care of women
Hematologist. Diseases of the blood
Infectious diseases specialist. Infectious diseases, immunization
Internist. Diagnosis and nonsurgical treatment of disease in adults
Nephrologist. Kidney problems
Neurologist. Nerve specialist
Neurosurgeon. Treats nerve diseases surgically
Obstetrician. Specialist in pregnancy, delivery and infant care
Orthopedist. Surgically treats bone disorders and injuries
Oncologist. Cancer specialist
Ophthalmologist. Eye specialist
Otorhinolaryngologist. Ear, nose and throat specialist
Pathologist. Studies bodily fluids and tissues
Pediatrician. Childhood diseases and preventive care
Physiatrist. Treats disorders of the nervous and musculoskeletal systems
Preventive medicine specialist. Focus on preventing diseases and injuries
Psychiatrist. Diagnosis and treatment of mental conditions and diseases
Psychologist. Specializes in psychological assessment and counseling therapy
Pulmonologist. Lung specialist. Also treats sleep disorders
Radiologist. Uses imaging techniques to diagnose and treat disease
Rheumatologist. Problems of the joints, muscles and connective tissue
Surgeon. Surgical treatment of various conditions. Many subspecialties
Urologist. Disorders of the urinary and urogenital tracts

Other Health Care Providers

Nurse. If you're in the hospital, you'll probably see nurses more frequently than doctors because nurses provide most of the care. The nurses observe symptoms and listen to you describe them, help carry out the treatment plan and evaluate the results.

The initials *R.N.* after a nurse's name mean registered nurse. To be an R.N., a person must complete a bachelor's degree in nursing or a similar program, and then pass a licensing examination in the state where he or she plans to practice. Some registered nurses have postgraduate degrees.

The initials *L.P.N.* mean licensed practical nurse. The L.P.N. course of study is shorter, and the L.P.N. generally works under the supervision of an R.N.

Some nurses specialize. For instance, they might focus on pediatrics or cardiology. Some not only specialize but also become a nurse practitioner (N.P.). A nurse practitioner usually has at least a master's degree and performs many of the same basic tasks as a doctor — examining and treating people as well as writing prescriptions. A nurse practitioner usually works in group practices, helping doctors manage the heavy load of office visits by diagnosing and treating people with the more common and less serious health problems.

Most N.P.s specialize in a particular area of health care, such as family medicine, adult health, pediatrics, neonatal care or geriatric care.

Occupational therapist. If you're injured or disabled, an occupational therapist helps you regain your ability to carry out everyday tasks, such as the activities required to make a living. The word *occupational* is misleading because the therapy isn't aimed solely at helping you get back to work, but at regaining the ability to do daily tasks wherever you are, at home or on the job: eating, dressing, bathing, homemaking and recreational skills. This therapist may recommend physical changes to your home or workplace — such as rearranging furniture or adding ramps and railings — to make it easier for you to get around and carry out your tasks.

Pharmacist. Your pharmacist is a good source of information about your medicine, whether it's prescription or nonprescription drugs. Since the pharmacist keeps a record of all prescriptions you buy at his or her pharmacy, it's helpful to use the same pharmacy for all your prescription drugs. This provides a double-check, to make sure you don't take a medication that reacts with something else you're taking. The pharmacist can also help you select nonprescription drugs that are best for you. But if you're taking prescription medicine, check with your main doctor before taking nonprescription drugs that are new to you.

Physical therapist. Like an occupational therapist, a physical therapist also helps injured and disabled people regain lost physical functions, using techniques such as exercise, massage and ultrasound. The focus here is to maximize physical ability and compensate for physical functions that have been lost.

Health care problems among older adults that may require physical therapy include:

- Arthritis
- Deconditioning
- Incontinence
- Joint replacements
- Osteoporosis
- Parkinson's disease
- Spinal cord injuries
- Stroke and other neurologic conditions

Physician assistant. Like a nurse practitioner, a physician assistant (P.A.) often helps relieve some of the patient care load of a doctor by diagnosing and treating people with some of the more common health care problems. Most P.A.s have at least a bachelor's degree. They generally work under the supervision of a doctor, performing work assigned by the doctor. Working as part of the health care team, they take medical histories, treat minor injuries that may require stitches or casting, order and interpret lab tests and X-rays, and make diagnoses. In most states they can also write prescriptions.

In some clinics most of the routine care is given by P.A.s. You may not see the doctor unless you have a major problem.

Selecting a Surgeon

Your primary doctor will help you find a good surgeon should you ever need an operation. If you need a joint replacement, for example, you'll probably be recommended to an orthopedic surgeon, who specializes in operations involving joints, muscles and bones. When choosing a surgeon, try to select one who has performed a lot of the kind of surgery you'll be having.

Given the potential risks and costs of many surgeries, it often makes good sense to get a second opinion. Either you or your primary doctor can make the decision to get that second opinion. So don't feel you need to be secretive about visiting a second surgeon. Keep your main doctor informed.

Questions to Ask Before Surgery

Whether your regular doctor or a surgeon recommends surgery, you'll want to ask several questions:

What is done during the operation? Ask for a clear description of the operation. If necessary, perhaps you could ask the doctor to draw a picture to help explain exactly what the surgery involves.

Are there alternatives to surgery? Sometimes surgery is the only way to correct the problem. But one option might be watchful waiting, to see if the problem gets better or worse.

How will surgery help? A hip replacement, for example, may mean you'll be able to walk comfortably again. To what extent will the surgery help and how long will the benefits last? You'll want realistic expectations.

What are the risks? All operations carry some risk. Weigh the benefits against the risks. Ask also about the side effects of the operation, such as the degree of pain you might expect and how long that pain will last.

What kind of experience have you had with this surgery? How many times has the doctor performed this surgery, and what percentage of the patients had successful results? To reduce your risks, you want a doctor who is thoroughly trained in the surgery and who has plenty of experience doing it.

Where will the surgery be done? Many surgeries today are done on an outpatient basis. You go to a hospital or a clinic for the surgery and return home the same day.

Will I be put to sleep for the surgery? Your surgery may require only local anesthesia, which means that just part of your body is numbed for a short time. General anesthesia puts you to sleep.

How long will recovery take? You'll want to know when most people are able to resume their normal activities, such as doing chores around the house and returning to work. You may think there would be no harm in lifting a sack of groceries after a week or two. But there might be. Follow your doctor's advice as carefully as possible.

What will it cost me? Health insurance coverage varies. You may not have to pay anything. You might have a deductible to meet. Or perhaps you'll have to pay a percentage of the cost. The doctor's office can usually give you information about this, but also check with your insurance company.

Be certain to know if you are responsible for a flat co-pay — a set amount for the surgery — or if you have to pay a percentage of the bill. There is a big — and expensive — difference.

Dealing With the Health Care System

Managed care organizations (MCOs), such as health maintenance organizations (HMOs) and preferred provider organizations (PPOs), are health insurers and networks of health care providers. They are alternatives to the traditional system of medical care in which you or your insurance company pays a fee for the service you receive.

In traditional fee-for-service plans, also known as indemnity plans, you pay a monthly premium to an insurance company. You also pay a percentage of the cost for health care services you receive.

Run by MCOs, managed care plans can save you money over traditional fee-for-service plans. Here's how they work:

- You pay a fixed, monthly premium and receive all your health care — doctor and hospital services, outpatient surgery, home health care, and some nursing home services — from providers who participate in the MCO networks. Some plans require a copayment for each doctor, emergency room or hospital visit.
- Your choice of providers is usually limited, but in some cases you may have broader coverage (for preventive care, for example). You'll likely pay less out-of-pocket for copayments or coinsurance if you use network providers.
- Network doctors who provide your care have agreed to accept a discount for their services. The discount may be in the form of a percentage off their usual charges, a fixed fee schedule per service, or even a fixed salary, regardless of how many office visits, tests or other services you receive (or don't receive). The MCO is your "bargaining agent" or health care contractor. Doctors join MCO networks in the hope of getting more business from patients who have a financial incentive to obtain care from the network (because patients in a managed care plan pay less out-of-pocket if they see a network doctor).

Types of Managed Care Plans

There are three main types of managed care plans:

1) **Preferred provider organization (PPO)** — This type of health plan contracts with independent doctors, hospitals and urgent care centers to provide care for plan subscribers. In return for bringing together subscribers and contract doctors, a PPO pays lower fees for the doctor's services. You may be allowed to see doctors outside this network in exchange for higher out-of-pocket expenses.

2) **Health maintenance organization (HMO)** — This type of plan provides health care in return for a fixed payment from you or your employer. There are many types of HMOs. A common feature is that you're limited to receiving your care from doctors, hospitals and urgent care centers affiliated with the HMO. In addition, many HMOs require that your HMO primary care doctor refer you if you want to see a specialist or surgeon. Many HMOs pay most of the cost of prescription drugs and preventive care, but traditional plans may not.

3) **Point of service plan (POS)** — Many HMOs offer an option known as a POS plan. This option allows you to seek care outside of the plan's network. For this option, you'll usually pay a higher percentage of the cost of your care to the out-of-network provider (in other words, at the point of service).

■ Pros and Cons of Managed Care Organizations

Managed care plans can save you money over traditional health insurance, and they often save you paperwork. Here is an overview of the benefits:

- **Less expensive** — You usually pay lower premiums and lower copayments, coinsurance or deductibles.
- **Broader coverage** — Most managed care plans pay the greater cost of prescription drugs and preventive care, such as regular checkups, whereas most traditional plans don't.

But there are drawbacks to managed care plans as well:

- **Limited choice** — If you live in an area well supplied with doctors, the managed care plan will probably have a reasonable number of primary care physicians from which to choose. However, if you live in a small town or rural area with relatively few physicians, you'll have a more limited choice.
- **Conflict of interest** — Some managed care plan physicians are strongly encouraged to hold expenses down. This can lead to reduced ability to get an appointment, rushed office visits, limited use of diagnostic tests, reluctance to refer you to a specialist, and shorter than ideal hospital stays to recover.
- **Convenience** — Most people have to travel less than 10 miles to receive their medical care. However, before you join a managed care plan, ask for its directory listing the names and locations of its hospitals, doctors and other health care facilities.
- **Waiting periods** — You may have to wait to see a doctor and to get medical tests. Before you join, ask for an estimate of how long you'll have to wait for both routine and urgent care.
- **Reimbursement for emergency or out-of-town care** — Some managed care plans have complicated rules for emergency services that are provided at night, on weekends or away from home.
- **Reliability** — Most managed care organizations are profitable, but some are in financial trouble. Make sure the organization you choose has been in business at least 3 years.

How Does Your Health Plan Rate?

The National Committee for Quality Assurance (NCQA) offers a Health Plan Report Card that rates health plans in five key areas, including accessibility and customer service, and quality of providers and care. Plans that meet NCQA standards receive accreditation from the nonprofit organization. For more information about the Health Plan Report Card, visit NCQA's Web site at *www.ncqa.org* or call 202-955-3500.

■ Making the Most of Your Insurance

To take maximum advantage of your health insurance policy, you first have to understand it. But like most legal descriptions, policy language can be confusing. It helps to anticipate the types of services you may need, and then to talk to your insurance representative. Be sure to ask whether there is a copay or deductible. Your goal is to maximize benefits and reduce your out-of-pocket expenses. Here are some tips to help you choose a private or supplemental health insurance policy:

- **Buy group insurance.** You usually get broader benefits and lower premiums and deductibles. Also, you're usually not required to prove insurability, and pre-existing health conditions will probably be covered. If your employer offers a choice of plans, consult your employer's benefits manager for help in making an informed choice. (Some professional associations offer health insurance at group rates for elgible members.)

- **Buy from a well-known, reputable insurance company or agent.** Get the name and address of your agent and the company he or she is representing. Agents are required by law to give you an outline of coverage and benefits. Be sure you get one of these documents.

- **Read the policy carefully before you buy.** It's just as important to know what's not covered as what is covered. Many policies do not cover pre-existing conditions; cosmetic surgery; eyeglasses, dental visits and other preventive care; prescription drugs; pregnancy and elective Caesarean section; and mental illness, substance abuse problems and attempted suicide.

- **Don't over-insure or buy duplicate coverage.** One comprehensive policy is enough, and you probably won't be able to collect full benefits even if you have two policies or more. If both you and your spouse work, carefully consider all options for family coverage from both employers, and choose the best combination for your family. Your secondary insurance covers the difference of what your primary insurance doesn't.

- **Avoid disease-specific or accident insurance.** This probably duplicates insurance you already have.

- **Follow the rules.** Find out if your policy has managed care requirements for reimbursement before you have a medical test or procedure. Then remember to get approval from your insurer beforehand.

- **Pay premiums yearly.** Most policies have discounts if you pay your annual premium on time and in full, not in installments.

- **File claims promptly, keep a copy and note the date you mail your claim.** Your insurer should send your payment promptly. If you have a complaint and don't receive a satisfactory answer from your insurer, contact your state insurance commissioner. To locate your state commissioner, contact the National Association of Insurance Commissioners (816-842-3600, or *www.nclnet.org*)

Home Medical Testing Kits

Your pharmacy or drugstore has kits that can be used to perform medical tests at home, without the involvement of a physician or health care provider.

Like most tests in a laboratory, home tests use urine, blood or stool. Some of them are relatively inexpensive and can be performed more than once.

Types of Kits
- **Pregnancy tests** to determine whether you are pregnant.
- **Ovulation prediction tests** to help determine the best time for intercourse that may lead to conception.
- **Sugar tests,** of either urine or blood, to determine whether diabetes is present or well controlled.
- **Cholesterol tests** to determine your total cholesterol level; 200 milligrams per deciliter of blood or lower is desirable.
- **Other urine tests**, such as for excess protein, which may signal a kidney problem.
- **Tests to detect blood** in the stool, which may indicate a tumor in the colon.
- **Human immunodeficiency virus (HIV) tests** check for antibodies to HIV, the virus that causes AIDS. The test involves placing a drop of blood on a test card with an identification number. You mail the card to the designated certified laboratory, then call for results in about 1 week.

Disadvantages of Home Tests
- **There is the risk of simply doing the test wrong** and, therefore, getting a misleading result. You must follow the instructions exactly or the test will not work properly. Professionals in a medical laboratory are less likely to make a mistake because they have more experience and better equipment.
- **Medical tests do not always work correctly.** This is true for tests done at home and for tests performed in a medical laboratory. A certain percentage of test results suggest that something is present when it is not (false positive). For example, a false-positive test result would indicate that you do have hidden blood in the stool when in fact you do not, or that you are pregnant when you are not.
- **False-negative results** can be found. A certain percentage of test results indicate that something is not present when it is, which is called a false negative. For example, a false-negative test result would indicate that your blood glucose concentration is normal when it is not, or that you are not pregnant when you are. A physician is in a better position to judge false-negative and false-positive test results on the basis of other medical evidence, training and experience.
- **You may interpret the result incorrectly.** Changes in the appearance of the test result, such as the color, may be confusing. Often, you need to see your physician or have the test repeated by a medical laboratory no matter what the result.
- **Indecision** is a factor. After performing the test, it is often difficult to decide what to do next. For example, if you are certain there is blood in your stool but the test indicates otherwise, should you still see your physician?

Caution

When used appropriately, many home testing kits can be accurate. Nevertheless, use them carefully. They are not a substitute for appropriate medical care, especially when you think you may be at risk of a serious medical condition. Follow up worrisome, unexpected test results with your health care provider.

Healthy Consumer

Your Family Medical Tree

Family gatherings are an ideal time to catch up on family news. They are also an opportunity to learn more about your family health history.

Some 10 to 15 percent of people with colon cancer have a family history of the disease. Up to one-fourth of children of alcoholics are themselves likely to become alcoholics. And a family history of high blood pressure, diabetes, some cancers and certain psychiatric disorders significantly increases all family members' odds of developing the condition.

If blood relatives have had a particular disease or condition, are you destined to get it? Usually not. But it may mean you are at an increased risk.

Many major diseases have a hereditary component. But when you know you are at increased risk for a disease, you may be able to take steps to prevent it—or at least detect it early, when the odds for a cure may be in your favor.

Medical trees reveal patterns of hereditary illness. With this kind of information, your doctor may prescribe tests or recommend lifestyle changes. In fact, one study showed that 25,000 medical trees identified 43,000 people who were at risk for hereditary illnesses. And the people who were evaluated proved to be excellent candidates for preventive treatment.

Creating a Family Medical Tree

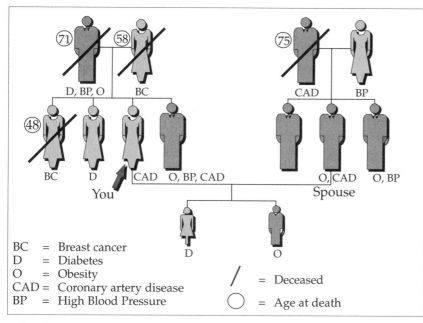

BC = Breast cancer
D = Diabetes
O = Obesity
CAD = Coronary artery disease
BP = High Blood Pressure

/ = Deceased
○ = Age at death

A family tree showing how you can chart a family medical history.

- **Learn who's who.** Research your parents, siblings and children. Then add information about grandparents, aunts and uncles, cousins and nieces and nephews. The more relatives you include, the better.
- **Dig for details.** Interview relatives by phone, or mail them questionnaires.
- **Look into the past.** Information about any ailment—from allergies to limps—could prove helpful. Pay special attention to serious but potentially preventable conditions, such as cancer, high blood pressure, heart disease, diabetes, depression and alcoholism. Note the age of the relative when the illness was diagnosed. What kind of lifestyle did the person lead (smoker? activity level?).
- **Put it all together.** Organize your chart so you can view the health histories of several relatives at once (see the illustration). Assign each medical condition a letter, and then write this letter next to the person's name or figure. Note the person's age when he or she died.
- **Talk it over.** Ask your physician to review your medical tree.

Medications and You

No matter what your age or condition, there are fundamental rules to follow when taking medications.

- **Advise your physician about any over-the-counter drugs** you are taking, including laxatives or antacids; aspirin or acetaminophen; cough, cold or hay fever medicines; mineral and vitamin supplements, or herbal medications. Nonprescription drugs can be potent, and some can cause serious reactions when mixed with prescription drugs.
- **Read labels carefully.** Ask your physician and pharmacist about potential side effects, about any dietary restrictions you should follow, whether you should avoid alcohol while taking the drug or about other concerns you have. If you get a prescription refilled and it appears different from what you had been taking, ask your pharmacist why.
- **Follow instructions.** Anyone who uses more than the recommended dosage is in danger of an overdose. The "more is better" theory does not apply to drugs.
- **Do not stop taking a prescribed drug** just because your symptoms seem to lessen. Take your medication for the entire length of time prescribed, even if symptoms have disappeared, unless instructed otherwise by your physician.
- **Keep a record** of what you take if you are taking numerous medications on a daily basis. Carry it in your purse or wallet. Also, list your allergies and any intolerance to drugs.
- **Inform your physician of side effects.** Be alert to headache, dizziness, blurred vision, ringing in your ears, shortness of breath, hives and other unexpected effects.
- **Have prescriptions filled at one pharmacy.** Using one pharmacy can help you avoid problems with drug interactions. Your pharmacist can help monitor the mix of medications, even if they are prescribed by different physicians.
- **Properly store medications.** Most require a dry, secure place at room temperature and out of direct sunlight. Some drugs need refrigeration. A bathroom cabinet is often a poor place to store medications because of temperature and moisture variations.
- **Discard outdated drugs.** Medicine deteriorates over time and can sometimes become toxic. Never take leftover medicine.
- **Be concerned for children.** Keep prescription and nonprescription drugs safely away from the reach of children. Buy childproof packages, especially if you have young children, grandchildren or very young guests.
- **Keep medicines in their original containers.** If the label gets separated from a medicine container and there is any doubt as to its contents, discard the medicine immediately. Prescription containers are designed to protect medications from light and moisture.
- **If you have trouble opening a container** with a safety cap, ask your pharmacist for a special nonsafety cap.
- **Don't lend or share prescription drugs.** What helps you might harm others.
- **Don't take a medication in the dark.**
- **Avoid mixing medications and alcohol.** This combination can cause a harmful interaction.

◼ Pain Relievers: Matching the Pill to the Pain

Although the packaging and promises are different, all nonprescription pain relievers contain one of these five chemicals—aspirin, acetaminophen, ibuprofen, naproxen sodium and, most recently, ketoprofen. For pain relief, the differences among products are more subtle than significant.

Pain relievers are called analgesics (from the Greek words *an*, meaning "without," and *algos*, meaning "pain"). Over-the-counter (OTC) analgesics relieve mild to moderate pain associated with headache, colds, toothache, muscle ache, backache, arthritis and menstrual cramps. They also reduce fever. OTC analgesics fall into two main categories: those that also decrease inflammation and those that don't.

- **NSAIDS:** Aspirin, ibuprofen, naproxen sodium and ketoprofen reduce inflammation and are called nonsteroidal anti-inflammatory drugs (NSAIDs). They're most helpful when a painful condition also involves inflammation (some forms of arthritis, tendinitis). Common side effects include stomach upset, ulcer and bleeding (see page 265).
- **Acetaminophen** doesn't relieve inflammation. Because it's relatively free of side effects at recommended doses, it may be a good alternative for long-term use or when taking NSAIDs presents a risk.

All regular-strength doses of OTC pain relievers provide comparable relief for everyday pain such as headache or sore muscles. For menstrual pain, ibuprofen, naproxen sodium and ketoprofen may offer better relief.

Separating Help From Hype

OTC pain medications come in a great variety of forms. Sometimes a less expensive generic form is all you need. If you have questions, ask a pharmacist or your doctor.

Here's a guide for sorting through different forms of drug delivery:

- **Buffered:** A buffered analgesic contains an antacid to reduce acidity. It's controversial whether these products actually protect your stomach.
- **Enteric-coated:** A special coating allows pills to pass through your stomach and dissolve in the small intestine. This helps reduce stomach irritation. Consider an enteric-coated product if you need daily relief for chronic pain. Because the coating delays absorption, it's not the best choice for quick relief (such as for a headache).
- **Timed-release:** Also called extended-release and sustained-release, these products dissolve slowly. They prolong relief by maintaining a constant level of analgesic in your blood. Use them if you need lasting, not immediate, relief.
- **Extra-strength:** A single dose of these preparations contains more pain-relieving medicine than regular-strength products—typically 500 milligrams of aspirin or acetaminophen vs. 325 milligrams. They're more convenient when it takes more than one regular-strength dose to improve your symptoms, but you should take them less often.
- **Combination formulas:** Some products are paired with caffeine or an antihistamine to boost their effect. Studies show that the addition of caffeine to aspirin or acetaminophen does improve pain relief.
- **Tablet, caplet, gelcap, gum or liquid:** If you have trouble swallowing a round tablet or oval caplet, a smooth gelcap might work better. Other options include taking aspirin as an effervescing pain reliever plus antacid (Alka-Seltzer) or chewing aspirin as a gum (Aspergum).
- **Generic:** Generic pain relievers almost always cost less than brand name drugs, but they're just as effective.

- **Know your special risks.** In general, don't take NSAIDs if you also take a blood thinner, or if you have kidney disease, ulcers, a bleeding disorder or an allergy to aspirin.
- **Avoid drug interactions.** If you take other OTC or prescription medications, talk with your doctor or pharmacist about which pain reliever is best.
- **Don't exceed the recommended dose**—unless your doctor advises it.
- **Avoid alcohol.** Mixing alcohol with aspirin, ibuprofen or naproxen sodium increases the chance of stomach upset and bleeding. In combination with higher-than-recommended doses of acetaminophen, alcohol increases the risk of serious damage to your liver.
- **Take NSAIDs with milk and food** to help minimize stomach upset.
- **Don't take longer than necessary.** Periodically reevaluate your need for pain relievers.
- Always read and follow label instructions.

Over-the-Counter Pain Relievers

	Aspirin	Acetaminophen	Ibuprofen	Naproxen Sodium	Ketoprofen
Sampling of brand names	Anacin, Ascriptin, Bayer, Bufferin, Ecotrin, Empirin	Excedrin (Aspirin Free), Panadol, Tylenol	Advil, Ibuprin, Motrin-IB, Nuprin	Aleve	Orudis KT, Actron
Reduces pain and fever	Yes	Yes	Yes	Yes	Yes
Reduces inflammation	Yes	No	Yes	Yes	Yes
Side effects	Gastrointestinal (GI) bleeding, stomach upset and ulceration	None when taken as directed for short periods (days to weeks)	GI bleeding, stomach upset, ulceration and pain	GI bleeding, stomach upset, bloating and dizziness	GI bleeding, ulceration
Special cautions	Don't take if you have allergy to aspirin, asthma, bleeding disorder, gout or ulcers	Overdoses can be toxic to the liver. Alcohol enhances toxic effects of high doses	Don't take if you have allergy to aspirin, asthma, heart failure, kidney problems, ulcers	Don't take if you have allergy to aspirin, asthma, heart failure, kidney problems, ulcers	Don't take if you have allergy to aspirin, asthma, heart failure, kidney problems, ulcers
Children's use	Can cause Reye's syndrome* in children with chickenpox, the flu or other viral illness	Available for children. Dosages based on age and weight. Consult your physician	Available for children. Dosages based on age and weight. Consult your physician	Do not give to children younger than 12 except on advice of a doctor	Not recommended. Safety and effectiveness have not been studied

*Reye's syndrome is a potentially fatal swelling of brain tissues. Note: This list is not comprehensive and is not an endorsement. We have not tested these products but rely on data supplied by the manufacturers.

Healthy Consumer

■ Cold Remedies: What They Can and Cannot Do

There is no cure for the common cold. Yet drugs used to treat the effects of the common cold—runny nose, fever, congestion and cough—are the largest segment of the over-the-counter market for America's pharmaceutical industry. Some of these medications also are formulated as allergy medicines to treat itchy eyes and sneezing.

Most people don't need any medication for a cold. With the possible exception of zinc lozenges (see page 115), none of the various cold remedies will make your cold resolve more rapidly. But if your cold symptoms are particularly bothersome, careful use of over-the-counter cold medicines may provide some relief. If used at the wrong time, they can make you feel worse.

Cold Remedies

	Antihistamines	Decongestants	Cough Medicines	Cough/Cold Combinations

Products and brand names	Benadryl
	Chlor-Trimeton
	Tavist
	Teldrin
	Generics
		Neo-Synephrine
		Afrin
		Propagest
		Sudafed
		Generics
			Expectorants
			  Robitussin
			  Generics that
			  contain
			  guaifenesin
			Antitussives
			  Robitussin-DM
			  Generics that
			  contain
			  dextromethorphan
				Actifed
				Chlor-Trimeton D
				Contac
				Dimetapp
				Drixoral
				Sudafed Plus
				Tavist D
				Generics

Symptoms relieved	Sneezing, runny nose, itchy eyes, congestion due to allergies	Congestion, stuffiness	*Expectorants* loosen mucus in the chest, making it easier to cough *Antitussives* reduce the frequency of coughing	Cough, stuffy nose, general discomfort
Side effects and cautions	Drowsiness, dry mouth, may dry secretions making mucus harder to clear, may increase the effects of alcohol	Insomnia, jitters, palpitations, may raise blood pressure	Antitussives may have a sedating effect because some include narcotic-like substances	Many do not contain enough antihistamine for significant benefit, may combine three or more products
Time of maximal benefit	Early in a cold when sneezing and watery, runny nose are common	When nose is stuffed up. Use for only a few days; the effect often wears off after 3 to 4 days of use	When mucus is thick and cough is prominent	Use individual products instead, when they will have the most benefit

Here's some helpful advice on the use of cold medicines:

- **Always read the labels** to determine the active ingredients and side effects of the particular medicine.
- **A single-symptom medicine is often better** than a combination medication.
- **Most combination cold medications contain some form of analgesic** such as aspirin, ibuprofen or acetaminophen (see page 257). Therefore, you don't need to take a separate analgesic.
- **Don't mix** various cold medications or take with other medications without consulting your physician or pharmacist.
- **Avoid alcohol** when taking cold medications.
- **Consult your physician** before giving any cold medicine to a child.

■ Home Medical Supplies

When an emergency or medical problem occurs in the home, you often don't have time to search for supplies. Keep your medical supplies in a place that is easily accessible to adults but out of the reach of children. And remember to replace items after their use to make sure the kit is always complete. Here's what you need to be properly prepared for accidents and common illnesses that are mentioned in this book:

- **For cuts:** Bandages of various sizes, gauze, adhesive tape, an antiseptic solution to clean wounds and an antiseptic cream to prevent infection.
- **For burns:** Cold packs, gauze, burn spray and an antiseptic cream.
- **For aches, pain and fever:** Aspirin (for adults only) or another nonsteroidal anti-inflammatory drug, and acetaminophen for children or adults.
- **For eye injuries:** Eyewash, an eyewash cup and eye patches.
- **For sprains, strains and fractures:** Cold packs, elastic wraps for wrapping injuries and a triangular bandage for making an arm sling.
- **For insect bites and stings:** A tweezers to remove stingers and hydrocortisone cream to relieve itching. If a family member is allergic to insect stings, also include a kit containing a syringe and epinephrine (adrenaline).
- **For ingestion of poisons:** Syrup of ipecac to induce vomiting. Use it only after contacting a poison control center or medical professional (keep the number of your local poison control center on a sticker on your telephone).
- **For general care:** Thermometer, sharp scissors, cottons swabs, tissues, soap or cleansing pads, gloves for use if blood or body fluids are present and a first aid manual.

Vitamin and Mineral Supplements

Vitamins and minerals are substances your body needs in small amounts for normal growth, function and health. Together, vitamins and minerals are called micronutrients. Your body can't make most micronutrients, so you must get them from the foods you eat or, in some cases, from supplements.

You need vitamins for normal digestion, mental alertness and resistance to infection. They enable your body to process proteins, carbohydrates and fats. Certain vitamins also help you produce blood cells, hormones, genetic material and chemicals of your nervous system. Unlike carbohydrates, proteins and fats, vitamins and minerals don't provide fuel (calories). However, they help your body release and use calories from food.

There are 14 vitamins, which fall into two categories:

- The fat-soluble vitamins are vitamins A, D, E and K. They're stored in your body's fat. Because they're stored, excess fat-soluble vitamins can accumulate in your body to toxic levels. Your body is especially sensitive to too much vitamin A and vitamin D.
- The water-soluble vitamins are vitamin C, choline, biotin and the seven B vitamins: thiamin (B-1), riboflavin (B-2), niacin (B-3), pantothenic acid (B-5), pyridoxine (B-6), folic acid (B-9) and cobalamin (B-12). They're stored to a lesser extent than fat-soluble vitamins.

Your body also needs 16 minerals. Major minerals include calcium, phosphorus, magnesium, sodium, potassium, chloride and sulfur. Calcium, phosphorus and magnesium are important in the development and health of bones and teeth. Sodium, potassium and chloride, known as electrolytes, are important in regulating the water and chemical balance in your body. In addition, your body needs smaller amounts of chromium, copper, fluoride, iodine, iron, manganese, molybdenum, selenium and zinc. These are all necessary for normal growth and health.

Having the right balance of vitamins and minerals in your body is essential. Prolonged vitamin or mineral deficiencies can cause specific diseases or conditions, such as night blindness (vitamin A deficiency), pernicious anemia (vitamin B-12 deficiency) and anemia (iron deficiency). Too much of some vitamins and minerals can cause toxic reactions.

■ Whole Foods Are Your Best Source

You can get your entire daily requirement of vitamin C by just popping a pill. You can get the same amount by eating an orange. So which is better? In most cases, the orange — a "whole food."

Benefits of Whole Foods

Whole foods — fruits, vegetables, grains, lean meats and dairy products — have three main benefits you can't find in a pill:

- **Whole foods are complex.** They contain a variety of the nutrients your body needs — not just one — giving you more "bang" for your nutrition "buck." An orange, for example, provides vitamin C but also beta carotene, calcium and other nutrients. A vitamin C supplement lacks these other nutrients. Similarly, a glass of milk provides you with protein, vitamin D, riboflavin, calcium, phosphorus and magnesium. If you take only calcium supplements and skipped calcium-rich foods, such as dairy products, you miss all the other nutrients you need for healthy bones.

- **Whole foods provide dietary fiber.** Fiber is important for digestion and in preventing certain diseases. Soluble fiber — found in certain beans and grains and in some fruits and vegetables — and insoluble fiber — found in whole-grain breakfast cereals and in some vegetables and fruits — may help prevent heart disease, diabetes and constipation.
- **Whole foods contain other substances that may be important for good health.** Fruits and vegetables, for example, contain naturally occurring food substances called phytochemicals, which may help protect you against cancer, heart disease, osteoporosis and diabetes. It's not yet known precisely what role phytochemicals play in nutrition. However, if you depend on supplements rather than trying to eat a variety of whole foods, you miss the potential health benefits of phytochemicals.

Benefits of Supplements Uncertain

Only long-term, well-designed studies can sort out which nutrients in food are beneficial — and whether taking them in pill form provides the same benefit.

In fact, some nutrients may actually be harmful to your health when taken as a supplement. In one study, researchers found an increased risk of prostate cancer among men who drank alcohol and took beta carotene supplements. In an earlier study, they found that smokers who took beta carotene supplements had an increased risk of lung cancer. It's possible that alcohol and tobacco change the way your body absorbs and uses beta carotene. In addition, it's known that large amounts of beta carotene can alter blood levels of other similar natural food pigments called carotenoids, some of which may actually be more beneficial to you than beta carotene.

The Bottom Line

Concentrate on getting your nutrients from food, not supplements. Whole foods provide an ideal mix of nutrients, fiber and other food substances. It's likely that all these work in combination to keep you healthy.

■ Should You Take Supplements?

The American Dietetic Association and other major medical organizations all agree that the best way to get the vitamins and minerals you need is through a nutritionally balanced diet. However, sometimes a supplement may be appropriate.

Even if you don't have a vitamin or mineral deficiency, a vitamin or mineral supplement may be appropriate for you if:
- **You're a postmenopausal woman.** It can be difficult to obtain the recommended amounts of calcium and vitamin D without supplementation. Both calcium and vitamin D supplements have been shown to protect against osteoporosis.
- **You don't eat well.** If you don't eat the recommended five servings a day of fruits

and vegetables, taking a multivitamin supplement may be reasonable. However, your best course of action would be to adopt better eating habits.

- **You're on a very low-calorie diet.** If you eat fewer than 1,000 calories a day, you may benefit from a vitamin-mineral supplement. However, remember: A very low-calorie diet limits the types and amounts of foods you eat and, in turn, the types and amounts of nutrients you receive. Very low-calorie diets should only be undertaken with guidance from your doctor.
- **You smoke.** Tobacco decreases absorption of many vitamins and minerals, including vitamin B-6, vitamin B-12, vitamin C, folic acid and niacin.
- **You drink alcohol excessively.** Alcoholics have impaired digestion and absorption of thiamin, folic acid and vitamins A, D and B-12. Altered metabolism also affects minerals such as zinc, selenium, magnesium and phosphorus. If you drink excessively, you also may substitute alcohol for food, resulting in a diet lacking in essential nutrients. (Excessive drinking is defined as more than one drink a day if you're a nonpregnant woman and more than two drinks a day if you're a man.)
- **You're pregnant or breast-feeding.** During these times, you need more of certain nutrients, especially folic acid and iron. Folic acid helps prevent neural tube defects in your baby, such as spina bifida. Iron helps prevent fatigue by helping you make the red blood cells you need to deliver oxygen to your baby. Your doctor can recommend a supplement. It's important to start taking a supplement before becoming pregnant.
- **You eat a special diet.** If your diet has limited variety because of intolerance or food allergy, you may benefit from a vitamin-mineral supplement. If you're a vegetarian who eliminates all animal products from your diet, you may need additional vitamin B-12. In addition, if you don't eat dairy products and don't get 15 minutes of sun each day on your hands and face, you may need to supplement your diet with calcium and vitamin D.
- **You're age 65 or older.** As you get older, health problems can contribute to a poor diet, making it difficult for you to get the vitamins and minerals you need. You may lose your appetite, as well as some of your ability to taste and smell. Depression or problems with dentures can also inhibit eating. If you eat alone, you also may not eat enough to get all the nutrients you need from food. In addition, as you get older, your body may not be able to absorb vitamins B-6, B-12 and D like it used to, making supplementation more necessary. There's also evidence that a multivitamin may improve your immune function and decrease your risk of some infections if you're older.

■ Vitamins and Minerals: How Much Do You Need?

You may be confused about how much of a specific vitamin or mineral you need. Here's how to figure out what you need:

- **Recommended Dietary Allowances (RDAs)** describe the average amount of each vitamin and mineral needed each day to meet the needs of nearly all healthy people. They're determined by the Food and Nutrition Board of the Institute of Medicine, part of the National Academy of Sciences. RDAs for some vitamins and minerals vary according to your sex or age, or both.
- **Daily Values (DV)** are used on food and supplement labels. They have their origin in the Recommended Dietary Allowances (RDAs), but they're set by the Food

and Drug Administration (FDA). The FDA bases DVs on a 2,000-calorie-per-day diet. Of course, the 2,000-calorie-per-day standard is just a guideline. Individual needs may vary. Many women and older adults may actually need only about 1,600 calories a day. Active women and most men need about 2,200 calories a day. Active men may need about 2,800 calories a day. If your calorie needs are greater or less than 2,000 per day, your DVs for various nutrients generally rise or fall accordingly.

- **Percent Daily Value (%DV)** tells you what percent of the DV one serving of a food or supplement supplies — that is, how it measures up as a percentage of the daily recommendation. For example, if the label on your multivitamin bottle says that your multivitamin provides 30 percent of the DV for vitamin E, you have 70 percent still needed to meet the recommended goal. The higher the %DV, the greater its contribution to meeting nutrient goals.

■ Choosing and Using Supplements

Supplements are not substitutes. They can't replace the hundreds of nutrients in whole foods you need for a nutritionally balanced diet. However, if you do decide to take a vitamin or mineral supplement, here are some factors to consider:

- **Avoid supplements that provide 'mega-doses.'** In general, choose a multivitamin-mineral supplement that provides about 100% DV of all the vitamins and minerals instead of one that supplies, for example, 500% DV of one vitamin and only 20% DV of another. The exception to this is calcium. You may notice that calcium-containing supplements do not provide 100% DV. If they did, the tablets would be too large to swallow. Doses above 100% DV don't give extra protection in most cases, but they do increase your risk of encountering toxic side effects. Most cases of nutrient toxicity stem from high-dose supplements. Some specific conditions are treated with large doses, such as Hartnup disease, a genetic condition treated with large doses of niacin. These are uncommon, however.
- **Consider buying generic.** Generic brands are generally less expensive and equally effective as name brands. Compare the list of ingredients and the %DV to make sure the brands are comparable.
- **Look for 'USP' on the label.** This ensures that the supplement meets the standards for strength, purity, disintegration and dissolution established by the testing organization, U.S. Pharmacopeia (USP).
- **Beware of gimmicks.** Synthetic vitamins are the same as so-called natural vitamins. Don't give in to the temptation of added herbs, enzymes or amino acids — they add nothing but cost.
- **Look for expiration dates.** Supplements can lose potency over time, especially in hot and humid climates. If a supplement doesn't have an expiration date, don't buy it.
- **Store all vitamin and mineral supplements out of the sight and reach of children.** Put them in a locked cabinet or other secured location. Don't leave them sitting out on the counter or rely on child-resistant packaging. Be especially careful with any supplements containing iron. Iron overdose is a leading cause of poisoning deaths among children.
- **Explore your options.** If you have difficulty swallowing, ask your doctor whether liquid or children's vitamin and mineral supplements might be right for you.

- **Play it safe.** Before taking anything other than a standard multivitamin-mineral supplement of 100% DV or less, check with your doctor or a registered dietitian. This is especially important if you have a health problem or are taking medication. High doses of niacin, for example, can aggravate a stomach ulcer. In addition, supplements may interfere with medications. Vitamin E, for example, isn't recommended if you're taking blood-thinning medications (anticoagulants) because it can complicate the proper control of blood thinning. If you're already taking an individual vitamin or mineral supplement and haven't told your doctor, discuss it at your next checkup.

Supplements and Digestive Health Problems: What You Need to Know

If you have a digestive health problem, such as a disease of your liver, gallbladder, intestine and pancreas, or you've had surgery on your digestive tract, you may not be able to digest and absorb nutrients properly. Therefore, your doctor may recommend that you take a vitamin or mineral supplement. Some conditions that may require you to take supplements include:

- **Crohn's disease**. A chronic inflammation of the intestine. It mainly involves the ileum (the lower part of the small intestine). However, it can also affect your colon or any other part of your digestive tract. Your ability to absorb adequate nutrients often is limited with Crohn's disease, particularly if the disease affects large portions of your small intestine or if you've had portions of your small intestine removed surgically. If you have Crohn's disease, doctors advise that you take a standard multivitamin that provides 100% DV. Your doctor may also advise specific replacement of certain vitamins or minerals, if there is evidence of deficiency. If you have Crohn's disease, you may not be able to absorb vitamin B-12. Left untreated, a deficiency of this vitamin can lead to pernicious anemia. If this occurs, you can get the vitamin B-12 you need with monthly injections.

- **Primary biliary cirrhosis**. A condition characterized by chronic inflammation and scarring of the microscopic bile ducts within the liver. This inflammation and scarring can cause bile flow to become blocked, which can interfere with your body's absorption of fat-soluble vitamins (A, D, E and K). If you have primary biliary cirrhosis, your doctor may prescribe supplements for these vitamins in a special form that is easier to absorb.

- **Pancreatitis**. An inflammation of the pancreas. The inflammation may be acute or chronic. With chronic pancreatitis, your pancreas gradually becomes less able to secrete the enzymes you need to properly digest dietary fats. This pancreatic insufficiency therefore also affects your ability to absorb fat-soluble vitamins. If you have chronic pancreatitis, your doctor may prescribe pancreatic enzyme supplements to help improve digestion and absorption. In addition, a multivitamin or specific vitamins or mineral supplements may be recommended, if there is evidence of deficiency.

Alternative Medicine and Your Health

Complementary and alternative treatments have become more popular as Americans seek greater control of their own health. According to a study published in the *Journal of the American Medical Association*, Americans made more visits to complementary and alternative practitioners between 1990 and 1997 than they did to primary care physicians. Many of these people paid for the services without using medical insurance, spending more out-of-pocket for complementary and alternative treatments than they did for hospital care.

What Is Complementary and Alternative Medicine?

Most of what we call complementary and alternative treatments aren't new. Many have been practiced for thousands of years.

The National Center for Complementary and Alternative Medicine, a division of the National Institutes of Health, defines complementary medicine as unconventional treatments used *in addition to* treatments by your physician. An example is using tai chi (see page 281) in addition to prescription medication to manage anxiety.

In contrast, alternative medicine includes treatments used *in place of* traditional medicine. This might include seeing a homeopath or naturopath instead of your regular physician.

The Promise — and Peril — of New Treatment Options

This is one of the most exciting and challenging times in health care history. You have many treatment options — conventional, complementary and alternative. You also face greater risk of confusion and even harm.

You can't always accept the claims of complementary and alternative medicine practitioners at face value. True, the vast majority of these practitioners are well intentioned, and many have specialized training. Yet quack treatments have always existed, and some unscrupulous people may falsely claim to be experts in complementary and alternative medicine. Even practitioners with the best of intentions may be undertrained, uninformed or both.

Arm Yourself With Two Strategies

If you decide to use complementary and alternative treatments, protecting your health — and your wallet — requires you to do two things.

First, learn about these treatments. Find out what they are and what benefits their practitioners claim to provide. Learn about the five major groups of complementary and alternative medicine treatments:
- Herbal treatments
- Healing through manipulation and touch
- Mind-body connection
- Restoring natural energy forces
- Systems that combine treatments

Second, take responsibility for your own care. Before choosing a treatment, evaluate the benefits and risks. For tips, see Five Steps in Considering Any Treatment, starting on page 283.

■ Check Out Claims of Treatment Success

Ask your doctor for information on research results to help you make an informed decision about using a treatment. You can also find information on your own, but it's important to understand the quality of research. If you dig into the medical literature for studies about complementary and alternative treatments, you'll see several terms that describe different types of research. For example:

- *Clinical studies* are those that involve human beings as subjects — not animals. They're usually preceded by studies that demonstrate safety and effectiveness of the treatment in animals.
- In *randomized, controlled trials,* participants are usually divided into two groups. The first group receives the treatment under investigation. The second is a control group — they receive standard treatment, no treatment or an inactive substance called a placebo. Participants are assigned to these groups on a random basis. This helps to ensure that the groups will be similar.
- In *double-blind studies,* neither the researchers nor the human subjects know who will receive the active treatment and who will receive the placebo.
- *Prospective studies* are forward-looking. Researchers establish criteria for study participants to follow and then measure or describe the results. Information from these studies is usually more reliable than retrospective studies. Retrospective studies involve looking at past data (for example, asking participants to recall information), which leaves more room for errors in interpretation.
- *Peer-reviewed journals* only publish articles that have been reviewed by an independent panel of medical experts.

Identify the Best Research

Prospective double-blind studies that have been carefully controlled, randomized and published in peer-reviewed journals provide the "gold standard." When these involve large numbers of people (several hundred or more) studied over several years, they gain even more credibility. Doctors also like to see studies that are replicated — repeated by different investigators with generally the same results.

To date, few complementary and alternative treatments have been researched according to rigorous standards. For the majority of unconventional treatments, the jury is still out on whether they're helpful.

Why People Seek Alternative Medicine

(National phone survey of 2,055 adults)

Five Leading Reasons	Alternative Therapies Most Commonly Used
1. Back problems	Chiropractic care, massage therapy
2. Allergies	Herbal medicine, relaxation techniques
3. Fatigue	Relaxation techniques, massage therapy
4. Arthritis	Relaxation techniques, chiropractic care
5. Headaches	Relaxation techniques, chiropractic care

Source: Trends in alternative medicine in the United States, 1990 to 1997: Results of a follow-up national survey, *Journal of the American Medical Association*, Nov. 11, 1998.

Herbal Treatments

One of the biggest competitors to conventional medical care is herbal medicine. Walk into the vitamin aisle of any pharmacy, chain discount store or even your local grocery store, and you'll find them — herbal remedies such as St. John's wort, echinacea, ginkgo and garlic. Manufacturers claim that each herb treats one ailment or another.

Herbs, vitamins and minerals are all considered dietary supplements by the Food and Drug Administration (FDA). Some people use herbal treatments in addition to conventional medical care. Others use it instead of conventional treatments.

Although popularly thought of as "natural" and less risky than prescription drugs, herbal supplements aren't subject to the same rigorous quality control as drugs.

Limited FDA Regulation

In 1994, Congress passed the Dietary Supplement Health and Education Act (DSHEA). This law limited the FDA's control over products labeled dietary supplements. The DSHEA stated that manufacturers don't have to prove a product is safe or effective before it goes on the market.

As a result, in the United States herbs can be marketed with limited regulation. Vendors can make health claims about products based on their own review and interpretation of studies — without FDA authorization. However, the FDA can pull a product off the market if it's proved dangerous.

Use Herbs Safely

If you plan to make herbal treatments part of your health care plan, keep these points in mind:

- **Follow directions.** Like over-the-counter (OTC) and prescription drugs, herbal products have active ingredients that can affect how your body functions. Don't exceed the recommended dosages. Some herbs can be harmful if taken for too long a time period. Get advice from your doctor and other reputable resources.
- **Tell your doctor what you're taking.** Some herbs may interfere with the effectiveness of prescription or OTC drugs or have other harmful effects. (See Avoid Herb-Drug Interactions on page 227.) In addition, make sure you don't have an underlying medical condition that calls for treatment by your doctor.
- **Keep track of what you take.** Take one type of supplement at a time to try to determine its effect. Make a note of what you take, how much and how it affects you. Does it do what it claims to do? Do you experience any side effects, such as drowsiness, sleeplessness, headache or nausea?
- **Read the label for content.** Quality and strength can vary greatly by brand. Look for the letters USP (United States Pharmacopeia) or NF (National Formulary), which indicate the supplements meet certain standards of quality.
- **Avoid herbs if you're pregnant or breast-feeding.** Unless your doctor approves, don't take any medications — prescription, OTC or herbal — when you're pregnant or breast-feeding. They can harm your baby.
- **Be very cautious about using herbal products manufactured or purchased outside the United States.** In general, European herbs are well regulated and standardized. However, toxic ingredients (including lead, mercury and arsenic) and prescription drugs (such as prednisone) have been found in some herbal supplements manufactured in other countries, particularly China and India.

- **Avoid dangerous herbs altogether.** According to the FDA, these include belladonna, broom, comfrey, lobelia and pennyroyal. Goldenseal is another controversial herb that can cause serious side effects. And there may be others. Overdoses of any of these herbs can be fatal.

The effectiveness of many herbs still hasn't been established. And few studies have investigated the risks of taking several different herbs at the same time.

Of all the unconventional treatments, herbal therapies may present the greatest potential for harm. This is especially true when people self-prescribe herbs, or products are mislabeled or contaminated.

What the Research Shows

If you're thinking about using **herbal supplements**, read information on clinical studies about safety and effectiveness. From the examples below, you'll see why it's important to tell your doctor if you're using herbal products so that you can work out an effective treatment plan.

- In 1996, the *British Medical Journal* published a review of 23 European clinical studies on **St. John's wort**. Researchers concluded that this herb seemed to be useful for mild to moderate depression and that it had fewer side effects than some prescription antidepressants. However, studies also show that St. John's wort is not effective in treating major depression. And it can cause serious problems when taken with various types of prescription medications, such as antidepressants, digoxin, warfarin (Coumadin), cyclosporine and other drugs. If your depression is serious, don't try to treat this condition yourself. See your doctor.

- In 1998, researchers with the Department of Veterans Affairs reviewed more than a dozen studies involving **saw palmetto** and concluded that this herb may help reduce symptoms of noncancerous enlargement of the prostate gland (benign prostatic hyperplasia). However, studies are inconclusive as to whether saw palmetto can interfere with the results of the prostate-specific antigen (PSA) test, a tool that helps detect prostate cancer.

- Studies indicate that **feverfew** may reduce the frequency and severity of migraines because of an active ingredient, called parthenolide. However, feverfew products vary widely in the amount of parthenolide they contain. Avoid feverfew if you're using aspirin or warfarin (Coumadin). Don't take feverfew or any other herbs if you're pregnant.

Avoid Herb-Drug Interactions

Although "natural" and therefore popularly considered harmless, herbal supplements contain ingredients that may not mix safely with prescription or over-the-counter (OTC) drugs. In addition, some medical problems may increase your risk of adverse effects if you take herbal products.

Talk to your doctor before taking any herbal products if you're pregnant or nursing. Also see your doctor before you take herbs if you have any of the following conditions:
- High blood pressure
- History of stroke
- Blood-clotting problems
- Thyroid problems
- Diabetes
- Heart disease

- Epilepsy
- Parkinson's disease
- Glaucoma
- Enlarged prostate gland
- HIV, AIDS or other diseases of the immune system
- Depression or other psychiatric problems

In addition, herbal supplements can be just as dangerous as prescription and OTC drugs when used with anesthesia. If you're anticipating surgery, tell your doctor about any drugs you're taking — including herbal supplements.

Stop taking herbal supplements at least 2 to 3 weeks before surgery to allow them to clear from your body. If this isn't possible, bring the herbal product in its original container to the hospital so the anesthesiologist knows exactly what you're taking.

Healing Through Manipulation and Touch

One attraction of many complementary and alternative treatments is that they involve human touch. Examples are chiropractic treatment, osteopathy and massage.

Chiropractic Treatment

Chiropractic care has come a long way since the days of its founders, who pointed to misaligned vertebrae as the source of all disease. Today, chiropractors sometimes even work with medical doctors.

Although they can't prescribe drugs or perform surgery, chiropractors use many standard medical procedures. And the services of chiropractors are sometimes cov-

Five Tips if You Seek Chiropractic Care

To get the most out of chiropractic care or other treatments that rely on spinal manipulation, here are some tips:
1. Ask your primary doctor to refer you to an appropriate provider. This could be a chiropractor, osteopath or physical therapist.
2. If you seek chiropractic care without a referral, do so carefully. Find someone who is licensed and who completed the training program (usually 3 to 4 years long) at a school accredited by the Council on Chiropractic Education.
3. See only chiropractors who are willing to send a report to your doctor, give you a written treatment plan and allow your doctor to observe chiropractic treatments (if desired).
4. Avoid chiropractors who order frequent X-rays or ask to extend your treatment indefinitely.
5. Avoid chiropractors who view spinal manipulation as a cure for "whatever ails you." There is no evidence to support this idea.

Healthy Consumer

ered by medical insurance.

Most chiropractors use a hands-on type of adjustment called spinal manipulative therapy or spinal manipulation. According to chiropractic theory, misaligned vertebrae can restrict your spine's range of motion and affect nerves that radiate out from your spine. In turn, the organs that depend on those nerves may function improperly or become diseased. Chiropractic adjustments aim to realign your vertebrae, restore range of motion and free up nerve pathways.

People other than chiropractors do spinal manipulation. Many osteopathic doctors and physical therapists are trained in this treatment. And there is no evidence that chiropractors do better spinal manipulation than other health care providers. Some chiropractors hold tightly to the theory that spinal manipulation can treat disease other than back pain, but no scientific evidence supports this.

What the Research Shows

Chiropractic treatment. Although research results sometimes conflict, studies indicate that spinal manipulation can effectively treat *uncomplicated* low back pain, especially if the pain has been present for less than 4 weeks.

After reviewing many studies, the Agency for Healthcare Research and Quality concluded that spinal manipulation may provide temporary relief from acute low back pain. However, the agency limited its conclusions to short-term treatment. There was little evidence that long-term treatment was effective. And most acute low back pain resolves without treatment in 4 to 6 weeks.

In another review of medical studies, Dutch researchers found evidence that spinal manipulation can effectively treat low back pain. However, the low quality of many of the studies prevented the researchers from making strong conclusions about spinal manipulation.

Osteopathic Manipulation

Osteopathy is a recognized medical discipline that has much in common with conventional medicine and chiropractic treatment. Like traditional physicians, doctors of osteopathy go through long training in academic and clinical settings. Osteopaths are licensed to perform many of the same therapies and procedures as traditional doctors. They can perform surgery and prescribe medications. Osteopaths may also specialize in various areas of medicine, such as gynecology or cardiology.

Osteopathy does differ from conventional medicine in one area: manipulation to address joint and spinal problems. Similar in this respect to a chiropractor, an osteopath may perform manipulations to release pressure in your joints, align your muscles and joints, and improve the flow of body fluids. Interestingly, a 1995 survey of osteopath family physicians found that they used spinal manipulation only occasionally.

Massage

Massage is often used as part of physical therapy, sports medicine and nursing care. It may be used, for example, to relieve muscle tension or promote relaxation, helping people as they undergo other types of medical treatment. It's also accepted as a simple means for healthy people to relieve stress and just feel good.

Massage is the kneading, stroking and manipulation of your body's soft tissues — your skin, muscles and tendons. Your massage will vary depending on the rhythm, rate, pressure and direction of these movements.

You shouldn't get massage over an open wound, skin infection, phlebitis or areas of weakened bones. In addition, don't get a massage if any of your joints are inflamed. And if you've been injured, consult your doctor first. Don't rely exclusively on massage to repair damaged tissues.

Generally, a massage should feel good or cause very little discomfort. If this is not the case, speak up promptly.

■ Mind-Body Connection

These treatments are based on the idea that mind and body function as a unified field. Practitioners who take this approach may hold that negative thoughts and feelings can produce symptoms in your body. Treatment often aims to help you detach from these thoughts and feelings, or to actively change them.

Biofeedback

This practice uses technology to teach you how to control certain body responses. During a biofeedback session, a trained therapist applies electrodes and other sensors to various parts of your body. The electrodes are attached to devices that monitor your responses and give you visual or auditory feedback. For example, you might see patterns on a monitor that display your levels of muscle tension, brain wave activity, heart rate, blood pressure, breathing rate or skin temperature.

With this feedback, you can learn how to produce positive changes in body functions, such as lowering your blood pressure or raising your skin temperature. These are signs of relaxation. The biofeedback therapist may use relaxation techniques to further calm you, reducing muscle tension or slowing your heart rate and breathing even more.

You can get biofeedback treatments in several settings — physical therapy clinics, medical centers and hospitals.

Hypnosis

Hypnosis produces a state of deep relaxation, but your mind stays alert. During hypnosis, you can receive suggestions designed to decrease your perception of pain or to help you stop habits such as smoking. No one knows exactly how hypnosis works, but experts believe it alters your brain wave patterns in much the same way as other relaxation techniques.

The success of hypnosis depends on the expertise of the practitioner, your understanding of the procedure and your willingness to try it. You need to be strongly motivated to change. Some people eventually develop the skills to hypnotize themselves.

Psychiatrists and psychologists occasionally practice hypnosis. There are also professional hypnotists, but beware, because this field is poorly regulated.

By the way, don't worry about what you see in movies and on television: You can't be forced under hypnosis to do something that's truly against your will.

Yoga

People do yoga for many reasons. For some, yoga is a spiritual path. For others, yoga is a way to promote physical flexibility, strength and endurance. In either case, you may find that yoga helps you to relax and manage stress.

Healthy Consumer

Americans generally associate the term *yoga* with one particular school of this ancient discipline — hatha yoga. In most cases, hatha yoga combines gentle breathing exercises with movement through a series of postures called asanas.

Yoga teachers commonly offer instruction in meditation. According to one of the most ancient yoga texts, the purpose of yoga is to calm the mind in preparation for meditation.

One principle of meditation is that stress comes with a racing mind. Meditators observe the flow of thoughts without judging them, a process that helps the mind to slow down naturally.

What the Research Shows

Biofeedback. According to a 1995 consensus statement from the National Institutes of Health (NIH), there is evidence that biofeedback can help to relieve many types of chronic pain, including tension and migraine headaches. And based on a research review, the Agency for Healthcare Research and Quality recommends biofeedback to help adults with urinary incontinence control their pelvic muscles.

Hypnosis. The 1995 consensus statement from the NIH cited strong evidence that hypnosis can reduce chronic pain associated with cancer and other conditions, such as irritable bowel syndrome and tension headaches. And according to another analysis of several studies, hypnosis can enhance the effects of therapy for phobia, obesity and anxiety.

Yoga. There are few recent studies of yoga in the medical literature. In one study, people who used yoga and relaxation techniques in addition to a wrist splint experienced more relief from carpal tunnel syndrome than people who used the splint alone. In another study, people with osteoarthritis of the hands who took yoga classes had less finger pain and tenderness during activity than the control group.

■ Restoring Natural Energy Forces

Acupuncture

Acupuncture is a part of Chinese traditional medicine that has been around for at least 2,500 years. According to this Eastern philosophy:
- Health depends on the free circulation of blood and a subtle energy called chi (pronounced "chee" and sometimes written Qi).
- Chi flows through your body along pathways called meridians.
- Inserting needles into points along the meridians promotes the free flow of chi.

Medical researchers are skeptical about these claims. Even so, acupuncture is one of the most well-researched and accepted practices in complementary and alternative medicine. Pain specialists at Mayo Clinic have used acupuncture since 1974 as part of their pain treatment program.

Depending on your reasons for seeking acupuncture, you'll have one or several hair-thin needles inserted under your skin. Some may go in as deep as 3 inches, depending on where they're placed in your body and what the treatment is for. Others will be placed superficially. The needles usually are left in for 15 to 30 minutes. Once inserted, needles are sometimes stimulated with an electrical current.

Expect to have several sessions. If you experience no relief after six or eight sessions, acupuncture probably isn't for you.

There are about 10,000 licensed acupuncturists in the United States, and 3,000 of them are physicians. To find a qualified practitioner, ask for a referral from your doctor or contact the American Academy of Medical Acupuncture (AAMA). Visit the AAMA Web site at *www.medicalacupuncture.org* or call 323-937-5514. AAMA's members are all licensed physicians with more than 200 hours of special training in acupuncture.

In a 1997 consensus statement, the National Institutes of Health concluded that acupuncture can be a useful treatment for nausea and vomiting after surgery and chemotherapy, and for pain after dental surgery. In addition, acupuncture can play a useful role in treatment for headaches, menstrual cramps, tennis elbow, fibromyalgia, myofascial pain, osteoarthritis, low back pain and carpal tunnel syndrome. According to this statement, future research will likely uncover more areas where acupuncture will be useful.

Getting Safe Acupuncture Treatment

Adverse side effects from acupuncture are rare, but they do occur. Hepatitis B has been transmitted from needles that aren't properly sterilized. Make sure your acupuncturist uses disposable needles.

You should feel little or no pain from the needles. You might even find their insertion to be relaxing. Significant pain from the needles is a sign that the procedure is being done improperly.

Tai chi

One sophisticated and enjoyable method to improve physical and emotional balance is an ancient form of exercise called tai chi (TIE-chee). Originally developed in China, tai chi involves slow, gentle, dancelike movements that relax and strengthen muscles and joints. Many people who practice tai chi view it as a form of meditation in motion.

You'll find tai chi classes offered in cities throughout the United States. To locate a class in your community, contact your local senior center, YMCA or health club.

Research indicates that tai chi can prevent falls in older adults by improving strength and balance. In one large study, those who practiced tai chi reduced their risk of falls by about 47 percent. Another study indicated that tai chi can help to reduce blood pressure.

Therapeutic Touch

Therapeutic touch resembles the religious concept of "laying on of the hands," where healing power is believed to flow from a minister's hands to a patient. However, therapeutic touch is not necessarily based on a religious concept. Instead, it comes from the idea that your body is surrounded by a field of energy. Illness results from disturbances in that field.

Some practitioners of therapeutic touch attempt to get rid of these disturbances by moving their hands back and forth across your body. Practitioners believe that by transferring healing energy through their hands to your body, they can reduce pain, stress and anxiety. Many conventional health care providers are skeptical of therapeutic touch, which is not supported by solid research.

Healthy Consumer

■ Systems That Combine Treatments

Homeopathy

Homeopathy (ho-me-OP-uh-the) is a very controversial treatment. It's based on two beliefs:

- *The law of similars.* When given to a healthy person in large quantities, some plant, animal and mineral substances produce symptoms of disease. But when given to a sick person, much smaller doses of the same substances can (theoretically) relieve the same symptoms.
- *The law of infinitesimals.* Literally, infinitesimal means too small to be measured. According to this belief, substances treat disease most effectively when they are highly diluted, often in distilled water or alcohol.

The law of similars is sometimes stated as "like cures like" — a capsule summary of homeopathy. Vaccination, a conventional practice, is based on a similar idea: Injecting a small dose of a modified infectious agent stimulates the body's immune system to fight diseases caused by that agent.

However, homeopathy in general departs widely from conventional medicine. Modern drug therapy primarily uses substances to reverse symptoms, not produce them. In addition, medical doctors find it difficult to accept the law of infinitesimals — especially when homeopathic treatments are so diluted that no trace of the original substance remains. Although highly diluted substances may not help you, they probably won't harm you either.

People who practice homeopathy (homeopaths) may also recommend changes in diet, exercise and other health-related behaviors. But avoid practitioners who encourage you to use homeopathic remedies instead of the medications that your doctor prescribed.

Many studies of homeopathy examine whether the benefits claimed for this treatment result from a placebo effect — that is, from the belief of patients in the treatment rather than the treatment itself. One analysis of over 100 controlled, randomized studies concluded that homeopathy appeared to have results that went beyond the placebo effect. However, researchers determined there was not enough evidence to conclude that homeopathic treatment was effective. There is little published evidence that homeopathy can effectively treat specific diseases or conditions.

Ayurveda

One of the oldest systems of health care comes from Hindu medicine practiced in India since ancient times. It's called ayurveda (AH-yoor-vay-duh), a Sanskrit word that means "the science of life."

Ayurveda begins with the premise that people differ both physically and psychologically. So treatments take these differences into account.

According to ayurvedic practitioners, there are three main types of energy (doshas) that create differences between people and govern health:

- Vata is the energy of movement. People dominated by vata are alert, creative and physically active.
- Pitta is the energy of digestion and metabolism. People with this primary dosha have larger appetites, warmer bodies and more stable temperaments than vata-dominated people.
- Kapha is the energy of lubrication. People dominated by kapha generally have

---

oily skin. They easily gain weight and tend to be less physically active. In addition, kapha types are usually calm, patient and forgiving.

It's believed that one of these energies can go to extremes, creating a lack of balance. For example, kapha types can become lethargic. Treatment in this case might include recommendations to exercise regularly, avoid naps and stay away from fatty, oily foods.

Naturopathy

Naturopathic care is one of the least organized of the complementary and alternative treatment approaches. It didn't emerge from the ideas of a single founder. Nor do people who practice naturopathy (naturopaths) go through standardized training.

Based on their belief in the healing power of nature, early naturopaths prescribed hydrotherapy — literally, water treatment. They recommended soaks in hot springs, walking barefoot on grass or through cold streams, and other water-related treatments.

Traditionally, naturopaths emphasized lifestyle — including plenty of fresh air, clean water and exercise — as the foundation of health. Today, naturopaths draw on many complementary and alternative practices. They typically counsel patients to avoid prescription drugs and surgery. However, don't stop taking your prescription medications without talking to your doctor first.

■ Five Steps in Considering Any Treatment

1. Gather Information About the Treatment

The Internet offers an ideal way to keep up with the latest on complementary and alternative treatments — a fast-changing field. If you don't have Internet access at home or work, then contact public libraries. Many of them have computer labs that are open to the public. But beware — the Internet is also one of the greatest sources

Steer Clear of Misinformation on the Internet — Apply the Three D's

You can find thousands of Web sites devoted to health. But — be careful. The material you'll find ranges from solid research to outright quackery. Carefully evaluate any information you find on the Internet. Remember to look for these three features:

- *Dates.* Search for the most recent information you can find. Reputable Web sites include a date for each article they post.
- *Documentation.* Check for the source of information. Notice whether articles refer to published medical research. Look for a board of qualified professionals who review content before it's published. Be wary of commercial sites or personal testimonials that push a single point of view or sell miracle cures.
- *Double-checking.* Visit several health sites and

compare the information they offer. And before you follow any medical advice, ask your doctor for guidance.

Some Web sites post a logo from the Health on the Net (HON) Foundation. Sites that display this logo have agreed to abide by the HON Code of Conduct.

Brooks Edwards, M.D., medical editor of MayoClinic.com, also recommends staying aware of privacy and security issues: "Before you share information with a Web site about a condition you have, be sure they don't sell data that can identify individuals. Remember that e-mail is not secure, and information about your medical history could be traced back to you through your e-mail address."

Healthy Consumer

of misinformation.

Begin with Web sites created by major medical centers, national organizations, universities or government agencies. Sites from the U.S. government include:

National Center for Complementary and Alternative Medicine
http://nccam.nih.gov

National Institutes of Health
http://www.nih.gov

National Library of Medicine MEDLINEplus Health Information
http://www.nlm.nih.gov/medlineplus

Office of Dietary Supplements
http://dietary-supplements.info.nih.gov

Also, look to Mayo Clinic for the latest health news:

Mayo Clinic Health Information
http://www.MayoClinic.com

2. Find and Evaluate Treatment Providers

After gathering information about a treatment, you may decide to find a practitioner who offers it. Choosing a name from the classified section of the phone book is risky if you have no other information about the provider. Check your state government listings for agencies that regulate and license health providers. These agencies may list names of practitioners in your area and offer a way to check credentials.

Organizations such as the American Academy of Medical Acupuncture also can give you names of certified practitioners in your area. To find addresses and phone numbers for these associations, visit your local library. Or use the Internet

Too Good to Be True — Signs of Medical Fraud

The Food and Drug Administration and the National Council Against Health Fraud recommend that you watch for the following claims or practices. These are often warning signs of potentially fraudulent herbal products or other "natural" treatments:

- The advertisements or promotional materials include words such as breakthrough, magical or new discovery. If the product were in fact a cure, it would be widely reported in the media and your doctor would recommend it.
- Promotional materials include pseudo-medical jargon such as detoxify, purify or energize. Such claims are difficult to define and to measure.
- The manufacturer claims that the product can

treat a wide range of symptoms, or cure or prevent a number of diseases. No single product can do this.

- The product is supposedly backed by scientific studies, but references aren't provided, are limited or are out of date.
- The product promotion mentions no negative side effects, only benefits.
- The manufacturer of the product accuses the government or medical profession of suppressing important information about the product's benefits. There is no reason for the government or medical profession to withhold information that could help people.

Mayo Clinic Guide to Self-Care

to find associations' Web sites. But many official sounding organizations may not be reputable. Talk with your doctor or another trusted health care professional to get advice.

Talk to people who've received the treatment you're considering and ask about their experience with specific providers. Start by asking friends and family members. Before you agree to treatment, call the provider to schedule an informational interview.

There are risks and side effects with many types of treatment, both conventional and unconventional. With any treatment you consider, find out if the benefits outweigh the risks.

3. Consider Treatment Cost

Many complementary and alternative approaches are not covered by health insurance. Find out exactly how much the treatment will cost you. Whenever possible, get the amount in writing before you start treatment.

4. Check Your Attitude

When it comes to complementary and alternative medicine, steer a middle course between uncritical acceptance and outright rejection. Learn to be open-minded and skeptical at the same time. Stay open to various treatments but evaluate them carefully. Also remember that the field is changing: What's alternative today may be well accepted — or discredited — tomorrow.

Alternative Medicine: Comments From a Mayo Clinic Physician

Brent Bauer, M.D., currently directs Mayo Clinic's efforts to develop research and education in complementary and alternative care.

Here at Mayo Clinic there is no official point of view on complementary and alternative medicine. Yet this is an important issue for Mayo because so many of our patients are using such therapies.

In the past, conventional medicine tended to make two errors:
- Lumping all complementary and alternative treatments together into the category of "snake oil" and closing down dialogue with patients. This is unsatisfactory. As physicians, we want what's best for our patients. If we're to be their advocates as they sail the murky waters of complementary and alternative medicine, people must feel free to come to us and discuss their questions.
- Embracing some complementary and alternative treatments too quickly and uncritically. This led to foolish expectations, and in some cases, harm.

We should avoid being either total skeptics or uncritical embracers of complementary and alternative medicine. Instead, we can hold to the middle ground, where scientific evidence and reason determine our responses.

The Mayo approach to assessment of complementary and alternative medicine is to apply the same standards that we do to all other treatment claims:
- Do sound and scientific research to investigate claims of safety and effectiveness.
- Educate ourselves and others about the results.
- Bring the best of our new knowledge to patient care.

This effort is well under way. Already Mayo has done several studies that helped dispel exaggerated claims of certain cancer cures. Other ongoing studies are looking at the roles of some herbs in treating chronic and common health problems.

In short, Mayo Clinic recognizes the interest our patients have in alternative treatments. Through research, education and open communication, we can help them make informed decisions.

5. Opt for Complementary Over Alternative Medicine

Research indicates that the most popular use of unconventional medical treatments is to *complement* rather than *replace* conventional medical care. Ideally, the various forms of treatment should work together.

You can use complementary treatments to maintain good health and to relieve some symptoms. But continue to rely on conventional medicine to diagnose a problem and treat the sources of disease. And tell your medical doctor about all the treatments you get — both conventional and unconventional.

Be sure to seek conventional treatment if you have a sudden, severe or life-threatening health problem. If you break a bone, get injured in a car accident or develop food poisoning, then make the emergency room your first stop.

Also, remember that your lifestyle choices make a difference. Most practitioners — conventional, complementary and alternative — will tell you that nutrition, exercise, not smoking, stress management and safety practices are your keys to a longer life and better health.

The Healthy Traveler

Becoming ill away from home poses a special set of problems. This chapter suggests ways to deal with common conditions that plague travelers. For people with chronic health problems, it's always a good idea to talk with your physician before you leave home.

◼ Planning Your Trip

Even if you're just taking a short trip, it pays to be prepared when you travel.

The first item to pack is always common sense. Think ahead about the conditions you'll encounter at your destination. And remember that traveling doesn't mean taking a vacation from your doctor's orders, especially if you're on prescribed medications, a special diet or an exercise program.

- **Get a physical examination.** If you've recently had surgery, a heart attack, a stroke, a bone fracture or another significant health problem, your doctor can advise you how soon you may travel, especially by air.
- **Update immunizations.** Even if you're just traveling to a nearby country, be sure your immunizations are up-to-date (see page 291).
- **See your dentist.** Don't let the excruciating pain of a toothache spoil your trip as you fly in a pressurized airplane or bite into an unfamiliar delicacy. Have cavities filled, poorly fitting dentures adjusted and other dental work done before you go.
- **Plan ahead when you pack.** You never know when your stay might be extended or what unexpected circumstances might happen at your destination. Pack more of your medications than you'll need, and get your prescription filled before you go. If you wear eyeglasses, pack an extra pair. Include a pair of sturdy, comfortable shoes and clothes that are appropriate for all weather variations at your destination. Make sure you take a first-aid kit.
- **Be aware of health precautions at your destination.** High altitudes and severe air pollution (often a problem in large cities overseas) may be a particular health risk for older adults and people with high blood pressure, anemia or respiratory or cardiovascular problems. Talk to your doctor ahead of time about how to handle these health concerns.
- **Check on your insurance needs.** Check with your current health insurance carrier to see which travel-related medical expenses, if any, are covered. Also, be aware of what its policies are for obtaining medical care in another city. If you're taking a long trip, consider buying travel insurance. Your regular insurance policy may have a travel clause that covers personal injury and loss of baggage. But certain restrictions may apply for medical emergencies. Travel insurance policies are available from many U.S. carriers, including associations for older adults and major credit plans. Review the policy carefully to make sure you know what it covers.

Traveler's Diarrhea

Diarrhea affects up to 50 percent of people who travel to developing countries. To reduce your risk:

- Eat foods that are well cooked and served hot.
- Drink bottled water, sodas, beer or wine served in their original containers. Beverages from boiled water, such as coffee and tea, are also usually safe.
- Use bottled water even for brushing your teeth. Keep your mouth closed while you shower.
- Avoid salads, buffet foods, raw or undercooked meats, raw vegetables, grapes, berries, dairy foods, tap water and ice cubes.
- Ask your physician whether you should take diarrhea medication with you.

Heat Exhaustion

In hot climates, a day of sightseeing can leave you weak, dizzy, nauseated and perspiring faster than you can replenish lost fluids. To prevent heat exhaustion:

- Pace yourself. Go slow the first few days after arriving in a warm climate.
- Plan regular breaks in the shade.
- Don't overeat.
- Drink liquids before you feel thirsty. Avoid alcoholic beverages.
- Wear lightweight, light-colored clothing and a broad-brimmed hat.
- At the first sign of heat exhaustion, get out of the sun and rest in the shade or an air-conditioned building.

Blisters

Blisters can be an unwelcome reminder to slow down. To avoid them:

- Wear comfortable shoes.
- Wear cotton or wool socks dusted inside with talcum powder.
- Use moleskin as a cushion.

Altitude Sickness

Decreased oxygen in the air at higher altitudes can cause altitude sickness. Symptoms can include headache, breathlessness with mild exertion, fatigue, nausea and disturbed sleep. To avoid this:

- **Start slowly.** Begin at an altitude below 9,000 feet.
- **Allow time to adjust.** Rest a day after arriving to adjust to the altitude.
- **Take it easy.** Slow down if you're out of breath or tired.
- **Limit ascent.** Don't climb more than 3,000 feet a day (or 1,000 feet if you're at 12,000 feet or above).
- **Sleep at a lower altitude.** If you're above 11,000 feet during the day, spend your nights at 9,000 feet or lower.
- **Avoid cigarettes and alcohol.**
- **Consider medication.** Ask your doctor about acetazolamide (Diamox) or other prescription medications that may help prevent or lessen symptoms.

■ Motion Sickness

Any type of transportation can cause motion sickness. It can strike suddenly, progressing from a feeling of restlessness to a cold sweat, dizziness and then vomiting and diarrhea. Motion sickness usually quiets down as soon as the motion stops. The more you travel, the more easily you'll adjust to being in motion.

You may escape motion sickness by planning ahead.

- If you're traveling by ship, request a cabin in the middle of the ship, near the waterline. If you're on a plane, ask for a seat over the front edge of a wing.
  Once aboard, direct the air vent at your face. On a train, take a seat near a window, and face forward. In an automobile, drive or sit in the front passenger's seat.

If you're susceptible to motion sickness:
- Focus on the horizon or a distant, stationary object. Don't read.
- Keep your head still, rested against a seat back.
- Don't smoke or sit near smokers.
- Avoid spicy foods and alcohol. Don't overeat.
- Take an over-the-counter antihistamine such as meclizine or dimenhydrinate before you feel sick. Expect drowsiness as a side effect.
- Consider scopolamine, available in a prescription adhesive patch. Several hours before you're in motion, apply the patch behind your ear for 72-hour protection. Talk to your doctor before using the medication if you have health problems such as asthma, glaucoma or urine retention.
- If you become ill, eating dry crackers or drinking a carbonated beverage may help settle your stomach.

■ A Word of Caution

As a tourist, you may be an especially obvious and tempting target to thieves at your destination. But if you use the same common sense that you would at home, you can enjoy your trip and not become the victim of a crime. Here's a checklist to keep in mind.
- Dress modestly, with minimum jewelry.
- Avoid areas where you may be victimized. Don't use shortcuts, narrow alleys or poorly lit streets.
- Don't travel alone at night.
- Don't carry large amounts of cash. Take traveler's checks and a few major credit cards instead. Know how to report the loss of both of these.
- When you carry your cash, credit cards and other valuables with you, you may want to conceal them in several places rather than putting them all in one wallet or purse. Money belts worn underneath clothing are one of the safest places to store valuables.
- Avoid public demonstrations and civil disturbances.
- Keep a low profile, and avoid loud conversations or arguments. Don't discuss travel plans or personal matters with strangers.
- Beware of pickpockets. They often have an accomplice who will jostle you or distract you—such as asking you for directions or trying to start a conversation with you.
- Wear the strap of your shoulder bag across your chest and walk with the bag away from the curb to deter thieves.

- Try to appear purposeful when you move about — even if you're lost. When possible, ask directions only from police or other authority individuals.
- Let someone know when you'll return if you'll be out late at night.
- If you're confronted, don't fight back. Give up your valuables. They can be replaced. You can't.
- Keep your hotel room locked at all times. Meet visitors in the lobby.
- Don't leave money and other valuables in your hotel room while you're out. Use the hotel safe.
- If you're alone, don't get on an elevator with a suspicious-looking person.

■ Traveling Abroad

Before traveling overseas, especially if you have a health condition or take medications, review your plans with your doctor. Summarize your destination, length of stay and anticipated levels of activities.

If your plans include travel to a relatively remote location, consider consulting a specialist in travel medicine. Ask your doctor for a referral to a clinic or physician specializing in this area.

- **Get a head start on immunization updates.** Immunizations you may need depend on your destination, the length of your visit and your medical history. See your doctor at least 4 to 6 weeks — and preferably 6 months — before your departure to schedule the immunizations you'll need. Some vaccinations require several injections spaced days, weeks or even months apart.

Information on immunizations and health precautions for travelers is available from your local health department, your doctor and the Centers for Disease Control and Prevention (see Travel Information Sources, page 294).

- **Get medical clearance.** Depending on your circumstances, your doctor may clear you for travel even if you have an unstable health condition. Get this clearance in writing in case transportation authorities or other officials question your ability to travel.
- **Take your medical history summary.** Make multiple copies. In case of an emergency, you may need copies for the medical professionals caring for you. If you have a history of heart problems or wear a pacemaker, ask for a copy of a recent electrocardiogram (ECG).
- **Know where medical care will be available.** Take with you a list of the names, addresses and telephone numbers of the recommended English-speaking physicians and hospitals at your destination. Your doctor, local or state medical society, the International Association for Medical Assistance to Travelers (IAMAT) or the U.S. State Department's Office of Overseas Citizens Services (see Travel Information Sources, page 294) can help you make your list.
- **Take copies of your prescriptions.** Request typewritten prescriptions (they're easier to read). Take your eyeglasses prescription too.
- **Pack medication carefully.** Keep your prescription medications in their original containers, with typed labels, in your carry-on luggage. Always fill your prescriptions before you leave home and bring more than you think you'll need. If you're taking a controlled substance, such as prescription narcotics, spare yourself an embarrassing encounter with customs agents by obtaining a letter of authorization on your physician's letterhead stationery. Know the laws of the countries you'll be in.

- **Double-check your health insurance.** Find out ahead of time how your health insurance plan handles medical care abroad.
- **Learn about the countries you plan to visit.** Before you go, read up on the culture, people and history. For up-to-date information, obtain a consular information sheet from the Office of Overseas Citizens Services. This provides information on health and security conditions.

Vaccines for International Travel

In addition to making sure you've had your primary vaccine series (measles, mumps, rubella, diphtheria, pertussis, tetanus, polio), the Centers for Disease Control and Prevention recommends that you consider these additional vaccines:

Booster Vaccines or Additional Doses
- **Tetanus and diphtheria:** A booster dose of adult tetanus-diphtheria is recommended every 10 years.
- **Polio:** Unless you've had a polio booster as an adult, you may need an additional single dose if you're traveling to Africa, Asia, the Middle East, India and neighboring countries, and most of the former republics of the Soviet Union.
- **Measles:** If you were born in 1957 or after, consider a measles vaccine booster.

Additional Vaccines
- **Yellow fever:** Recommended if you're traveling to certain parts of Africa and South America.
- **Hepatitis B vaccine:** Consider if you'll be staying 6 months or longer in areas with high rates of hepatitis B (Southeast Asia, Africa, the Middle East, islands of the South and Western Pacific and the Amazon region of South America).
- **Hepatitis A vaccine (or immune globulin):** Recommended for travelers to all areas except Japan, Australia, New Zealand, Northern and Western Europe and North America (excluding Mexico).
- **Typhoid:** Recommended if you'll be staying 6 weeks or longer in areas where food and water precautions are recommended (such as many developing countries).
- **Meningococcal vaccine:** Recommended if you'll be traveling to sub-Saharan Africa.
- **Japanese encephalitis:** Consider if you'll be staying long-term in Southeast Asia where this disease is common.
- **Rabies vaccine: Recommended if you'll be staying 6 months or longer (or in a rural region) in a developing country**

Air Travel Hazards

The fastest way to travel—by airplane—is also one of the safest. Yet by placing you thousands of feet in the air, moving at a speed of hundreds of miles per hour, air travel does subject your body to special challenges. Here are common problems that you might experience during air travel:

Dehydration

The pressurized cabin of an airplane has extremely low humidity, only 5 to 10 percent. This may cause you to become dehydrated. To prevent dehydration, drink liquids such as water and fruit juices during your flight. Limit alcohol and caffeine.

Blood Clots

Sitting during a long flight causes fluid to accumulate in the soft tissues in your legs. This increases your risk of a blood clot (thrombophlebitis). To improve circulation back to your heart:

- Stand up and stretch periodically after the "wear your seat belt" sign is turned off. Take a walk through the cabin once an hour or so.
- Flex your ankles or press your feet against the floor or seat mountings in front of you.
- If you're prone to swollen ankles or have varicose veins, consider wearing support hose.

Ear Pain

To avoid ear pain during ascent or descent, try this exercise to equalize the pressure in your ears:

- Take a deep breath; hold it for 2 seconds.
- Slowly exhale about 20 percent of the air while gradually pursing your lips.
- With your lips tightly closed, try to gently blow air as though you were playing a trumpet. Don't blow too hard.
- After about 2 seconds, exhale normally.
- To avoid light-headedness, limit your pressure breaths to no more than 10.
- Yawning, chewing gum and swallowing also help during ascent or descent.

Jet Lag

If you've ever traveled by air to a different time zone, you're probably familiar with what it's like to get jet lag—that dragged-out, out-of-sync feeling. Not all jet lag is the same. Flying eastward—and therefore resetting your body clock forward—is often more difficult than flying westward and adding hours to your day. Most peoples' bodies adjust at the rate of about 1 hour a day. Thus, after a change of four time zones, your body will require about 4 days to resynchronize its usual rhythms.

- **Reset your body's clock.** Begin resetting your body's clock several days in advance of your departure by adopting a sleep-wake pattern similar to the day-night cycle at your destination.
- **Drink plenty of fluids and eat lightly.** Drink extra liquids during your flight to avoid dehydration, but limit beverages with alcohol and caffeine. They increase dehydration and may disrupt your sleep.

■ Questions & Answers

Flying When You Have a Cold

QUESTION: **Can flying make a head cold worse?**

Answer: Air travel probably won't make your cold worse. But landing with a cold can cause severe ear pain. The problem is air pressure. At high altitudes, air pressure is low. But as you descend, it increases.

When you have a cold, the tiny tube (the eustachian tube) that connects your throat and middle ear is often blocked. Normally, the eustachian tube equalizes air pressure in your middle ear with the increasing outside pressure. Blockage in the tube leaves a vacuum in your middle ear, leading to a buildup of painful pressure on your eardrum. Your body's attempt to fill the vacuum causes fluid and sometimes blood to enter the middle ear.

To prevent ear pain when you fly with a cold, take a decongestant at least an hour before landing. Also, use a decongestant nasal spray before descent. These over-the-counter medicines help keep your eustachian tubes open. Sipping a non-alcoholic drink on takeoff and landing also helps keep these tubes open.

Drink plenty of fluids (non-alcoholic) when you fly, but especially when you have a cold. Liquids keep your throat and sinus membranes from drying and keep sinus secretions thin and easy to clear.

Melatonin and Jet Lag

QUESTION: A friend suggested that I take melatonin supplements to prevent jet lag. Do they work?

Answer: They might, but Mayo Clinic physicians generally don't recommend them.

Melatonin is sometimes called the "hormone of darkness" because it's produced naturally in your brain at night. It helps control your body's schedule for sleeping and waking.

For that reason, it's been explored as a way to prevent jet lag. Some studies suggest you may be able to gradually move your bedtime ahead or back by taking small doses of melatonin (often less than 1 milligram) at different intervals during the day. That may make it easier to adjust once you arrive at your destination. Although some studies suggest this is effective, other studies have found that melatonin doesn't help jet lag or may even make it worse.

Despite a recent flurry of books and articles about melatonin, much remains unknown about this hormone and its effects on your body, particularly when it's used long-term or with other medications. There are also concerns about the quality and purity of the supplements. Because melatonin isn't considered a drug, the Food and Drug Administration doesn't regulate the safety of supplements before they go on the market.

Travel After a Heart Attack

QUESTION: My husband has had a heart attack. Are there any special precautions we should take when traveling?

Answer: If you have cardiovascular disease, chest pain (angina) or a history of a heart attack or stroke:

- Be alert to the symptoms of a heart attack or stroke. At the first warning, seek emergency care. Know in advance where this medical care is available.
- Check the expiration date of nitroglycerin tablets. Get a new supply if they're older than 6 months.
- Don't drive for more than 4 hours without a rest.
- Stay out of the midday sun if you're traveling in a hot, humid climate.
- Limit or avoid alcohol. It reduces your heart's pumping action.
- If you wear a pacemaker, have your doctor check the battery before you go.

■ Travel Information Sources

International Association for Medical Assistance to Travelers (IAMAT)
417 Center Street
Lewiston, NY 14092
(716) 754-4883
Internet address: http://www.sentex.net/~iamat
    IAMAT offers a free list of English-speaking physicians

Centers for Disease Control and Prevention (CDC)
Atlanta, Georgia
(800) 311-3435
Internet address: http://www.cdc.gov
    The CDC offers 24-hour recordings on specific countries, detailing diseases and how to prevent them. In addition, its Internet site also offers this information, along with immunization recommendations for regions of the world. The CDC book *Health Information for International Travel* is available for purchase for $14 (call the telephone number listed above, or write to the Superintendent of Documents, U.S. Government Printing Office, Washington, DC 20402).

National Insurance Consumer Help Line
(800) 942-4242
    This organization offers a helpline for general travel insurance information, including a brochure listing companies and their travel insurance offerings.

Mayo Clinic
Internet address: http://www.MayoClinic.com
    Mayo Clinic's award-winning Internet site offers a variety of health information articles for travelers.

U.S. Department of State Office of American Citizens Services
Room 4811
2201 C Street NW
Washington, DC 20520
(202) 647-5225
Fax: (202) 647-3000
Internet address: http://travel.state.gov
    This office of the U.S. State Department offers a list of English-speaking doctors available in the countries in which you'll be traveling. Consular information sheets, travel warnings and public safety announcements are also available by recording at (202) 647-5225. You can obtain this information by faxing your request to the telephone number listed above or by sending a written request for information, along with a self-addressed, stamped envelope, to the Office of Overseas Citizens Services. The Bureau of Consular Affairs also offers a flyer called "Medical Information for Americans Traveling Abroad." It's available by faxing your request to the number above or by sending a written request and a self-addressed, stamped envelope to the Bureau of Consular Affairs, U.S. Department of State, Room 6831, Washington, DC 20520-4818.

Traveler's First-Aid Kit

Accidents and minor injuries can happen away from home. Be prepared to treat yourself and any companions for minor medical mishaps. Include these basic supplies:

Adhesive tape
Antacid
Antibacterial cream
Antidiarrheal tablets
Antihistamine
Bandages (including the elastic type)
Cotton swabs
Decongestant
Laxative

Moist towelettes
Moleskin (for blisters)
Over-the-counter heartburn medicine
Over-the-counter pain relievers
Scissors
Skin cream
Sunscreen (sun protection factor of at least 15)
Thermometer
Tweezers

Index

Joint pain
- arthritis, 161–164
- big toe, 92
- bursitis, 90
- in children, 86
- elbow, 93
- fibromyalgia, 91
- finger, 95
- gout, 92
- hip, 97
- knee, 100–101
- shoulder, 92–93
- tendinitis, 90–91
- thumb, 97
- wrist, 95

K

Kegel exercises, 150
Keloids, 23
Ketoprofen, 265
- forms of, 264
- and gastritis, 61
- and ulcers, 67
Kidney infections, 142
Knee braces, 101
Knee pain, 100–101

L

Lactose, 60
Laryngitis, 134, 136
Laxatives, 58
LDL cholesterol, 212–214
Lead poisoning, 227
Leg pain
- cramps, 98–99
- hamstring muscle, 98
- knee, 100–101
- shin splint, 99
Leg swelling, 99–100
Lescol (fluvastatin), 213
Leukoplakia, 139
Lice, 126
Lidocaine, 137
Lifting properly, 54, 232–233
Ligaments, 88
Light-headedness, 34–35
Lighthouse Inc., The, 81
Lipitor (atorvastatin), 213
Listening skills, 241–242
Little League elbow, 94
Lopid (gemfibrozil), 213

Loss of voice, 136
Lovastatin (Mevacor), 213
Low back pain, 51–52
Low blood pressure, 180
LSD, 194
Lump in throat, 135
Lump on wrist or hand, 95
Luvox (fluvoxamine), 148
Lyme disease, 16

M

Macular degeneration, 80
Mallet toe, 104
Mammograms, 145
Managed care, 258
Marijuana, 194
Massage, 278
Mastitis, 146
Mayo Clinic weight pyramid, 211
Measles, 125, 223
Meclizine, 289
Medical history, 262
Medications
- acetaminophen, 265
  - and arthritis, 163
  - and chronic pain, 43
  - and fever, 38
  - forms of, 264
  - and headache, 83
- Actifed, 266
- Afrin, 266
- allergies, 13
- aluminum chlorhydrate, 46
- aluminum sulfate, 46
- antihistamines, 116, 123, 160, 266
- aspirin, 265
  - and arthritis, 163
  - and asthma, 165
  - and children, 38
  - and chronic pain, 43
  - forms of, 264
  - and gastritis, 61
  - and headache, 83
  - and heart attack, 175, 177
  - and muscle strains, 87
  - reactions to, 13
  - and tinnitis, 72
  - and ulcers, 67

bacitracin ointment, 119
Bactroban (mupirocin ointment), 123
Benadryl (diphenhydramine hydrochloride), 123, 125, 137
benzoyl peroxide lotion, 118
Biaxin, 67
bupropion zybar, 192
calamine lotion, 15, 29, 123, 125, 128
cefixime, 184
ceftriaxone, 184
Chlor-Trimeton (chlorpheniramine maleate), 123, 266
Chlor-Trimeton D, 266
ciprofloxacin, 184
clot-dissolving drugs, 5
clotrimazole, 122
coal tar, 120, 127
Colestid (colestipol), 213
Contac, 266
cortisone, 13, 91, 97, 105, 163
cromolyn sodium, 160, 167
cyclosporine, 127
Depo-Provera (medroxy progesterone acetate), 148, 152
dextromethorphan, 266
dimenhydrinate, 289
Dimetapp, 266
Drixoral, 266
Effexor (venlafaxine), 148
epinephrine, 11, 15, 16
erythromycin, 123
expectorants, 108, 266
Famvir (famciclovir), 128, 183
Fenteramin, 208
fluconazole, 132
griseofulvin, 132
guaifenesin, 266
hydrocortisone cream, 15, 29, 46, 62, 121, 124, 127
hydrogen peroxide, 22, 137
ibuprofen, 265
- and chronic pain, 43
- and fever, 38
- forms of, 264
- and gastritis, 61
- and headache, 83

Naps, 45
Narcotics, 194–195
Narcotics Anonymous, 195
Nasal sprays, 160
National Cancer Institute
Information Service, 171
National Council on Alcoholism
and Drug Dependence, 189
National Digestive Diseases
Information Clearinghouse, 67
National Domestic Violence
Hotline, 201
National Eye Institute, 81
National Institute of Allergy and
Infectious Disease, 167
National Institute of Drug Abuse
Hotline, 195
National Mental Health
Association, 197, 200
National Organization for
Victim Assistance, 201
National Sleep Foundation, 45
Naturopathy, 283
Nausea and vomiting, 66
Nearsightedness, 81
Neck and back pain, 51–55, 244
Nedocromil sodium, 167
Neo-Synephrine, 266
Neosporin, 22
Neurodermatitis, 121
Neuropathic pain, 41
Niacin and triglycerides, 213,
214
Nicotine replacement therapy,
191–192
Nicotine withdrawal, 192
Nicotrol, 191
Night driving, 80
Night terrors, 45
Nightmares, 45
Nighttime sweating, 46
Noise and hearing loss, 74, 234
Nonoxynol-9, 182
Nose
colds, 115
deviated septum, 114
loss of sense of smell, 112
nose drop addiction, 114
nosebleeds, 113
object in nose, 112
runny nose, 115

sinus infection, 116
stuffiness, 114
NSAIDs, 264–265
and arthritis, 165
and asthma, 165
Nuprin (ibuprofen), 265
Nutrition, 170, 209–210

O
Opium and opioids, 194
OPV vaccine, 223
Oral contraceptives, 152
Oral thrush, 139
Orchitis, 140
Orudis KT (ketoprofen), 265
Osteoarthritis, 53, 161–164
Osteopathy, 278
Osteoporosis, 53, 149
Otitis media, 70–71

P
Pain. See also specific parts of
the body
anatomy of, 40
and cancer, 170–171
chronic, 40–43
in joints (See Joint pain)
Pain relievers, 43, 264–265
Palpitations, 111
Panadol (acetaminophen), 265
Panic attacks, 197
Pap test, 151
Paroxetine (Paxil), 148
Passing gas, 60
PCP (phencyclidine), 194
Peak flowmeter, 167
Pedialyte, 66
Penicillin, 13, 123, 134, 184
Pepcid, 61, 64, 67
Perceived exertion scale, 218
Phlebitis, 100
Phototherapy, 127
Pinkeye, 78
Plantar fasciitis, 105–106
Plantar warts, 130
PMS (premenstrual syndrome),
147–148
Pneumonia, 115, 223
Poison ivy, oak, sumac, 29
Poisoning, 9
Polyps, 62

Polysporin, 22
Popliteal cyst, 101
Postherpetic neuralgia, 128
Postural hypotension, 34
Pravachol (pravastatin), 213
Precordial catch, 111
Prednisone, 163
Preeclampsia, 154
Pregnancy
anemia, 154
backache, 155
constipation, 155
general, 153
heartburn, 155
hemorrhoids, 155
home tests, 153
morning sickness, 154
sleep problems, 155
swelling, 154
vaginal bleeding, 153
varicose veins, 154
and working, 246–248
Presbycusis, 75
Presbyopia, 81
Prescription drug rules, 263
Prevacid, 67
Prilosec, 67
Proctoscopy, 222
Propagest, 258
Prostate
cancer, 141
enlarged, 141
Protonix, 67
Prozac (fluoxetine), 148
PSA (prostate-specific antigen)
test, 141
Psoriasis, 127
Psyllium, 65, 155
Pubic lice, 126
Puncture wounds, 23
Pyloric stenosis, 66

Q
Questran (cholestyramine), 213

R
Rabies, 14
Radon, 228
Rashes, 124–125
Rectal bleeding, 62
Reflux, 64

Index

Sudafed, 266
Sudafed Plus, 266
Suicide warning signs, 200
Sumatriptan (Imitrex), 83
Sunburn, 19
    in children, 129
Sunglasses, 19
Sunscreen, 19
Sweating, excessive, 46
Swelling
    feet, 105
    hands and wrists, 95
    legs, 99–100
    in pregnancy, 154
    testicles, 140
Swimmer's ear, 72
Syphilis, 184

T

Tagamet, 61, 64, 67
Tai chi, 281
Taking temperature, 39
Tavist, 258
Tavist D, 258
"Technophobia," 243
Teeth grinding, 45
Teldrin, 258
Temperature (fever), 38–39
Tendinitis, 90–91
Tennis elbow, 94
Tension headache, 82–84
Terbinafine hydrochloride, 132
Testicles
    cancer, 140
    pain, 140
    self-exam, 140
    swelling, 140
Tetanus vaccine, 23, 223
Theophylline, 167
Therapeutic touch, 281
Third-degree burns, 17
Throat problems
    hoarseness, 136
    laryngitis, 136
    lump in, 135
    sore, 133–134
    strep, 133, 134
Thumb pain, 97
Tick bites, 16
Time management tips
    personal, 236
    at work, 240

Tinnitus, 72
Tiredness, 36–37
Tobacco, 190–193
Toenail, ingrown, 132
Tonsillitis, 133
Tooth decay, 30
Tooth loss, 30
Toothache, 30
Torsion, testicular, 140
Toxic shock syndrome, 156
tPA (tissue-plasminogen
    activator), 5
Transient ischemic attack (TIA), 7
Trauma, 31–32
Travel
    abroad, 290–291
    air travel, 291–292
    altitude sickness, 288
    crime, 289–290
    Elderhostel, 250
    first-aid kit, 295
    information sources, 294
    traveler's diarrhea, 288
    trip planning, 287
Trenchmouth, 139
Trichomoniasis, 150
Trichotillomania, 131
Trigger finger, 96
Triglycerides, 213, 214
Tubal ligation, 152
Twitching eyelid, 79
Tylenol (acetaminophen), 257
Type 1 diabetes, 172
Type 2 diabetes, 172

U

Ulcers, 67
Undecylenic acid, 122
Urgent care
    allergic reactions, 12–13
    bites, 14–16
    bleeding, 10
    breathing problems, 2–4
    burns, 17–19
    choking, 4
    CPR, 2–3
    cuts and scrapes, 22–23
    dislocations, 31
    eye injuries, 24–25
    fractures, 31
    frostbite, 20

head injury, 32
heart attack, 5–6
heat-related problems, 28
Heimlich maneuver, 4
hypothermia, 21
object in eye, 25
poison ivy, oak, sumac, 29
poisoning, 9
shock, 11
sprains, 32
stroke (brain attack), 7–8
tooth loss, 30
trauma, 31–32
wounds, 22–23
Urinary tract infections
    in men, 142
    in women, 150
Urination problems
    frequent, in men, 141
    frequent, in women, 150
    incontinence, 150
    leakage, 150
    painful, in men, 142
    painful, in women, 150
    slow, in men, 141

V

Vaccines. See Immunizations
Vaginal bleeding, 147
Vaginal discharge, 150
Vaginitis, 150
Varicose veins in pregnancy, 154
Vasectomy, 143
Vasomotor rhinitis, 114
Venereal disease. See Sexually
    transmitted diseases
Venlafaxine (Effexor), 148
Ventricular fibrillation, 5
Vertebrae, 50
Vertigo, 34–35
Vibrio vulnificus, 27
Vision problems
    cataracts, 80
    contact lenses, 81
    farsightedness, 81
    floaters, 77
    glare sensitivity, 79
    glasses, 81
    glaucoma, 80
    macular degeneration, 80
    night driving, 80

NOTES